EXERCISES FOR HEALTH PROMOTION

A Prescriptive Approach

David Ash, MPT, ATC, CSCS
Exercise/Health Consultant
Howell, New Jersey

Caren J. Werlinger, PT
Partner, Director of Clinical Services
Physical Evaluation and Rehabilitation Center
Winchester, Virginia

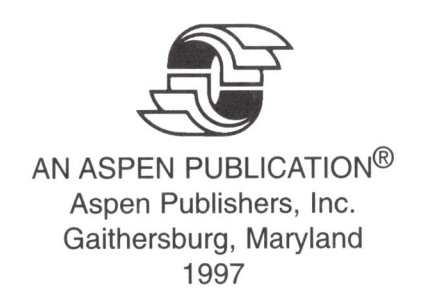

AN ASPEN PUBLICATION®
Aspen Publishers, Inc.
Gaithersburg, Maryland
1997

Library of Congress Cataloging-in-Publication Data

Ash, David.
Exercises for health promotion: a prescriptive approach/
David Ash, Caren J. Werlinger.
p. cm.
Includes bibliographical references and index.
ISBN 0-8342-0869-5
1. Exercise therapy. 2. Health promotion.
I. Werlinger, Caren J. II. Title.
RM725.A84 1997
613.7'1—dc21 96-49908
CIP

Copyright © 1997 by Aspen Publishers, Inc.
All rights reserved.

Aspen Publishers, Inc., grants permission for photocopying for limited personal or internal use. This consent does not extend to other kinds of copying, such as copying for general distribution, for advertising or promotional purposes, for creating new collective works, or for resale. For information, address Aspen Publishers, Inc., Permissions Department, 200 Orchard Ridge Drive, Suite 200, Gaithersburg, Maryland 20878.

Orders: (800) 638-8437
Customer Service: (800) 234-1660

About Aspen Publishers • For more than 35 years, Aspen has been a leading professional publisher in a variety of disciplines. Aspen's vast information resources are available in both print and electronic formats. We are committed to providing the highest quality information available in the most appropriate format for our customers. Visit Aspen's Internet site for more information resources, directories, articles, and a searchable version of Aspen's full catalog, including the most recent publications: **http://www.aspenpub.com**
Aspen Publishers, Inc. • The hallmark of quality in publishing
Member of the worldwide Wolters Kluwer group

The authors have made every effort to ensure the accuracy of the information herein. However, appropriate information sources should be consulted, especially for new or unfamiliar procedures. It is the responsibility of every practitioner to evaluate the appropriateness of a particular opinion in the context of actual clinical situations and with due considerations to new developments. Authors, editors, and the publisher cannot be held responsible for any typographical or other errors found in this book.

Editorial Resources: Jane Colilla
Library of Congress Catalog Card Number: 96-49908
ISBN: 0-8342-0869-5

Printed in the United States of America

1 2 3 4 5

There are in fact two things, science and opinion; the former
begets knowledge, the latter ignorance.

—*Hippocrates c. 460–377 BC*

To the faculty and staff of the West Virginia University Division of
Physical Therapy: Just a reminder that your faith and your commitment
in teaching us reach far beyond the classroom to touch the lives of
those whom we, in turn, treat and teach.

Caren J. Werlinger, PT

This book is dedicated to these extraordinary teachers: Dan Foster,
John Streif, Bill Dervrich, Ted Lambrinides, and most of all my parents,
M.L. and Elizabeth Ash.

David Ash, MPT, ATC, CSCS

Table of Contents

Preface ix

PART I—PRINCIPLES OF EXERCISE 1

Chapter 1—A Preventive Approach 3
David Ash

    Introduction 3
    Evolution of Preventive Exercise 4
    Benefits of Exercise 5
    Benefits in the Workplace 5
    Chapter Summary 5

Chapter 2—The Client Education Process 9
David Ash

    The Client Interview 9
    Common Exercise Misconceptions 10
    Medical Approval To Exercise 14
    Strategies To Facilitate Motor Learning 14
    Specificity 15
    Recording Exercise Data 16
    Intensity (Difficulty) of Resistive Exercise 16
    Muscle Contraction Following Rapid Stretch 17
    Chapter Summary 19

Chapter 3—Client Motivation and Compliance 21
David Ash

    Motivation 21
    Facilitation of Compliance 21
    Chapter Summary 22

Chapter 4—Resistive Exercise: Characteristics, Goals, and Principles 23
David Ash

    Characteristics of a Resistive Exercise Program 23
    Principles of Resistive Exercise 24

Exercise Prescription Case Study 28
Chapter Summary 29

Chapter 5—Aerobic Exercise 31
Caren J. Werlinger

Benefits 31
Metabolic Pathways 31
Training Intensity 32
Determining Target Heart Rate 32
Duration of Exercise 33
Weather Considerations 34
Aerobic Activities 34
Longevity Factors 36
Research Findings 36
Chapter Summary 36

Chapter 6—Flexibility 39
Caren J. Werlinger

Physiology of Stretch 39
Specific Stretches 40
Research Findings 40
Chapter Summary 41

Chapter 7—Posture 43
Caren J. Werlinger

Postural Muscles 43
A Postural Base for Exercise 43
Postural Changes with Exercise Equipment 44
Dynamic Posture Control 44
Posture and Aging 44
Postural Exercises 44
Chapter Summary 45

Chapter 8—Safety 47
Caren J. Werlinger

Guidelines 48
Chapter Summary 48

Chapter 9—Recovery and Overtraining 49
David Ash

Signs and Symptoms of Overtraining 49
Resistive Exercise: How Many Sets and Repetitions? 50
Overtraining and Recovery in Aerobic Activities 51
Chapter Summary 52

Chapter 10—Exercise Dependence 53
David Ash

Exercise Dependence Defined 53
Intervention 54
Chapter Summary 54

Chapter 11—Exercise for Children 55
David Ash

    Introduction 55
    Benefits of Youth Exercise 55
    Specific Activities and Injury Trends 56
    Recommendations 57
    Prevention of Patellofemoral Dysfunction 58
    Chapter Summary 61

Chapter 12—Exercise for Older Persons 63
David Ash

    Introduction 63
    Research 63
    Functional Benefits 63
    Falling in Older Persons: Exercise as Prevention 65
    Exercise and Self-Efficacy 68
    Exercise Programming for Older Persons 68
    Chapter Summary 68

Chapter 13—Home Exercise 71
Caren J. Werlinger

    Aerobic Exercise 71
    Strength Training 71
    Stretches 72
    Safety 72
    Chapter Summary 72

Chapter 14—Alternative Resistive Exercise Movements: Use of a Biomechanical Model 73
David Ash

    Purpose 73
    Example Exercise Movements 78
    The Future 83

PART II—EXERCISES 85

Chapter 15—Resistive Exercise Movements 87
David Ash

    Resistive Exercise Terminology 87
    Resistive Exercise Movements 87

Chapter 16—Flexibility Exercise Movements 181
Caren J. Werlinger

    Flexibility Program 181
    Activity-Specific Stretches 181

Appendix A—The Recommended Quantity and Quality of Exercise for Developing and Maintaining Cardiorespiratory and Muscular Fitness in Healthy Adults 187

Appendix B—Individual Guidelines for Cardiovascular Exercise 198

Appendix C—Physical Activity, Health, and Well-Being: An International Scientific Consensus Conference Consensus Statement. 199

Appendix D—American College of Obstetricians and Gynecologists Exercise Guidelines during Pregnancy and the Postpartum Period. 200

Appendix E—Physical Activity and Health: Summary of a Report of the Surgeon General 205

Appendix F—Physical Activity and Public Health 210

Appendix G—Sample Exercise Programs 219

Appendix H—Recording Sheet 222

Index 225

About the Authors 231

Preface

The 21st century will cull a health professional with the ability to adapt to rapidly evolving health care needs. The desire to remain abreast of and to utilize the latest research literature, the flexibility to become proficient at new and yet unknown skills, and the communication skills to motivate clients will be characteristics of the effective health care practitioner. The emphasis on prevention of injury, dysfunction, and disease, as opposed to remediation, will proliferate.

This book is for health professionals involved in the prescription of preventive exercise. It is unique in its integration of research and practical application. As stated in Chapter 1, many of the exercise guides on the market have, at best, a minimal basis in scientific research. Frequently, the only qualification of the author is that he or she is an exercise enthusiast. Many exercise books are essentially a compilation of personal opinions, anecdotes, and favorite exercises. One well-designed research study is worth a thousand "expert" opinions. At the other end of the spectrum are research-based texts, which may not develop the clinical applications that can be derived from that research.

The value of a wealth of information is questionable if it cannot be synthesized into guidelines for daily use. This text couples research with practical application. The inferred importance of challenging unproven doctrine and of substantiating action with research is not coincidental. A comprehensive approach to exercise, as well as the characteristics of safety, productivity, and time efficiency, are emphasized throughout.

The book is divided into two parts. Part I is comprised of information to be used by the professional. Part II is a collection of exercise movements to be reproduced for the exercise client and following the evaluation of individual exercise needs and goals.

The illustrations in Chapters 14 and 15 are by Caren J. Werlinger.

The authors wish to express their appreciation to Stephen Zollo of Aspen Publishers, Inc.; to photographer Beth Skinner; to John Scheetz, owner, Downtown Athletic Club, Winchester, Virginia, for facility use; and to David Sims, PhD, PT, and Camilla Wilson, PhD, PT, for their support.

PART I
Principles of Exercise

CHAPTER 1

A Preventive Approach

David Ash

CHAPTER OUTLINE

I. Introduction
II. Evolution of Preventive Exercise
III. Benefits of Exercise
IV. Benefits in the Workplace
V. Chapter Summary

INTRODUCTION

Aristotle said, "A man falls into ill health as a result of not caring for exercise." Since the landmark Framingham studies[1,2] indicated that active lifestyles can play a role in prevention of cardiovascular disease, the list of diseases and dysfunctions for which exercise has an identified preventive effect has grown considerably. As health care evolves, emphasis on preventive exercise will continue to increase based on its cost efficiency. Physical therapists, exercise physiologists, and athletic trainers, with their strong education regarding the musculoskeletal system and physiology of exercise, are well aligned to assume a leadership role in this aspect of preventive health care.

Many of the exercise guides on the market contain, at best, minimal basis in scientific research. Frequently, the only qualification of the author is that he or she is an exercise enthusiast. Many exercise books are essentially a compilation of personal opinions, anecdotes, and favorite exercises. One well-designed research study is worth a thousand expert opinions. At the other end of the spectrum are research-based texts, which may not develop the clinical applications that can be derived from such research. The usefulness of a wealth of information is questionable if it cannot be synthesized into guidelines for daily use. Therefore, this text couples research with practical application. For the purpose of this text, preventive exercise is operationally defined as exercise for the purpose of preventing disease, illness, dysfunction, or injury in individuals who are free of existing pathology. Emphasis is placed on comprehensive exercise, defined here as exercise containing aerobic, resistive, and range of motion components.

Consider the following scenario, which may soon become commonplace. An individual with an interest in beginning an exercise program approaches an exercise professional and asks, "I've heard about the importance of exercise in the prevention of disease and injury. I am interested in beginning an exercise program but am confused by all the conflicting information and advertising regarding the subject. I have 45 minutes, 4 days per week in which to exercise. I would like to include a balance of various types of exercise in the program. What do you recommend?" The exercise professional's response, based on scientific research, includes the following:

1. Designing a comprehensive exercise program that emphasizes safety, productivity, and time efficiency.
2. Educating the client regarding the goals and principles of the program.
3. Educating and demonstrating resistive exercise, which addresses each of the major muscular structures of the body; an aerobic component, with emphasis on specific progression and overuse injury prevention; and a comprehensive range of movement sequence.
4. Adapting the program to equipment accessible to the exerciser.
5. Adapting the program to the exerciser's time constraints.
6. Educating the client regarding expected physiological responses and adaptations to exercise, individual po-

tential for adaptations, and the anticipated time frames involved.
7. Motivating the client effectively.

Another situation that is quite common is that as a result of exposure to exercise as a patient, an individual may for the first time feel and see the benefits of exercise. Upon completion of rehabilitation, the patient expresses an interest in an ongoing, comprehensive preventive exercise program. This text serves as a reference to be used during the bridge between the rehabilitation program and the preventive exercise program. In both situations described above, the material herein will assist exercise professionals in providing accountable information to the exercise consumer.

EVOLUTION OF PREVENTIVE EXERCISE

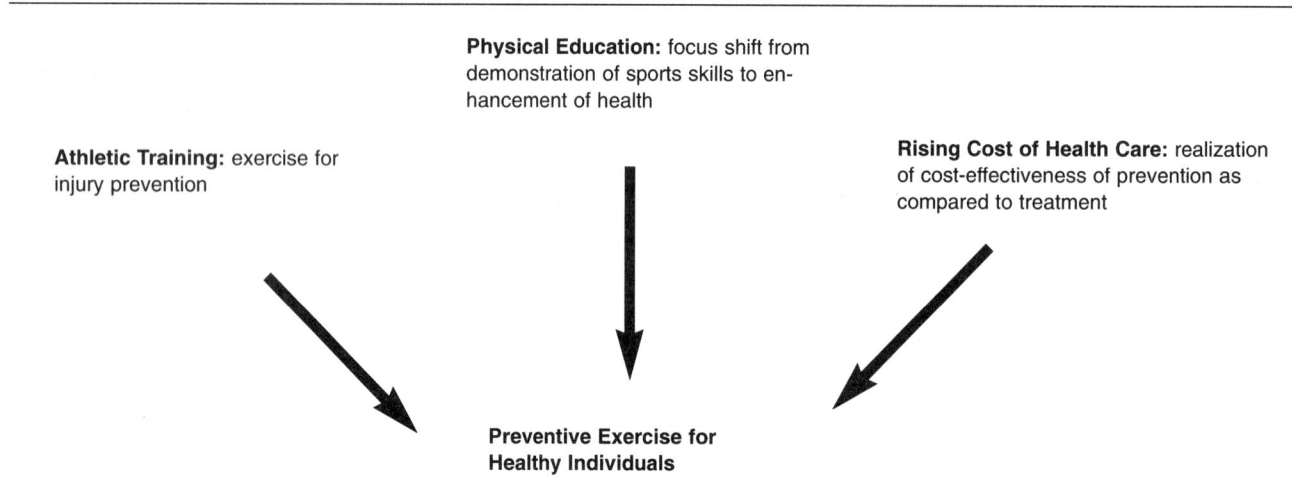

The evolution of preventive exercise (see Figure 1–1) has been influenced by several disciplines. The desire to prevent athletic injuries, the belief that physical education programs can have an important impact on general health, and most recently the realization that disease/injury prevention is much more cost-effective than treatment/rehabilitation have all contributed to the evolution of preventive exercise. The earliest sports developed as a result of the value societies placed on competition. With the rise of the Greek civilization, the Pan Hellenic Games evolved from religious festivals to sports competitions. The most famous of these events was the Olympic games. The games led to the development of coaches, trainers, and physicians to assist athletes with preparation for performance.[3] Herodicus is regarded as the greatest Greek athletic trainer, as well as the first sports medicine physician.[4] In addition to these accomplishments, Herodicus was the teacher of a student with a particular affinity for medical study. The student's name was Hippocrates. Throughout Roman times trainers emphasized the benefits of proper diet, rest, and exercise in preparation for such popular sports as boxing and wrestling. Three hundred years after Herodicus, Galen served as trainer to the gladiatorial school at Pergamum. Galen later became personal physician to Marcus Aurelius. With the fall of the Roman Empire, interest in sporting activities went through a period of decline. Not until the Renaissance did interest in sports slowly begin to return.

The proliferation of interscholastic and intercollegiate sports during the latter half of the 19th century led to increased interest in athletic training. Hitchcock, recognized as the founder of physical education in the United States, developed the first organized physical education program at Amherst College in 1854. In 1885, the American Alliance of Health, Physical Education, and Recreation was established to encourage research and information exchange throughout the exercise realm. The growth of competitive sports during the early 1900s influenced writers such as Bilek[5] to author books on prevention of sports injuries. The National Athletic Trainers Association was formed in 1950, followed by the establishment of the American College of Sports Medicine in 1954. The President's Council on Youth Fitness was created with the goal of upgrading school physical education programs.[4]

In 1968 the book *Aerobics*, by Kenneth Cooper, was published and espoused the value of preventive exercise. Preventive exercise continued to gain recognition in the 1980s as the President's Physical Fitness Awards Program was challenged by physical educators who favored a shift in emphasis from sports ability to exercise for health benefits. In 1990, resistive exercise was included in the American College of Sports Medicine position statement regarding exercise for developing and maintaining fitness in healthy adults.[6] Today, spiraling health care costs continue to facili-

Athletic Training: exercise for injury prevention

Physical Education: focus shift from demonstration of sports skills to enhancement of health

Rising Cost of Health Care: realization of cost-effectiveness of prevention as compared to treatment

Preventive Exercise for Healthy Individuals

Figure 1–1 The Evolution of Preventive Exercise

tate the awareness and growth of preventive exercise via cost containment measures such as capitation.

BENEFITS OF EXERCISE

Exercise, which includes aerobic, resistive, and range of motion components, can benefit many different body systems. Examples of systems that adapt favorably to exercise include the neuromuscular, skeletal, cardiovascular, and respiratory systems. Specific benefits of exercise are identified below:

- decreased blood pressure[7–9]
- decreased risk of cardiovascular disease[9–16]
- increased maximal oxygen consumption[17,18]
- increased cardiac output[18,19]
- decreased triglyceride level[20,21]
- increased stroke volume[19]
- improved glucose tolerance[7]
- decreased risk of osteoporosis[22–27]
- increased muscle strength[7,28–36]
- decreased risk of falls in the elderly[37–42]
- increased flexibility[7]
- increased fibrinolysis[43,44]
- increased high density lipoproteins[29,44,45]
- extended longevity[46]
- increased metabolic rate[47]
- increased lean body mass[17,48]
- improved posture[20]
- increased respiratory function[17]
- increased self-efficacy[49]
- increased bone density[50–52]
- increased gastrointestinal transit[52]
- improved work capacity[28]
- decreased resting heart rate[28]
- decreased total cholesterol[28]
- decreased risk of obesity[5,9,17,18,45,53]
- decreased platelet adhesiveness[54]
- reduced perceived exertion at a given work rate[18]
- decreased risk of colon cancer[55–57]
- beneficial effects on depression and psychological well-being[56–59]
- enhanced occupational performance[21]

The interaction of benefits of exercise may result in enhanced quality of life as depicted in the Exercise Cascade in Figure 1–2.

BENEFITS IN THE WORKPLACE

A relatively new and exciting field of study within the domain of preventive exercise is the investigation of exercise benefits as manifested in the workplace. A study was conducted to investigate the effectiveness of transcutaneous electrical nerve stimulation (TENS) when added to a standard exercise program for industrial workers with acute low back pain. The investigation revealed that exercise alone, when continued over four weeks, reduced disability and pain scores significantly. The addition of TENS to the exercise program resulted in no additional benefits.[60] Shephard,[61] in a review of "the economics of fitness and sport" comments, "likely benefits to a company include an improvement of corporate image, recruitment of premium employees, gains in the quality and quantity of production, decreased absenteeism and turnover, lower medical costs, and a reduced incidence of industrial injuries." Shephard also notes that current evidence suggests "exercise (particularly in the context of more general health promotion) is both cost-effective and cost-beneficial; the immediate return may be as much as $2 to $5 per dollar invested."

CHAPTER SUMMARY

As realization of the value of preventive exercise becomes more pervasive, there will be a corresponding increase in the demand for qualified professionals to provide expertise and guidance to individuals interested in exercise. Exercise professionals with a thorough educational background in the nervous, musculoskeletal, and cardiopulmonary systems, as well as the ability to extract practical application from the ever-growing research base, are well-positioned to accommodate this demand. The benefits of a preventive exercise program are extensive and diverse. Body systems for which exercise has a desirable effect include the cardiovascular, neuromuscular, skeletal, and pulmonary systems. Exercise may enhance the quality of life.

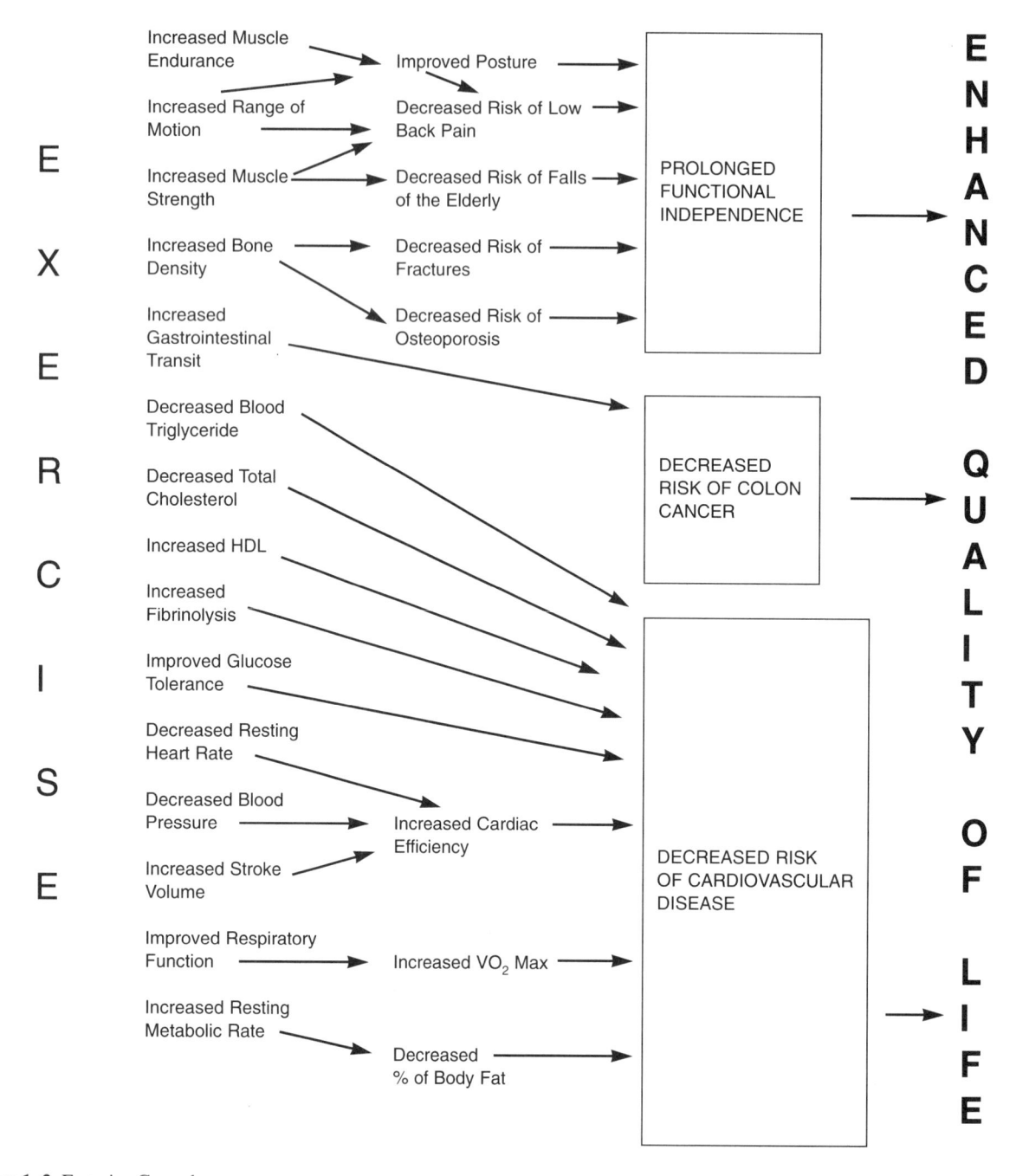

Figure 1–2 Exercise Cascade

REFERENCES

1. Dawber TR. *The Framingham Study*. Cambridge, MA: Harvard University Press: 1980:157–171.

2. Dawber TR, Meadors GF, Moore FEJ. Epidemiological approaches to heart disease: the Framingham Study. *Am J Public Health*. 1951; 41:279–286.

3. Arnheim DD. *Modern Principles of Athletic Training*. 7th ed. St. Louis, MO: Times Mirror/Mosby College Publishing; 1989:2–6.

4. American Academy of Orthopedic Surgeons. *Athletic Training and Sports Medicine*. 2nd ed. Park Ridge, IL: American Academy of Orthopedic Surgeons; 1991:4–12.

5. Bilek SE. *The Trainers Bible*. New York: TJ Reed Co; 1956.

6. American College of Sports Medicine. Position statement on the recommended quantity and quality of exercise for developing and maintaining fitness in healthy adults. *Med Sci Sports Exerc*. 1990;22: 265–274.

7. American Heart Association. Exercise standards: a statement for healthcare professionals from the American Heart Association. *Circ.* 1995;91:580–615.
8. Angotti CM, Levine MS. Review of 5 years of a combined dietary and physical fitness intervention for control of serum cholesterol. *J Am Diet Assoc.* 1994;9:634–638.
9. Bouchard C, Despres J. Physical activity and health: atherosclerotic, metabolic, and hypertensive diseases. *RQES.* 1996;66:268.
10. Bokovoy JL, Blair SN. Aging and exercise: a health perspective. *J Aging Phys Act.* 1994;2:243–260.
11. Goldberg AP. Aerobic and resistive exercise modify risk factors for coronary heart disease. *Med Sci Sports Exerc.* 1989;21:669–674.
12. O'Keefe JH, Lavie CJ, McCallister BD. Insights into the pathogenesis and prevention of coronary artery disease. *Mayo Clin Pro.* 1995;70:69–79.
13. Blair SN, Kohl HW, Barlow CE, Paffenbarger RS, et al. Changes in physical fitness and all cause mortality: a prospective study of healthy and unhealthy men. *JAMA.* 1995;273:1093–1098.
14. Young DR, Haskell WL, Jatulis DE, Fortmann SP. Associations between changes in physical activity and risk factors for coronary heart disease in a community based sample of men and women: the Stanford Five City Project. *Am J Epidemiol.* 1993;138:205–216.
15. Carroll JF, Pollock ML. Rehabilitation and lifestyle modification in the elderly. *Cardiovasc Clin.* 1992;22:209–227.
16. Brownson RC, Smith CA, Pratt M, Mack N. Preventing cardiovascular disease through community-based risk reduction: the Bootheel Heart Health Project. *Am J Public Health.* 1996;86:206–213.
17. Lowenthal DT, Kirschner DA, Scarpace NT, Pollock M, et al. Effects of exercise on age and disease. *South Med J.* 1994;87:s5–s12.
18. Astrand PO. Exercise physiology and its role in disease prevention and in rehabilitation. *Arch Phys Med Rehabil.* 1987;68:305–309.
19. Landin RJ, Linnemeier TJ, Chappelear J, Noble RJ. Exercise testing and training of the elderly. *Cardiovasc Clin.* 1985;15:201–218.
20. American Heart Association. Exercise standards: A statement for healthcare professionals from the American Heart Association. *Circ.* 1995;91:580–615.
21. Shephard RJ. Physical activity, health, and well-being at different life stages. *RQES.* 1996;66:298.
22. Allen SH. Primary osteoporosis. Methods to combat bone loss that accompanies aging. *Postgrad Med.* 1993;8:43–46,49–50,53–55.
23. Birge SJ. Osteoporosis and hip fracture. *Clin Geriatr Med.* 1993;9:69–86.
24. Vargo MM. Osteoporosis: strategies for prevention and treatment. *J Musculoskeletal Med.* 1995;12:19–30.
25. Orwoll ES, Bauer DC, Vogt TM, Fox KM. Axial bone mass in older women. *Ann Intern Med.* 1996;124:187–196.
26. Drinkwater B. Physical activity, fitness, and osteoporosis. In: Bouchard C, Shephard RJ, Stephens T, eds. *Physical Activity, Fitness, and Health.* Champaign, IL: Human Kinetics; 1994:724–736.
27. Vuori I. Exercise and physical health: musculoskeletal health and functional capabilities. *RQES.* 1995;66:276–285.
28. Barry HC, Eathorne SW. Exercise and aging: issues for the practitioner. *Sports Med.* 1994;78:357–376.
29. Nelson ME, Fiatarone MA, Morganti CM, Trice I, et al. Effects of high intensity strength training on multiple risk factors for osteoporotic fractures: a randomized controlled trial. *JAMA.* 1994;272:1909–1914.
30. Pyka G, Lindenberger E, Charette S, Marcus R. Muscle strength and fiber adaptations to a year-long resistance training program in elderly men and women. *J Gerontol.* 1994;49:M22–M27.
31. Roman WJ, Fleckenstein J, Stray-Gunderson J, Always SE. Adaptations in the elbow flexors of elderly males after heavy resistance training. *J Appl Physiol.* 1993;74:750–754.
32. McCartney N, Hicks AL, Martin J, Webber CE. Long term resistance training in the elderly: effects on dynamic strength, exercise capacity, muscle, and bone. *J Gerontol A Biol Sci Med Sci.* 1995;50:B97–B104.
33. Evans WJ. Effects of exercise on body composition and functional capacity of the elderly. *J Gerontol A Biol Sci Med Sci.* 1995;50:147–150.
34. Fiatarone MA, Marks CE, Ryan ND, Meredith CN, et al. High-intensity strength training in nonagenarians—effects on skeletal muscle. *JAMA.* 1990;263:3029–3034.
35. Hunter GR, Treuth MS, Weinsier RL, Kekes-Szabo T, et al. The effects of strength conditioning on older women's ability to perform daily tasks. *J Am Geriatr Soc.* 1995;43:756–760.
36. US Dept. of Agriculture. Agricultural Research Service. November 1994. 6303 Ivy Lane, Room 408, Greenbelt, MD 20770.
37. Tinetti ME, Baker DI, McAvay G, Claus EB, et al. A multifactorial intervention to reduce the risk of falling among elderly people living in the community. *N Engl J Med.* 1994;331:821–827.
38. Tideiksaar R. Preventing falls: how to identify risk factors, reduce complications. *Geriatr.* 1996;51:43–53.
39. Wolf SL, Barnhart HX, Kutner NG, McNeeley E, et al. Reducing frailty and falls in older persons: an investigation of Tai Chi and computerized balance training. *J Am Geriatr Soc.* 1996;44:489–497.
40. Lord SR, Ward JA, Williams P, Strudwick M. The effect of a 12-month exercise trial of balance, strength, and falls in older women: a randomized controlled trial. *J Am Geriatr Soc.* 1995;43:1198–1206.
41. Lord SR, Ward JA, Williams P. Exercise effect on dynamic stability in older women: a randomized controlled trial. *Arch Phys Med Rehabil.* 1996;77:232–236.
42. Province MA, Hadley EC, Hornbrook MC, Lipsitz LA, et al. The effects of exercise on falls in elderly patients: a pre-planned meta-analysis of the FICSIT trials. Frailty and injuries: cooperative studies of intervention techniques. *JAMA.* 1995;273:1341–1347.
43. Szymanski LM, Pate RR, Durstine JL. Effects of maximal exercise and venous occlusion on fibrinolytic activity in physically active and inactive men. *J Appl Physiol.* 1994;77:2305–2310.
44. Greendale GA, Bodin-Dunn L, Ingles S, Haile R. Leisure, home, and occupational physical activity and cardiovascular risk factors in postmenopausal women: the Postmenopausal Estrogens/Progestins Intervention (PEPI) Study. *Arch Intern Med.* 1996;156:418–424.
45. Rauramaa R, Tuomainen P, Vaisanen S, Rankinen T. Physical activity and health-related fitness in middle-aged men. *Med Sci Sports Exerc.* 1995;27:707–712.
46. Bokovoy JL, Blair SN. Aging and exercise: a health perspective. *J Aging Phys Act.* 1994;2:243–260.
47. Astrand PO. Physical activity and fitness. *Am J Clin Nutr.* 1992;55:1231s–1236s.
48. Lohman T, Going S, Pamenter R, Hall M, et al. Effects of resistance training on regional and total bone mineral density in premenopausal women: a randomized prospective study. *J Bone Mineral Res.* 1995;10:1015–1024.
49. McAuley E, Bane SM, Mihalko SL. Exercise in middle-aged adults: self-efficacy and self-presentational outcomes. *Prev Med.* 1995;24:319–328.
50. Block JE, Friedlander AL, Brooks GA, Steiger P, et al. Determinants of bone density among athletes engaged in weight-bearing and non–weight-bearing activity. *J Appl Physiol.* 1989;67:1100–1105.
51. Hartard M, Haber P, Ilieva D, Preisinger E. Systematic strength training as a model of therapeutic intervention. *Am J Phys Med Rehabil.* 1996;75:21–28.

52. Koffler KH, Menkes A, Redmond RA, Whitehead WE, et al. Strength training accelerates gastrointestinal transit in middle-aged and older men. *Med Sci Sports Exerc*. 1992;24:415–419.
53. Klesges RC, Klesges LM, Eck LH, Shelton ML. A longitudinal analysis of accelerated weight gain in preschool children. *Pediatr*. 1995;95:126.
54. Wang JS, Jen CJ, Chen HI. Effects of exercise training and deconditioning on platelet function in men. *Arterioscler Thromb Vasc Biol*. 1995;15:1668–1674.
55. Lee I. Exercise and physical health: cancer and immune function. *RQES*. 1995;66:286.
56. Shephard RJ. Exercise in the prevention and treatment of cancer: an update. *Sports Med*. 1993;15:258–280.
57. Potter JD. Risk factors for colon neoplasia—epidemiology and biology. *Eur J Cancer*. 1995;31A:1033–1038.
58. Biddle S. Exercise and psychosocial health. *RQES*. 1996;66:292.
59. Norvell N, Belles D. Psychological and physical benefits of circuit weight training in law enforcement personnel. *J Consult Clin Psychol*. 1993;61:520–527.
60. Herman E, Williams R, Stratford P, Fargas-Babjak A, et al. A randomized controlled trial of transcutaneous electrical nerve stimulation (CODETRON) to determine its benefits in a rehabilitation program for acute occupational low back pain. *Spine*. 1994;19:561–568.
61. Shephard RJ. Current perspectives on the economics of fitness and sport with particular reference to worksite programs. *Sports Med*. 1989;7:286–309.

CHAPTER 2

The Client Education Process

David Ash

CHAPTER OUTLINE

I. The Client Interview
II. Common Exercise Misconceptions
III. Medical Approval To Exercise
IV. Strategies To Facilitate Motor Learning
V. Specificity
VI. Recording Exercise Data
VII. Intensity (Difficulty) of Resistive Exercise
VIII. Muscle Contraction Following Rapid Stretch
IX. Chapter Summary

THE CLIENT INTERVIEW

The client interview is the initial meeting between the exercise professional and the client. The purposes of this meeting are to establish communication, allow the client to verbalize questions and goals, and initiate the client education process. The criticality of the client education process is underscored by one of Deming's favorite phrases: "You have one chance to train someone, you cannot repeat it!"[1] It is much more effective to invest time teaching correct principles of preventive exercise early—from the first meeting—than to attempt to erase and correct improper technique. It is recommended that an initial meeting of one hour's duration be held, in which the professional and client communicate on a one-on-one basis. During this session, no actual exercise is demonstrated or performed. The professional's focus is on teaching *principles,* as opposed to merely demonstrating how to use equipment. The client will recognize and appreciate this individualized education and professional attention. Generally the client will be prepared to move on to the teaching, demonstration, and practice of exercise movements by the second session.

Suggestions for the Client Interview

1. Always project a positive, upbeat, optimistic demeanor during interaction with your clients.
2. Emphasize the very reasonable time commitment involved, as well as the high benefit/cost ratio.
3. During your discussion of exercise principles, emphasize safety.
4. Convey that the client's results are a function of **how** exercise equipment is used rather than use of a particular **type** of equipment. Emphasize using a facility or equipment that are readily accessible.
5. Prior to the interview, prepare a personalized folder containing several research studies regarding the benefits of preventive exercise. During the interview, you may add to this folder based on the client's specific questions and areas of interest.

Maldonato et al, in a review of literature regarding the education of diabetic patients commented, "Education demands a lot from health care providers: specific training, teaching skills, good communication, supportive attitude, readiness to listen, and ability to negotiate." Additional keypoints identified by Maldonato et al are as follows: (1) a prerequisite of structured education is the identification of specific, precise short-term goals, (2) the attainment of these goals shall be verified, (3) objectives may be set at different levels (ie, technical knowledge, skills, capacity to integrate into everyday life), and (4) the most pertinent objectives apply to the therapeutic goals.[2] For the healthy exerciser, the most pertinent objectives apply to prevention of disease or dysfunction.

Questions and Answers

When considering answers to client questions, several points may be kept in mind. A subtle comment to the effect that your answers are based on peer-reviewed scientific research will enhance your credibility with the client. Present answers confidently, yet with a touch of humility. Every question is important. Responses to questions may be prefaced with comments such as, "That is a frequently asked question," or "I can understand how you might infer that." In addition to encouraging the client to ask further questions, comments such as these provide the professional with a lead in to briefly discussing research relevant to the client's particular query. When finished with the question/answer session, encourage the client to ask additional questions as they arise. Offer to update the client about any special interests he or she may have as you obtain new information regarding that topic. If you do not know the answer to a question, inform the client that you will conduct a review of research literature and have the results ready for him or her by the next scheduled exercise session.

Identifying Short-Term and Long-Term Goals

The client is asked to verbalize two or three specific goals to be met within six weeks and two or three specific goals to be met within six months. These goals are put in writing and a copy is given to the client for motivational purposes. A copy is kept on file for periodic evaluation of client progress toward goals, and for evaluation of program effectiveness. The goals must be relevant, specific, and measurable. They must also be *realistic*. A large gap between the expected and the attained is not conducive to maintenance of client motivation. The following are examples of goals.

- *Short-term goal*: The client will complete 20 consecutive minutes on the exercise bicycle at 10.0 METs within 3 weeks.
- *Long-term goal*: The client will achieve 15% body fat within 6 months as measured by underwater weighing.

COMMON EXERCISE MISCONCEPTIONS

A goal of the exercise professional is to teach the client to be a critical consumer of exercise information. Several misconceptions in the area of exercise are so prevalent that it is in the client's best interest for the exercise professional to address this topic during the initial interview. As stated above, the professional emphasizes the positive aspects and benefits of the growing base of exercise research. Avoid dwelling on the negativity of the misconception. This approach leaves the client with an appreciation for the information the professional has provided.

Misconception 1: More Is Better

We live in a society that generally embraces the belief that more is better. However, with exercise there is an optimal level of activity for each individual, which if exceeded leads to diminishing returns and possibly injury. Chapter 9 is devoted entirely to recovery and overtraining issues.

Misconception 2: Strength Is Defined as the Amount of Force That Can Be Exerted during a Single Maximal Effort

This statement may be one definition of strength, but it is not the only way to define strength. Strength is a *construct* that can be operationally defined by anyone in any manner. Lambrinides[3] discusses five different definitions of strength that have appeared in resistive exercise literature. He goes on to agree with Caldwell's[4] statement, "There are as many strengths as there are conditions of measurement...."

Misconception 3: Type of Equipment Is Important

It is common to hear equipment sales representatives advocate the benefits of a particular brand of resistive and/or aerobic exercise equipment. If the equipment is safe and can provide the basic requirements for the type of exercise desired (eg, for resistive exercise equipment an allowance of full range of movement and a means to vary the resistance), the equipment is adequate. Physiological adaptations are not a function of the type of equipment used but rather of *how* the equipment is used. If used in a safe, productive, time-efficient manner, the particular brand of equipment is insignificant.

A question frequently asked of the exercise professional regarding resistive exercise is, "Do you recommend free weights (plate-loaded bars and dumbbells) or machines (selectorized resistive exercise machines)?" Research indicates no difference in the results produced by use of either free-weight resistance or machine resistance.[5–8] It is recommended that the equipment to which the exerciser has access be used.

Misconception 4: Explosive Resistive Exercise Movements Facilitate Explosive Movements in Sport Skills

The fact that it is desirable to perform certain activities—specific sports skill movements for example—in a rapid fashion may lead one to infer that resistive exercise should also be performed in the same rapid fashion. Before relevant research studies are presented, a brief analogy will be used to illustrate that the aforementioned line of reasoning may be overly simplistic. Let us suppose an individual is performing a 100-meter sprint. Throughout the sprint, as the quadriceps rapidly contract, the antagonistic hamstrings must lengthen just as rapidly, and vice versa. If one held that rapid muscle contraction during the performance of a 100-meter sprint was justification for performing rapid muscular contraction during resistive exercise, would that person not be contradicting him- or herself if rapid range of motion exercise (stretching) was not also advocated, based on the fact that muscles lengthen very rapidly throughout the course of a 100-meter sprint? In actuality, slow, controlled stretching is recommended due to the potential of rapid or ballistic stretching to cause tissue trauma. Refer to Table 2–1 for a summary of research on the speed of movement during resistive exercise.

A common belief in sports training facilities involves the use of 300 to 400 degree/second isokinetic resistive training speeds. The rationale for training at these speeds is that they may facilitate the performance of rapid sport skill movements. It should be realized, however, that though speeds in this range may be the most rapid offered by an isokinetic device, the 300 to 400 degree/second speeds are much slower than actual movement speeds; elite baseball athletes exhibit peak shoulder internal rotation velocities of greater than 9000 degrees per second.[15,16] The angular velocity spectrum depicted in Exhibit 2–1 elucidates two important concepts.

1. Even the fastest isokinetic angular velocities (point C = 360°/second) are extremely slow when compared

Table 2–1 Research Regarding Speed of Movement during Resistive Exercise

Summary	Researchers/Authors
A study was conducted to investigate the effects of a rapidly performed hip extension resistive exercise movement as compared to a hip extension resistive exercise movement performed in a slower manner. It was hypothesized that the rapid movement speed would be more efficient in power development than the slower movement speed. Dependent variables were the Margaria-Kalamen power test, vertical jump, power clean, push press, and squat. At the conclusion of the study, no difference was found with respect to any of the dependent variables between the group that performed the resistive movement rapidly and the group that performed the movement in a slow, controlled manner.	Wenzel and Perfetto[9]
"It appears that mid-range isokinetic training speed carries over to both slower and faster speeds and that there are significant contralateral training effects."	Housh and Housh[10]
"Fifty-four college-aged males were randomly assigned to one of three experimental groups to determine the effects of slow, fast, and combination slow and fast speed dynamic concentric weight training on leg power. Dependent variables were vertical jump, Lewis formula leg power, and single repetition maximum squat. While each group improved in performance of the dependent variables, statistical analysis indicated that there existed no significant difference between groups. It was concluded that neither slow, fast, nor the combination slow and fast repetition training speeds was superior in developing leg power in untrained college-aged men."	Palmieri[11]
"The results suggest that the principal stimuli for the high velocity training response are the repeated *attempts* to perform ballistic contractions and the high rate of force development of the ensuing contraction. The *type* of muscle action (isometric or concentric) appears to be of lesser importance."	Behm and Sale[12]
"The purpose of the investigation was to examine the effects of dynamic constant external resistance (DCER) training on isokinetic peak torque (PT) and constant joint angle (CJA) torque at velocities from zero to 5.03 rad/second. The results indicate that DCER training significantly increased isokinetic PT and CJA torque values at velocities up to 3.53 radians/second *above the training velocity.*"	Weir, Housh, Evans, and Johnson[13]
A study was designed to examine the effects of using two different squat lift training velocities. Dependent variables were 1 RM squat, vertical jump, thigh muscle size, and squat position isometric force. Both groups demonstrated significant improvement in all dependent variables. There were no significant improvement differences between the two groups.	Young and Bilby[14]

Copyright © 1997, Aspen Publishers, Inc.
Exercises for Health Promotion

Exhibit 2–1 Angular Velocity Spectrum

```
                 Degrees per Second
ABC                                              D
 0 1000 2000 3000 4000 5000 6000 7000 8000 9000 10000

Legend: A = 120; B = 240; C = 360; D = 9000
```

to actual sport skill movements (point D = 9000°/second).

2. There is essentially no difference between the slowest (point A) and fastest (point C) isokinetic offerings when compared to actual sport skill movement speeds (point D).

Isokinetic devices at various velocities can be used as one of many tools to provide resistance. However, the rationale that the value of resistive training at the most rapid angular velocities offered by an isokinetic device is that these speeds are closer to sport movement velocity is overly simplistic.

For those wishing to increase their velocity during performance of a sport skill, it seems prudent to develop strength in the safest manner possible (using relatively slow, controlled movements) and then practice the sport skill at competition speed. This is the principle of "specificity."[17]

Misconception 5: Resistive Exercise Reduces Range of Motion

A misconception frequently heard is that resistive exercise will result in decreased range of movement. The only way this could occur is if the resistive movements were not performed throughout the full range of motion. The chronic performance of partial repetitions, seen when exercisers are attempting to use more weight than they can lift with proper technique, may lead to morphological shortening of tissues. However, if resistive exercise is performed through the full range of motion, flexibility can actually be enhanced by the phenomenon of reciprocal inhibition. For more information regarding reciprocal inhibition, refer to Chapter 6.

Misconception 6: Exercise Causes Female Masculinization

Females possess the hormone testosterone, but in small concentrations compared to their male counterparts. For this reason, increases in muscle mass will occur in females to a lesser degree than in males. The percentage of females possessing the genetic endowment to develop competition level physiques is very small. This population will be muscular whether or not they exercise.

Misconception 7: Split-Routines Are Better

Many of the exercise magazines one can purchase propose the practice of splitting the body's muscular structures into two or more different groups. Those who practice this method believe that if a given movement is not performed on successive days, the muscles that produce that movement are given a rest day or off day. Muscle groups can be split in various ways. Examples include dividing by body part (exercising upper body structures on one day and lower body structures on the following day) and dividing by movement (exercising flexion or pulling movements on one day and extension or pushing movements on the following day).

In actuality, the body does not function as segments isolated from each other. Multiple muscle groups function together to produce the resultant movement. To illustrate by example, the bench press movement elicits motor unit activity in many different muscle groups throughout the entire body (eg, the latissimus dorsi). Despite this fact, the muscles of the chest and back are commonly exercised on consecutive days by those who follow split routines. Consider also the variety of movements in which the low back muscles are used to stabilize the body. Are these muscles really getting a rest on their "off day"?

From the perspective of the endocrine system, it would seem likely that because hormones (insulin, growth hormone, testosterone) are produced only at specific sites in the body, their reserves would be drawn upon during resistive exercise, muscle group alternation notwithstanding. It is recommended here that resistive exercise be performed on nonsuccessive days to ensure recovery.

Misconception 8: Light Resistance and More Repetitions Decreases Body Weight; Heavy Resistance for Fewer Repetitions Increases Body Weight

A common misconception is that the use of light resistance and more repetitions will reduce body weight and that the use of heavier resistance for fewer repetitions will increase body weight. Whether one increases or decreases body weight is not a function of set-repetition combinations, but rather a function of caloric intake. If an individual exercises with heavy resistance and fewer repetitions but consumes fewer calories than he or she expends, that exerciser will lose body weight. Conversely, if an exerciser uses lighter resistance and performs more repetitions, while consuming more calories than expending, that individual will gain weight.

Misconception 9: Exercise Is Complicated

If one were to browse through exercise magazines it is understandable how he or she may become confused by the plethora of different routines, phases, formulas, and percentages of single repetition maximums. The exerciser is ad-

Table 2–2 Exercise Prescription Schema

Exercise Program Component	Exercise Base	Additional Exercise Based on Individual Needs/Goals
Aerobic Exercise	20 minutes, 3 days per week.	Additional activity specific exercise. For example, if a client's goal is participation in a sport which requires both sustained and brief intense activity (eg, basketball, soccer), the program may combine interval training with the aerobic base.
Resistive Exercise	One set of 8–12 repetitions. Eight to ten movements that condition the large mass muscle groups.* 2 sessions per week is the recommended minimum.	May add additional preventive exercises if client activity places high demand on particular muscle groups.
	Large mass muscle groups: (Alternate movements to maintain 8–10 movements per session.) Spinal flexors/ extensors, hip musculature, knee flexors/extensors, shoulder adductors/abductors, shoulder transverse adductors/abductors, shoulder extensors/flexors, shoulder elevators, shoulder rotators, elbow flexors/extensors, cervical musculature	Potential additional resistive exercise based on preventive needs of activity: Ankle eversion and dorsiflexion if high risk of ankle sprain. Wrist flexion, extension, and grip strength for tennis, golf.
Range of Motion (Flexibility) Exercise	All major muscle groups.	Additional range of motion exercise if specific morphological shortening is identified.

Note: *Refer to "Principles of Resistive Exercise" in Chapter 4. Prescription not to exceed specifications based on medical exam by physician.

vised to be conscious of the difference between exercise magazines and peer-reviewed journals. There is a difference between advertising and research. Table 2–2 illustrates that exercise prescription is not complicated. One could hypothesize that the sales of some of the exercise magazines may decrease if each month the central theme was safe, productive, time-efficient exercise rather than arcane programs endorsed by the genetically gifted.

Misconception 10: The Quick Fix Works

Physiological adaptations take time. Beware of claims touting immediate results or results comparable to champion physique athletes. Certainly everyone can improve body composition within an individual range with consistent exercise over time. The exerciser should realize that the upper limit of that range is predetermined genetically. If exercise is performed with patience and persistence, the exerciser will not be disappointed with the results.

Misconception 11: Spot Reduction Is Possible

It is common to see individuals performing countless sets of situps with the belief that they can isolate fat reduction in the abdominal region. Spot reduction is not a physiological phenomenon. When the body calls upon fat stores to be released for use as fuel, fat is mobilized from stores throughout the body, rather than only at the body segments where movement is occurring.

Misconception 12: Progress Is Evaluated from Single Repetition Maximums

Actually, each time an exerciser performs a set of resistive exercise, he or she is evaluating progress by comparing the resistance used and repetitions completed *today* to those completed *last week, last month, and last year.* Setting aside a particular day to do a single repetition maximum (RM) is not necessary to monitor progress. Rose and Ball[18] developed a prediction equation for college females' maximal single repetition bench press based upon the number of repetitions performed with a 20.4 kg (44.88 lb) bar. A high correlation ($r = 0.82$, $p < 0.05$) was identified between predicted 1 RM and actual 1 RM. Mayhew et al[19] and Brzycki[20] have also developed equations that predict single repetition maximums based on the number of repetitions performed with a submaximal load. While review of current and prior recording sheets would seem to provide a valid marker of progress toward specific goals, if additional evaluation is desired, use of prediction equations as described above is preferable to performing single repetition maximums.

Results of a 4-year study (1988–1992) conducted with members of the University of Connecticut men's varsity basketball team ($n = 29$) identified a low correlation between 1 RM bench press performance and playing time (r values ranging from -0.04 to 0.14). Rather, the coaches' evaluation of the player was the most valid predictor of playing time, explaining 56 to 86% of the variance in playing time.[21]

Of greater consequence, a study conducted by Smith[22] indicated that body mechanics deteriorated with maximal loads (1 RM) while performing a floor to waist lift. The author hypothesizes that 1 RM loads in *any* lifting movement will result in body mechanic deterioration, a common cause of injury.

Misconception 13: Exercise Programs for Males and Females Need To Be Different

In general, resistive exercise is gender independent. The same principles of exercise apply to females and males.

Misconception 14: Resistive Exercise Will Decrease Speed of Movement in Sport Skills

There is no reason to assume sport skill movement speed will decrease, provided sport skills are practiced at competition speed concurrently with the resistive exercise program. Resistive exercise principles include training agonist and antagonist muscle groups and emphasizing full range of motion.

Misconception 15: Strength and Speed Training Methods Practiced in Eastern Europe and the Commonwealth of Independent States Are Superior to Other Training Methods

"The United States has dominated Olympic track and field winning 218 gold medals since 1896. The best of the rest are Finland, 36; Russia, 34; Britain, 32; East Germany, 14; Sweden, 12; and Kenya, 10."[23]

MEDICAL APPROVAL TO EXERCISE

In addition to reviewing the client's history of physical activity both verbally and through a questionnaire, a physician's approval to participate in an exercise program is always secured prior to initiating teaching of exercise. A physician's approval should minimally contain the following information:

1. The general types of activities (ie, aerobic, flexibility, and resistive exercise) that have been deemed safe and appropriate for the client's participation.
2. Any activities that are contraindicated.
3. Any precautions that should be followed.
4. The intensity (difficulty level) that is not to be exceeded.

STRATEGIES TO FACILITATE MOTOR LEARNING

Optimization of the client learning process will enhance the performance of safe, productive, and time-efficient exercise. Several training strategies have been identified as being effective concerning motor learning. These techniques have been used successfully in teaching motor skills in rehabilitation settings with neurologic and orthopedic patients. Because the techniques enhance motor skill acquisition, it would seem appropriate to use these methods to teach the motor skills involved in preventive exercise to healthy individuals. Schmidt[24] recommends focusing on the following areas when teaching motor skills: design and preparation of practice, scheduling and organization of practice, and type of feedback. O'Sullivan and Schmitz[25] provide the following operational definitions.

- **Practice**
  1. *Massed practice:* A prolonged period of practice with infrequent rest periods.
  2. *Distributed practice:* An alternating sequence of rest and practice sessions in which the rest time equals or exceeds the practice time.
  3. *Constant practice:* Practice organized around one task performed repeatedly.
  4. *Variable practice:* Practice of several variations of the same task or within the same category or class of movements.

- **Feedback** is sensory information provided to the central nervous system from the production of movement. There are two types of feedback: intrinsic and extrinsic.
  1. *Intrinsic feedback:* The feedback normally received during the execution of a movement.
  2. *Extrinsic (augmented) feedback:* Feedback that is added to that normally received during a movement task. Types of information provided by extrinsic feedback include:

- *Knowledge of performance (KP):* Feedback that occurs during movement and allows for error detection and movement modification.
- *Knowledge of results (KR):* Feedback that occurs at the conclusion of movement and allows the appraisal of the overall success of the movement response.

- **Amount and frequency of feedback**
  1. *Summed feedback:* Feedback given after a set number of trials (eg, after every third trial).
  2. *Faded feedback:* Feedback given at first after every trial and then less frequently (eg, after every second trial progressing to every fifth trial).
  3. *Delayed feedback:* Feedback given after a time delay (eg, a 3-second delay).
  4. *Bandwidth feedback:* Feedback given only when performance is outside a given error.

- **Transfer of learning**
  1. *Parts to whole learning:* Practice of component parts before practice of the integrated whole.[25]
  2. *Whole-part-whole learning:* A variation of the parts to whole strategy, where the following sequence is followed:[26]
     - The desired skill is completed in its entirety to provide the learner with a big picture of the skill.
     - The component parts of the skill are practiced, with emphasis placed on components with which the learner has difficulty.
     - As soon as the learner demonstrates proficiency in performance of the components, the skill is practiced in its entirety.

Practical Application of Strategies To Facilitate Motor Learning

- *Strategy:* Before the exercise professional introduces a new skill to be learned, she or he explains that the next scheduled exercise session will begin with the client being expected to teach the new skill to the professional.
- *Rationale:* The learner is more likely to ask questions and make sure she or he understands the skill fully when the learner knows she or he will be required to teach the skill to others.

- *Strategy:* Prior to demonstration of a given movement, the exercise professional explains the movement verbally. The professional then demonstrates the movement in its entirety.
- *Rationale:* A prerequisite for correct performance of a task is the client's clear understanding of what she or he is being asked to do.

- *Strategy:* The client is initially asked to perform a particular movement, eg, the dumbbell lunge, in its entirety. If the exercise professional observes the client performing a component of the movement incorrectly (eg, allowing the torso to flex, or bumping the knees to the floor), performance of the total movement is stopped. Only that component of the movement that is not being performed correctly is practiced. As soon as possible, provided correct performance of the problematic component is demonstrated, the client returns to practicing the skill in its entirety.
- *Rationale:* This strategy uses the whole-part-whole method of learning.

- *Strategy:* Throughout the practice session verbal feedback is given to the client in varying amounts and frequencies.
- *Rationale:* For long-term retention (learning), varying the amount and frequency of feedback is recommended. Varied feedback requires an increased depth of cognitive processing, which is believed to enhance learning, though the initial acquisition of the skill may not occur as rapidly.[25]

- *Strategy:* The professional provides only relevant information. Constant chatter is avoided.
- *Rationale:* O'Sullivan and Schmitz[25] caution to avoid the common mistake of providing too much feedback. This can slow learning as the exerciser becomes distracted (if not irritated) as he or she is unable to concentrate on his or her own problem-solving skills.

- *Strategy:* Total practice time exceeds total rest time.
- *Rationale:* Gentile[27] recommends use of massed practice to facilitate learning.

- *Strategy:* The next exercise session begins with the client and exercise professional trading roles. The client must correctly teach the professional, who plays the role of a novice.
- *Rationale:* This strategy is a simple, effective procedure using role reversal to identify whether the client understands correct movement performance.

It is important to remember that different clients may respond better to different strategies of motor learning facilitation. Emphasize the techniques, identified through trial and error, that produce the best results for a particular client and a particular situation.

SPECIFICITY

In the context of motor skill teaching/learning, the distinction between *simulation* and *specificity* should be emphasized.

- *Simulation:* Performance of a movement or activity that *appears to resemble* the desired movement or activity (eg, performing throwing movements with a weighted baseball in hopes that it will improve throwing of a regulation baseball).
- *Specificity:* Performance of the desired movement or activity (eg, performing throwing movements with a regulation baseball in hopes that it will improve throwing of a regulation baseball).

Winstein[28] concurs, stating that with regard to physical therapy balance and locomotion retraining approaches, the notion of training carryover is an assumption. "It is generally accepted that practice of a motor skill from the 'lower' end of our imaginary skill continuum will enhance performance of a motor skill from the 'higher' end of the continuum. For example, common retraining protocols for certain locomotor deficits involve weight-shifting exercises in preparation for stepping and walking. From this, it would seem that physical therapists, for the most part, assume that practice of certain skills will carry over to the performance of other motor skills. In the motor skills literature, this concept is termed transfer of training." A study conducted with 61 subjects from Rancho Los Amigos Medical Center was conducted to investigate the question of whether routine standing balance and weight-shifting training has a facilitory effect on locomotor performance. The results of this study "provide no support for the notion that improved standing balance transfers to locomotor performance." In fact, the results support a *specificity of training* hypothesis.[28]

RECORDING EXERCISE DATA

Recording exercise data during each exercise session creates a valuable database. For resistive exercise, the recording of variables such as amount of resistance used, intensity, and number of repetitions performed provides an ongoing progress chart. This visual record can contribute to the client's compliance with the exercise program. The inclusion of sections on the recording form for all components of the program (resistive, aerobic, and range of motion) serves as a reminder that a balanced combination of these components is optimal for prevention of injury, illness, and disease. Furthermore, during the early stages of the program, the client may not recall the names of the exercises or the resistance used during the previous session. The recording form provides this information at one's fingertips.

INTENSITY (DIFFICULTY) OF RESISTIVE EXERCISE

When speaking of aerobic exercise, intensity is commonly understood to reflect heart rate or perceived exertion level. With reference to resistive exercise, however, the need to identify intensity and resistance often results in confusion regarding the definitions of these two variables. Operational definitions are as follows:

- *Resistance*: Objective, a quantity (eg, a five-pound dumbbell) used to perform a movement.
- *Intensity*: The subjective (perceived) difficulty of performance of a set of resistive exercise.

When teaching a client to record resistive exercise information, suggest that she or he consider the term intensity merely as a synonym for difficulty. The three categories in Exhibit 2–2 are then used by the client after each set of resistive exercise to identify the perceived level of difficulty for that set.

A common practice is to increase the amout of resistance used when a predetermined target number of repetitions is achieved. For example, a client may be instructed to increase the resistance used in a particular movement when he or she can perform 12 repetitions with correct form. A more accurate marker of the propriety of increasing resistance is to also consider the perceived difficulty during the performance of that set of 12 repetitions. The following example will elucidate that the amount of resistance used and the number of repetitions correctly performed provide necessary, but not sufficient, information to know when it is appropriate to increase resistance. Consideration of the perceived difficulty is also required.

Example: Suppose that on a given date (eg, 2-1-96), a client performs 10 repetitions of leg curls with 60 pounds. Upon completion of each set, the client is instructed to ask herself or himself "How difficult was that activity?" Let's say that the client perceives that the set was difficult. The information to be recorded includes:

- The exercise session was performed on 2-1-96.
- Leg curl was the movement performed.
- The resistance used was 60.
- The client performed 10 repetitions.
- This activity was perceived as being difficult.

On the section of the recording sheet (Exhibit 2–3) the client first records the exercise date. She or he then locates

Exhibit 2–2 Resistive Exercise Intensity (Difficulty) Scale

E	Easy
M	Moderate
D	Difficult

Exhibit 2–3 Sample Section of Recording Sheet: Difficult

	Date 2-1-96 R r D	Date 2-4-96 R r D	Date 2-6-96 R r D	Date 2-9-96 R r D	Date 2-12-96 R r D	Date 2-15-96 R r D
Exercise						
Leg Press						
Leg Curl	60 10 D	60				
Leg Extension						
Back Extension						
Abdominal Curl						

the row designated for the leg curl movement and follows it across the record form to the exercise date. Here, the client records three variables. Under "R," the client records the resistance used (60). Under "r," the client records that ten repetitions were performed. The third variable is perceived difficulty, denoted by "D." Under the "D," the client writes *D* because the activity was perceived as being difficult.

The fact that the client could perform the movement for ten correct repetitions indicates that the resistance is appropriate. The fact that completion was perceived as difficult indicates that the same resistance should be used during the next session in which that movement is performed.

Let's speculate that after performing the leg curl with a resistance of 60 for 4 sessions, the client performs 12 repetitions with correct form and subsequently characterizes the difficulty level as being moderate. Now it is appropriate to increase resistance as noted in Exhibit 2–4.

In addition to achieving a predetermined target number of repetitions, it is recommended that criteria for increasing resistance include the client's perception of the activity as progressing from difficult to moderate on a three-point scale of difficult, moderate, and easy. An entire sample exercise record form is provided in Exhibit 2–5.

MUSCLE CONTRACTION FOLLOWING RAPID STRETCH

Plyometrics is a term popularized by Verkhoshansky, a trainer of track and field athletes in the former Soviet Union. Based on the stretch reflex and elastic energy storage and release, Verkhoshansky believed the use of depth jumps (jumping from boxes of various heights), bounding on a single leg, and hopping exercises in training programs would improve athletic performance.[29,30] Over time, these jumping activities came to be collectively referred to as plyometrics. However, utilization of the stretch reflex and energy from elastic deformation are not specific to these activities. Such acts as closing a door, walking up a flight of stairs, and rising from a chair, for example, all utilize this mechanism. To ensure understanding in communication (among those who engage in these activities) regarding precisely the activity or movement to which is being referred, it is recommended that the activity be specifically described (eg, jumps from a 12-inch box, performing a chest pass with a weighted ball, bounding ten steps on each leg) rather than using the term plyometrics.

While it is agreed that the stretch reflex and utilization of energy from elastic deformation do exist, research has not

Exhibit 2–4 Sample Section of Recording Sheet: Moderate

	Date 2-1-96 R r D	Date 2-4-96 R r D	Date 2-6-96 R r D	Date 2-9-96 R r D	Date 2-12-96 R r D	Date 2-15-96 R r D
Exercise						
Leg Press						
Leg Curl	60 10 D	60 11 D	60 12 D	60 12 D	60 12 M	65
Leg Extension						
Back Extension						
Abdominal Curl						

Exhibit 2–5 Exercise Recording Sheet

Exercise Record

Name _____

Precautions _____

Contraindications _____

Comments _____

DIFFICULTY SCALE

E easy

M moderate

D difficult

	Date R r D	Date R r D	Date R r D	Date R r D	Date R r D
Pre-ex HR					
Resistive Exercise					
Abdominal Curl					
Back Extension					
Leg Press					
Lunge					
Knee Flexion					
Knee Extension					
Calf Raise					
Pull Up					
Shoulder Extension					
Sh. Trans AB					
Shoulder Flexion					
Shoulder Abduction					
Sh. Trans ADD					
Dumbbell Incline					
Shoulder Elevation					
Elbow Flexion					
Elbow Extension					
Wrist Flexion					
Wrist Extension					
(Perform 8–12 of the above movements. Address each major muscle group.)					
Aerobic Exercise	Duration/Difficulty				
Bike					
Swim					
U.B.E.					
Aerobics Class					
Flexibility					
(check when completed)					

Copyright © 1997, Aspen Publishers, Inc.
Exercises for Health Promotion

indicated that these phenomena can be trained to work more efficiently in the performance of sport skills.

Research regarding the effects of jumping from boxes, and performing various hopping activities has yielded contradictory findings.[31] Some studies indicate that depth jumps,[32] and a combination of depth jumps, hopping, and performing split squats[33] result in improved vertical jump performance. Other studies indicate that depth jumps and other activities called plyometrics do not have a significant effect on vertical jump or other dependent variables measured.[34–38]

CHAPTER SUMMARY

It is more efficient to invest time teaching correct principles of preventive exercise from the first meeting than to attempt to erase and correct improper technique. The initial session with the client is called the client interview. The purpose of this meeting is to establish communication, allow the client to verbalize questions and goals, and to initiate the client education process. Efficient and safe client education is enhanced by early education regarding common exercise misconceptions. A specific medical document indicating clearance to exercise is secured prior to the client initiating exercise. Training strategies that facilitate the motor skill learning process have been identified. The recording of exercise data provides a motivational tool and a readily available marker of client progress.

REFERENCES

1. Walton M. *The Deming Management Method*. New York: Putnam Publishing Group; 1986.
2. Maldonato A, Bloise D, Ceci M, Fraticelli E, et al. Diabetes mellitus: lessons from patient education. *Patient Educ Couns*. 1995;26:57–66.
3. Lambrinides T. Strength: what is it? *High Intensity Training Newsletter*. 1991;3:8–9.
4. Caldwell LS. The load-endurance relationship for a static manual response. *Hum Factors*. 1964;6:71–79.
5. Boyer BT. A comparison of the effects of three strength training programs on women. *J Appl Sport Sci Res*. 1990;4:88–94.
6. Stiggins CF. *Nautilus and Free Weight Training Program: A Comparison of Strength Development at Four Angles in the Range of Motion*. Salt Lake City, UT: Brigham Young University; 1978. Thesis.
7. Messier SP, Dill ME. Alterations in strength and maximal oxygen uptake consequent to Nautilus circuit weight training. *RQES*. 1985; 56:345–351.
8. Trappe SW, Pearson DR. Effects of weight assisted dry land strength training on swimming performance. *J Strength Conditioning Res*. 1994;8:209–213.
9. Wenzel RR, Perfetto EM. The effect of speed versus non-speed training in power development. *J Appl Sport Sci Res*. 1992;6:82–87.
10. Housh DJ, Housh TJ. The effects of unilateral velocity-specific concentric strength training. *J Orthop Sports Phys Ther*. 1993;17:252–256.
11. Palmieri GA. Weight training and repetition speed. *J Appl Sport Sci Res*. 1987;1:60.
12. Behm DG, Sale DG. Intended rather than actual movement velocity determines velocity-specific training response. *J Appl Physiol*. 1993; 74:359–368.
13. Weir JP, Housh TJ, Evans SA, Johnson GO. The effect of dynamic constant external resistance training in the isokinetic torque-velocity curve. *Intern J Sports Med*. 1993;14:124–128.
14. Young WB, Bilby GE. The effect of voluntary effort to influence speed of contraction on strength, muscular power, and hypertrophy development. *J Strength Conditioning Res*. 1993;7:172–178.
15. Dillman C. Biomechanics of pitching. Lecture presented at Olympic Training Center. March, 1989.
16. Pappas A, Zowacki R, Sullivan T. Biomechanics of baseball pitching, a preliminary report. *Am J Sports Med*. 1985;13:216–222.
17. Voigt M, Klausen K. Changes in muscle strength and speed of an unloaded movement after various training programmes. *Eur J Appl Physiol*. 1990;60:370–376.
18. Rose K, Ball TE. A field test for predicting maximum bench press lift of college women. *J Appl Sport Sci Res*. 1992;6:103–106.
19. Mayhew JL, Ware JR, Prinster JL. Using repetitions to predict muscular strength in adolescent males. *Natl Strength Conditioning Assoc J*. 1993;15:35–38.
20. Brzycki M. Strength testing: predicting a one rep max from reps-to-fatigue. *JOHPERD*. 1993;64:88–90.
21. Hoffman JR, Tenenbaum G, Maresh CM, Kraemer WJ. Relationship between athletic performance tests and playing time in elite college basketball players. *J Strength Conditioning Res*. 1996;10:67–70.
22. Smith RL. Therapists ability to identify safe maximum lifting in low back pain patients during functional capacity evaluation. *J Orthop Sports Phys Ther*. 1994;19:277–282.
23. The Washington Post 1992; August 5:F2.
24. Schmidt RA. *Motor Learning and Performance*. Champaign, IL: Human Kinetics; 1991.
25. O'Sullivan SB, Schmitz TJ. *Physical Rehabilitation: Assessment and Treatment*. 3rd ed. Philadelphia: FA Davis; 1994:239–249.
26. Poplin MS. Holistic/constructionist principles of the teaching/learning process: implications for the field of learning disabilities. *J Learn Disabil*. 1988;68:522–526.
27. Gentile AM. Skill acquisition: action, movement, and neuromotor processes. In: Carr JA, Shepherd RB, eds. *Movement Science: Foundations for Physical Therapy in Rehabilitation*. Gaithersburg, MD: Aspen Publishers; 1991:93–154.
28. Winstein CJ. Balance retraining: does it transfer? In: Duncan P, ed. *Balance: Proceedings of the APTA Forum*. American Physical Therapy Association; 1990:95–103.
29. Verkhoshansky YV. Depth jumping in the training of jumpers. *Track Technique*. 1973;51:60–61.
30. Verkhoshansky YV. Principles of planning speed and strength/speed endurance training in sports. *Natl Strength Conditioning Assoc J*. 1989;11:58–61.
31. Lundin P, Berg W. A review of plyometric training. *Natl Strength Conditioning Assoc J*. 1991;13:22–30.

32. Paceless R. *The Effect of Depth Jumping and Weight Training on Vertical Jump*. Ithaca, NY: Ithaca College; 1977. Thesis.
33. Adams K, O'Shea JP, O'Shea KL, Climstein M. The effect of six weeks of squat, plyometric, and squat-plyometric training on power production. *J Appl Sport Sci Res.* 1992;6:36–41.
34. Kramer JF, Morrow A, Leger A. Changes in rowing ergometer, weight lifting, vertical jump and isokinetic performance in response to standard and standard plus plyometric training programs. *Int J Sports Med.* 1993;14:449–454.
35. Blattner S, Noble L. Relative effects of isokinetic and plyometric training on vertical jumping performance. *Res Q.* 1979;50:583–588.
36. Durak E. Physical performance responses to muscle lengthening and weight training exercises in young women. *J Appl Sport Sci Res.* 1987;1:60.
37. Holcomb HR, Lander JE, Rutland RM, Wilson GD. The effectiveness of a modified plyometric program on power and the vertical jump. *J Strength Conditioning Res.* 1996;10:89–92.
38. Greenfield B, Catlin PA, Foltz M, Lawrence M, et al. *The Effect of Plyometric Training vs. Individualized, Dynamic, Variable Resistance Training in Healthy High School Baseball Players*. Atlanta, GA: APTA Combined Sections Meeting; 1996. Poster presentation. (Abstract in: *JOSPT.* 1996;23:83.)

CHAPTER 3

Client Motivation and Compliance

David Ash

CHAPTER OUTLINE

I. Motivation
II. Facilitation of Compliance
III. Chapter Summary

MOTIVATION

A characteristic of human nature is that people do what is important to them. A prerequisite for integration of exercise into an individual's lifestyle is that exercise becomes valuable to that individual. The exercise professional can use excellent communication and teaching skills to educate the exerciser about the value of a preventive exercise program. Client education emphasizes the many health benefits resulting from the very reasonable time investment involved in preventive exercise (benefit/cost ratio). As weeks pass and the exerciser begins to achieve desirable physical adaptations, intrinsic motivation often leads to ongoing interest in exercise.

It should be remembered that ultimately the work must be done by the exerciser. While the exercise professional continually provides support in the form of education, guidance, and positive reinforcement, the responsibility to actually carry out the program rests with the client.

FACILITATION OF COMPLIANCE

After a client has been motivated to begin an exercise program, there are multiple factors that affect long-term compliance with the program. Characteristics of exercise programs, as identified by Franklin,[1] that contribute to long-term compliance include:

- low probability of musculoskeletal injury (low to moderate intensity, duration, and frequency)
- group participation
- emphasis on variety and pleasure (use of games as exercise)
- setting of personal goals
- development of contracts
- assessment of response to training
- recruitment of friends
- support of family or spouse
- monitoring of progress (use charts to display changes visually)
- use of music
- positive feedback
- enthusiastic leadership
- role models

Additional factors that facilitate compliance include:

- reasonable exercise time commitment
- qualified supervision
- the professional's understanding of the client's goals[2,3]
- development of specific goals that have meaning and worth for the client[2]
- social support, which positively influences physical activity participation[3]
- maintenance of an exercise/activity journal to record progress toward fitness goals (enhances a sense of achievement)[4]
- confidence in the ability to be physically active[5]
- decreased perception of barriers to physical activity[5]
- enjoyment of activity[5]

A sampling of the research literature concerning exercise motivation and compliance is presented in Table 3–1.

Table 3-1 Sampling of Research Literature Concerning Exercise Motivation and Compliance

Summary	Researchers/Authors
A representative sample of Australian adults (N = 4404) served as subjects in a study using logistic regression analysis to investigate the relationship between exercise stage of change, sociodemographic variables, and beliefs about the benefits of exercise. Intention to do more exercise generally increased with level of education, but decreased with increasing age. Frequency of exercise participation was also associated with higher level of education, as well as the belief that exercise would help prevent heart disease. Based on this data, exercise recruitment efforts should target older adults and the less well-educated.	Booth, Macaskill, Owen, Oldenburg et al[6]
An investigation was designed to examine the exercise frequency of 949 employees during their first six months of membership to a worksite health promotion facility. Findings include: (1) the frequency of exercise declined, (2) the proportion of employees discontinuing the program increased, (3) men exercised more frequently and were less likely to drop out than were women ($p < .01$), (4) younger employees exercised more frequently than their older counterparts, (5) employees in the middle salary range had higher exercise frequencies than employees in the lower or upper salary ranges ($p < .01$), and (6) employees starting with lower exercise frequencies remained at lower frequencies throughout the duration of the study.	Lynch and Main[7]
One hundred outpatients with rheumatoid arthritis or osteoarthritis served as subjects in a study designed to identify factors that influenced exercise behaviors and aerobic fitness. Perceived benefits of exercise was a significant predictor of exercise participation. Subjects with less formal education, longer duration of arthritis, and higher impact of arthritis scores perceived fewer benefits of exercise. Subjects who reported exercising in their youth perceived more benefits of exercise.	Neuberger, Kasal, Smith, Hassanein et al[8]
Women who were overweight, shorter, had several physical complaints, and felt somewhat anxious were most likely to attend the exercise sessions. These variables accounted for 73% of the variance in sessions attended.	Klonoff, Annechild, and Landrine[9]
Behavioral techniques such as contracting, self-monitoring, and relapse prevention training assist in maintenance of physical activity.	Miller[10]
In a review of literature regarding the determinants of physical activity, factors are commonly grouped into the following three divisions: (1) personal characteristics (ie, education level, age), (2) psychological variables (ie, self-efficacy, goal-setting skills), and (3) environmental factors (ie, family support, proximity of exercise facility).	Marcus[3]

CHAPTER SUMMARY

Ongoing compliance is as important as client initiation of a preventive exercise program. Often, if the client can maintain the program for the initial six weeks, he or she will begin to see and feel desirable physical adaptations. While compliance is ultimately the client's responsibility, the exercise professional can provide support, guidance, and encouragement. Characteristics and factors that facilitate long-term compliance are presented.

REFERENCES

1. Franklin B. Program factors that influence exercise adherence: practical adherence skills for the clinical staff. In: Dishman R, ed. *Exercise Adherence: Its Impact on Public Health.* Champaign, IL: Human Kinetics; 1988:237–258.
2. Judge JO. Exercise programs for older persons: writing an exercise prescription. *Conn Med.* 1993;57:269–275.
3. Marcus BH. Exercise behavior and strategies for intervention. *RQES.* 1996;66:319.
4. Dishman RK. Motivating older adults to exercise. *South Med J.* 1994; 87:S79–S83.
5. Sallis JF, Hovell MF, Hofstetter CR, et al. A multivariate study of determinants of vigorous exercise in a community sample. *Prev Med.* 1989;18:20–34.
6. Booth ML, Macaskill P, Owen N, Oldenburg B, et al. Population prevalence and correlates of stages of change in physical activity. *Health Educ Q.* 1993;20:431–440.
7. Lynch WD, Main DS. Frequency of exercise and dropouts in a work-site program: correlates of 6-month activity patterns. *J Occup Med.* 1993; 35:1147–1151.
8. Neuberger GB, Kasal S, Smith KV, Hassanein R, et al. Determinants of exercise and aerobic fitness in outpatients with arthritis. *Nurs Res.* 1994;43:11–17.
9. Klonoff EA, Annechild A, Landrine H. Predicting exercise adherence in women: the role of psychological and physiological factors. *Prev Med.* 1994;23:257–262.
10. Miller NH. Physical activity: one approach to the primary prevention of hypertension. *AAOHN.* 1995;43:319–326.

Chapter 4

Resistive Exercise: Characteristics, Goals, and Principles

David Ash

CHAPTER OUTLINE

I. Characteristics of a Resistive Exercise Program
II. Principles of Resistive Exercise
III. Exercise Prescription Case Study
IV. Chapter Summary

Webster[1] defines productive as "having the quality or power of producing, especially in abundance." Productivity is a necessary, but not sufficient, characteristic of quality exercise. Exercise must also be safe and time efficient. While there is no single correct way to perform resistive exercise, the characteristics, goals, and basic principles are relatively consistent throughout sound resistive exercise programs.

CHARACTERISTICS OF A RESISTIVE EXERCISE PROGRAM

1. *Safety*. Safe exercise must be prescribed. There is no excuse for an exerciser to incur injury while performing resistive exercise. The purpose of engaging in the program in the first place was to decrease the risk of injury.
2. *Productivity*. Over time, the exerciser should strive to increase the number of repetitions and amount of resistance used.
3. *Time Efficiency*. A time-efficient program enhances the benefit/cost ratio and is a key to the permanent integration of exercise into one's lifestyle.

Quality exercise requires the presence of these three characteristics (see Figure 4–1).

The goals of a resistive exercise program are to decrease the risks of disease, dysfunction, and injury. Numerous studies (see Table 4–1) have indicated that resistive exercise may decrease the risk of musculoskeletal injury.

In addition, in the unfortunate event a disease or dysfunction does occur, an individual with increased muscular strength and endurance, increased bone density, increased ligament strength, and other physiological benefits of resistive exercise may experience more rapid recovery than a deconditioned counterpart, other factors being equal.

While the effects of resistive exercise on the prevention of injury have been documented, prevention of disease and illness have generally focused on exercise of the aerobic variety. Because resistive exercise produces many of the same physiological responses and adaptations as aerobic exercise, resistive exercise may be found to have preventive effects on disease and illness as well.

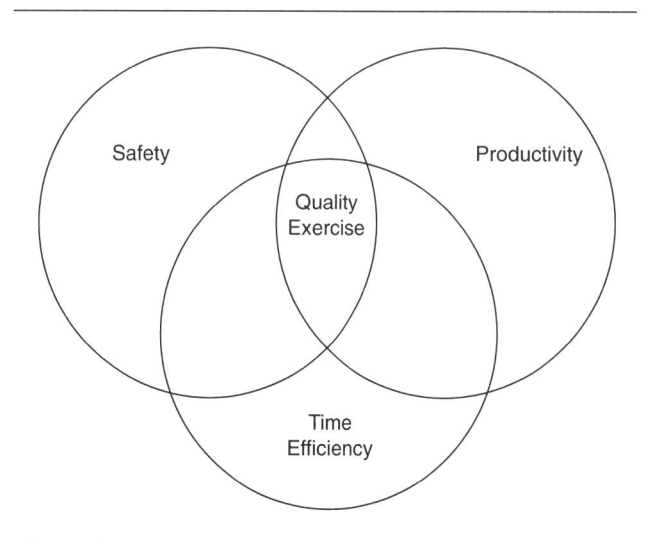

Figure 4–1 Characteristics of Quality Exercise

Table 4–1 Resistive Exercise and Injury Prevention

Summary	Researchers/Authors
"Screening of athletes for imbalances between agonist and antagonist muscle groups at particular joints can be utilized to locate athletes with imbalances suggesting a predisposition to injury. Resistance training can then be utilized to correct these imbalances. Examination of the scientific research indicates that resistance training can play a role in (preventing) musculoskeletal injuries."	Fleck and Falkel [2]
In a study conducted with high school wrestlers serving as subjects, the addition of a resistive exercise component decreased injury rate by almost one-third as compared to the wrestlers who did not perform resistive exercise. When injuries were incurred, the resistive exercise group required 50% less rehabilitation time than the wrestlers who did not perform resistive exercise.	Hejna, Rosenberg, Buturusis, and Krieger [3]
Twenty-six collegiate swimmers (13 male, 13 female) participated in the study as subjects. The experimental group performed resistive exercise three days per week for six weeks. The movements performed by the experimental group were as follows: (1) prone dumbbell transverse abduction, (2) prone dumbbell lateral rotation, (3) prone dumbbell medial rotation, (4) D2 with elastic tubing, and (5) push up with plus (protraction). The control group did not perform resistive exercise. The experimental (resistive exercise) group experienced a significantly ($p < .05$) lower incidence of shoulder pain.	Ashman, Swanik, Strapp, and Lephart [4]
A four-year study, performed with members of a college soccer team serving as subjects, was conducted to investigate the effect of strength training on injury rate. During the first two years, the subjects did not participate in any strength training program. During the final two years of study, all subjects participated in a year-round strength training program. The injury rate for the first two years of the study was 15.15 injuries per 1,000 exposures. The injury rate for years three and four was 7.99 injuries per 1,000 exposures.	Lehnhard, Lehnhard, Young, and Butterfield [5]

PRINCIPLES OF RESISTIVE EXERCISE

Physical Examination

A physical examination performed by a physician is a prerequisite to initiating any exercise program. A written approval to exercise, specifying the types of exercise (aerobic, resistive, etc.) allowed, the prescribed intensity of each activity, and any precautions and/or contraindications must be secured before the exercise program can be initiated.

Education and Guidance

The exercise professional provides the client with education and guidance regarding correct biomechanics, the importance of recovery, nutrition, full-body exercise, a balanced program (including resistive, aerobic, and range of motion exercise), and contemporary health/fitness issues. The exercise professional should demonstrate both proper and improper lifting and spotting techniques, and ensure that the client comprehends the difference. Questions are encouraged.

Supervision

An exercise professional should be present and actively engaged during every session.

Proper Posture and Breathing

The exerciser's posture and breathing pattern (diaphragmatic breathing as opposed to chest breathing) are analyzed during the first session and frequently thereafter. Often, as a result of dysfunctional posture characterized by decreased lumbar extension, anterior shoulders, and forward head, individuals resort to chest breathing. During chest breathing the shoulders are drawn upward by accessory respiratory muscles (trapezius, sternocleidomastoid, and pectorals) with each inspiration. In contrast to upward shoulder movement, diaphragmatic breathing involves anterior movement of the anterior abdominal wall with each inspiration as the shoulders maintain a relaxed, lowered position. Advantages of diaphragmatic breathing include greater minute ventilation and decreased risk of dysfunction from increased resting muscle tension in the accessory breathing muscles. Demonstration of the ability to monitor one's posture and breathing, and self-correct when necessary, is a prerequisite to progressing to the actual exercise program.

Breathing should follow a rhythmic pattern with exhalation occurring throughout concentric muscle action and inhalation occurring throughout eccentric muscle action. To avoid the adverse cardiovascular effects of the Valsalva maneuver the exerciser should at no time hold his or her breath while exercising.

Correct Form

Correct form while performing resistive exercise consists of two components: (1) relatively slow, controlled movements, and (2) performance of each movement through the full range of motion. The development of tension within the muscle is the stimulus for adaptation. Therefore, relatively slow movements (approximately three seconds concentric action and three seconds eccentric action, or two seconds concentric action and four seconds eccentric action) are recommended. The slow controlled movement applies to the eccentric muscle action as well as the concentric action. Faster movement speeds enable momentum to play a role in moving the resistance, effectively reducing the contribution required by the muscle. Also, faster movement speeds tend to encourage throwing, swinging, or bouncing the resistance, all of which have the potential to increase injurious forces.[6–10] If the resistance is moved in a ballistic manner, ligaments and the joint capsule may be needlessly overstretched as the body attempts to "catch" the resistance following eccentric action and prepare for the next throwing of the resistance. Generally for flexion and extension movements, when the position of maximal contraction is reached, that position is maintained for one full second before initiating eccentric muscle action. If a one-second pause at the point of full concentric contraction results in a locking out position in which muscles are allowed to decrease tension (leg press, bench press), the one-second pause is eliminated and replaced by a smooth yet continuous transition from concentric to eccentric action. Red flags that indicate that the resistance is excessive include: (1) lack of movement through full range of motion, (2) increased movement speed, and (3) bouncing or swinging the resistance by invoking compensatory movements.

The second component of correct form is full range of movement. Each repetition should begin with the agonist lengthened to the point of comfortable stretch followed by movement to the fully contracted position. In this manner, muscles are strengthened throughout the entire available range. In addition, using full range of motion while performing resistive exercise enhances flexibility. The starting position places the agonist in a lengthened position. The full contraction that follows places the antagonist in a lengthened position by the principle of reciprocal inhibition. For additional information regarding reciprocal inhibition, refer to Chapter 6.

Overload

The principle of overload states that the stimulus required to increase strength must be greater than that to which the structure is currently adapted.

Gradual Progression

When the exerciser can perform the upper limit of the repetition range (ie, 12 if the range is 8 to 12) with proper technique and, at most, moderate difficulty, the resistance should be increased. Increasing the resistance by small increments (ie, 5%) allows the exerciser to remain within the acceptable repetition range. The resistance maximum (rM) is defined here as the amount of resistance that allows the exerciser to achieve the lower limit of his or her repetition range. Therefore, it is the heaviest resistance the exerciser will use. For example, in the repetition range of 8 to 12, if 50 lbs is the most resistance that can be used while still completing eight repetitions correctly, the rM for that exerciser in that movement is 50 lbs.

Full-Body Exercise

It is advantageous to increase strength in the structures of the body as a whole. For example, budgeting available time to allow exercise of the trunk, lower extremities, and upper extremities is preferable to spending a disproportionate amount of time with the upper extremities. Using the agonist-antagonist guideline is a way to ensure that opposing muscle groups receive equal stimulation. Imbalance between reciprocal muscle groups may contribute to compromised posture and/or injury. For this reason, it is essential to perform an equal number of repetitions of resistance exercise for both agonist and antagonist. In the exercise setting it is common to see multiple sets of bench press and machine chest fly movements (transverse shoulder adduction) with few if any posterior deltoid (transverse abduction) movements. A rule of thumb is that agonist and antagonist receive an equal number of repetitions per session, week, and month.

The Volume-Intensity Relationship

Volume is the amount of work performed. Intensity is the difficulty of the work. High volume and high intensity are mutually exclusive. Intensity is a greater determinant of physiological adaptation than is volume. This is not to say that less than maximal intensity exercise is of no value. If performed on a regular basis, moderate and even low-intensity resistive exercise can yield desirable physiological adaptations. However, exercise of higher intensity results in greater effects. The intensity prescribed by the physician should not be surpassed.

Repetitions and Sets

A *repetition* is the process of performing an exercise movement one time. A *set* is a group of repetitions performed continuously, without resting. For example, if a low back exercise was performed 12 consecutive times followed by a brief recovery period, the exerciser has performed one set of 12 repetitions. One can find many different opinions regarding the optimal combinations of sets and repetitions. Research indicates that similar results are obtained when one or two sets per movement are performed, as compared to performance of additional sets.[9,11–15] The suggested repetition range is 8 to 12.[16]

Number of Different Movements per Session

Eight to ten different movements that address the body's major muscle groups are recommended.[16] An assortment of movements should be programmed within the different sessions of the weekly plan to take advantage of the benefits of each, and to provide variety. In general, proximal muscle groups are exercised prior to the smaller distal muscle groups to prevent the premature termination of an exercise due to the failure of a smaller muscle group.

Frequency of Resistive Exercise

The recommended minimum is two days per week.[16] To ensure recovery, three resistive exercise sessions per week is the recommended maximum.

Duration

The resistive exercise component of the program should not exceed 30 to 40 minutes. Recall that one of the characteristics of quality exercise is time efficiency. Westcott's 1990 studies,[17] which used brief, 20-minute exercise sessions resulted in 95% of the subjects committing to continue exercising after the conclusion of the experiment. Several common set/repetition protocols are examined in Table 4–2 to identify the following (see Figures 4–2 and 4–3 for a graphical representation of the data):

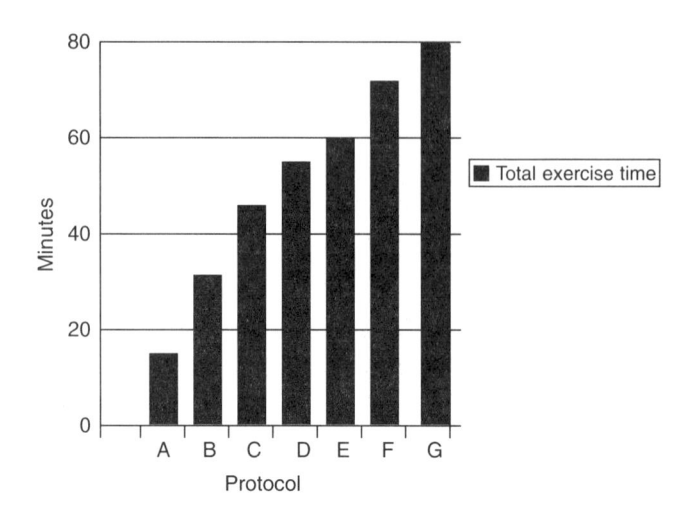

Figure 4–2 Exercise Time Presented Graphically

1. total exercise session time (minutes)
2. time spent exercising (minutes)
3. time spent resting between sets (minutes)

Table 4–3 provides a measure of time efficiency for common set and repetition schemes.

Rest Duration between Movements or Sets

The exerciser is encouraged to take as much time as necessary to feel prepared to advance to the next movement. It should be remembered that one of the characteristics of a quality exercise program is time efficiency. A study comparing intermovement or interset durations of 30 seconds, 2.5 minutes, and 8 minutes concluded that similar strength gains were achieved with each of the three different rest times.[18] Weir et al[19] concluded that no significant differences existed between rest intervals of 1, 3, 5, or 10 minutes between repeated bench press movements.

Table 4–2 Exercise Time for Common Set-Repetition Protocols

Protocol	Movements per Session	Sets per Movement	Repetitions per Set	Repetitions per Session	Time Spent Exercising* (Minutes)	Time Resting between Sets (Minutes)	Total Exercise Session Time (Minutes)
A	8	1	8	64	6.4	8	14.4
B	8	2	10	160	16	16	32
C	10	3	6	180	18	30	48
D	10	3	8	240	24	30	54
E	10	3	10	300	30	30	60
F	10	4	8	320	32	40	72
G	10	4	10	400	40	40	80

*Based on 10 repetitions per minute (1 repetition per 6 seconds)

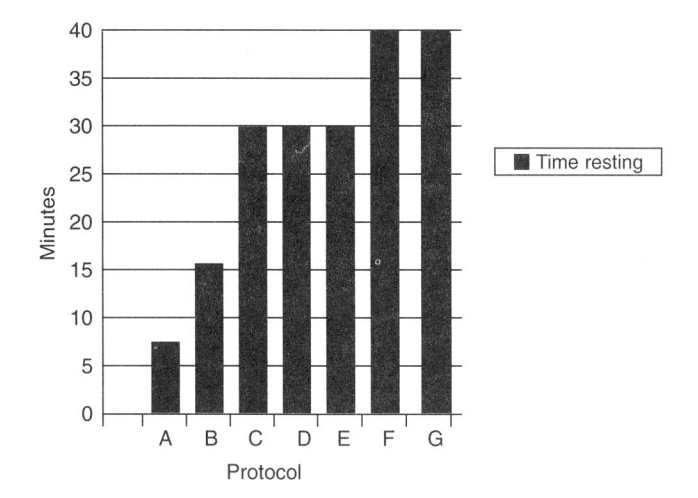

Figure 4–3 Resting Time Presented Graphically

Documentation of Exercise

Recording the results of the resistive exercises performed during each session is a quick and easy method to monitor progress over time. The increases in repetitions performed or resistance used can easily be displayed in chart form. A visible record of consistent progress over time is a strong motivation to continue exercising. For each exercise performed, the resistance used, repetitions completed, and difficulty (intensity) should be recorded. A method of documenting intensity is described in Chapter 2.

Variety

The use of variety allows the exerciser to reap benefits from different movements, decreases the likelihood of overuse stress, and prevents exercise from becoming monotonous. A commonly used phrase meaning variety in exercise is cross training.

Utilize Body Weight Exercises

With the wide variety of apparatus available at most commercial facilities, it may be easy to forget about exercises in which the weight of the body serves as resistance. Pullups, pushups, prone back extensions, and abdominal curls are valuable movements that can be performed at almost any place and time.

Correct Body Mechanics when Lifting an Object from the Floor

A prerequisite to any type of resistive exercise is the review of the proper technique to lift an object from the floor (or any level below the waist). In the exercise facility this skill will be used frequently as dumbbells or bars are commonly located in racks below waist level. The same technique applies to lifting a bag of groceries from the back seat of your car, or even picking up a light object, such as a pencil, from the floor.

To lift an object positioned below waist level, walk to the object and position yourself over the object as much as possible. Straddle the object if possible. This will minimize *reaching* so you can concentrate on proper *lifting*. Your feet should be wider than shoulder width. Bend at the knees. Contract your stomach and back muscles to hold your torso in a relatively erect posture. Do not bend forward at the waist. Think of sitting *back* on a chair. Do not allow your knees to move anterior to your ankles. Keep your heels in contact with the floor throughout the movement. As you bend at the knees your body will lower so that you can grasp the object. As you stand up, keep your lower back and torso muscles contracted for support. Lift with leg movement, not back movement. Think of pushing the floor away with 50% of your body weight on your heels and 50% on the balls of your feet. When you have the object in standing position, continue to use your stomach and back muscles to maintain erect posture. Do not hyperextend your low back when you

Table 4–3 Time-Efficiency Index of Resistive Exercise Protocols

Movements per Session	Sets per Movement	Repetitions per Set	Repetitions per Session	TEIRE (%)
8	1	8	64	100
8	2	10	160	40
10	3	6	180	36
10	3	8	240	25
10	3	10	300	21
10	4	8	320	20
10	4	10	400	16

Note: Time-efficiency index of resistive exercise = 1/[(movements/session) (sets/movement) (repetitions/set)/64] × 100. Based on American College of Sports Medicine recommended minimums of 8 repetitions and 8 movements.[16]

reach the standing position. To set the object down, reverse the procedure.

Warm-Up and Cool-Down

The initial five minutes of every exercise session should consist of light full-body activity (eg, brisk walking, jogging, bicycling) to serve as a warm-up. The warm-up allows the coronary arteries to dilate and perfuse the heart with blood. This preparation greatly reduces the stress to the heart during the initial stages of the exercise session. The cool-down consists of five minutes of light activity after the exercise session has been completed. The rhythmic muscle contractions during the cool-down activity serve as a pump to encourage venous return and prevent pooling of blood in the extremities. **Remember, Resistive Exercise Should Be Fun!**

EXERCISE PRESCRIPTION CASE STUDY

The results of a client interview provide the following data.

Exhibit 4–1 Sample Exercise Program

Monday	*Tuesday*	*Wednesday*	*Thursday*	*Friday*	*Saturday*	*Sunday*
RESISTIVE	RECOVERY	RESISTIVE	RECOVERY	RESISTIVE	RECOVERY	RECOVERY
4-way neck	walk	leg extension	walk	4-way neck	walk	
leg press	(optional)	seated leg curl	(optional)	dumbbell lunge	(optional)	
leg curl		low back machine		standing leg curl		
prone back extension		heels up		prone back extension		
abdominal curl		calf raise		abdominal curl		
pullup		supraspinatus raise		dumbbell row		
posterior deltoid		bench press		machine tricep extension		
machine chest fly		posterior deltoid		dumbbell incline press		
lateral raise		lat rowing		ankle dorsiflexion		
dumbbell tricep extension		dumbbell bicep curl		shoulder rotators		
AEROBIC		AEROBIC		AEROBIC		
bike		upper extremity ergometer		swim—intervals		
RANGE OF MOTION		RANGE OF MOTION		RANGE OF MOTION		
EXERCISE TIME		EXERCISE TIME		EXERCISE TIME		
Resistive Exercise = 27 minutes		Resistive Exercise = 27 minutes		Resistive Exercise = 27 minutes		
Aerobic Exercise = 20 minutes		Aerobic Exercise = 20 minutes		Aerobic Exercise = 20 minutes		
Range of Motion = 10 minutes		Range of Motion = 10 minutes		Range of Motion = 10 minutes		
Total Time **57 minutes**		**Total Time** **57 minutes**		**Total Time** **57 minutes**		

Total Weekly Exercise Time = 57 minutes × 3 = 171 minutes = 2 hours, 51 minutes.

RESISTIVE EXERCISE: 1–2 sets per movement
                                        8–12 repetitions per set

RESISTIVE EXERCISE TIME IS BASED ON THE FOLLOWING:
- Time to complete 1 repetition = approximately 6 seconds
- Time to complete 1 set = 6 seconds × 12 repetitions = approximately 72 seconds
- Recovery time = 90 seconds
- Time to complete 1 set + recovery time for that set = 72 + 90 = 162 seconds = 2.7 minutes
- Time to complete 10 sets of resistive exercise + recovery time = 2.7 minutes/set × 10 sets = approximately 27 minutes

Note: If 2 sets per movement are performed, add an additional 27 minutes to each exercise session. Precede each session with a 5-minute warm-up. Conclude each session with a 5-minute cool down.

1. The client wishes to participate in a combination of resistive, aerobic, and range of motion exercise. (Each of these types of exercise has been recommended without restriction by the client's physician).
2. The client has allotted one hour after work on Monday, Wednesday, and Friday for the exercise program.
3. The client enjoys evening walks with spouse when their schedules permit.
4. The client mentioned repeated prior attempts at a program consisting of running 3 to 4 times per week. The client stated that the program seemed to "increase my endurance." However, it has been repeatedly discontinued after approximately a month due to soreness behind the kneecaps.
5. The client would like the program to address the whole body (lower body, midsection, upper body).

Based on the interview and assessment, the exercise professional develops the exercise program shown in Exhibit 4–1. This is Sample Exercise Program A found in Appendix G. Refer to Appendix G for other sample programs.

CHAPTER SUMMARY

Characteristics of quality resistance exercise programs include safety, productivity, and time efficiency. Goals of the program include prevention of disease, illness, and injury, as well as decreased recovery time should pathology or dysfunction occur. Principles of resistance exercise include physician approval, education, guidance, correct form, overload, the volume-intensity relationship, full-body exercise, number of movements per session, frequency, duration, and recovery. An exercise prescription schema and case study have been included to facilitate practical application.

REFERENCES

1. *Webster's Ninth New Collegiate Dictionary*. Springfield, MA: Merriam-Webster; 1987:397.
2. Fleck SJ, Falkel JE. Value of resistance training for the reduction of sports injuries. *Sports Med*. 1986;3:61–68.
3. Hejna WF, Rosenberg A, Buturusis DJ, Krieger A. The prevention of sports injuries in high school students through strength training. *Natl Strength Conditioning Assoc J*. 1982;4:28–31.
4. Ashman KJ, Swanik CB, Strapp EJ, Lephart SM. Functional training effects on the incidence of shoulder pain and strength in intercollegiate swimmers. *J Athletic Training (Suppl)*. 1996;31:S12.
5. Lehnhard RA, Lehnhard HR, Young R, Butterfield SA. Monitoring injuries on a college soccer team: the effect of strength training. *J Strength Conditioning Res*. 1996;10:115–119.
6. Duda M. Elite lifters at risk for spondylolysis. *Physician Sports Med*. 1987;15:57–59.
7. Hall SJ. Effect of attempted lifting speed on forces and torque exerted on the lumbar spine. *Med Sci Sports Exerc*. 1985;17:440–444.
8. Hattin HC, Pierrynowski MR, Ball KA. Effect of load, cadence, and fatigue on tibio-femoral joint force during a half squat. *Med Sci Sports Exerc*. 1989;21:613–618.
9. Reid CM, Yeater RA, Ullrich IH. Weight training and strength, cardiorespiratory functioning, and body composition of men. *Br J Sports Med*. 1987;21:40–44.
10. Westcott W. Muscle development, safety make case for slow strength training. *J Phys Educ Program*. 1986;April:E14–16.
11. Jacobson BH. A comparision of two progressive weight training techniques on knee extensor strength. *Athletic Training*. 1986;21:315–318.
12. Messier SP, Dill ME. Alterations in strength and maximal oxygen uptake consequent to Nautilus circuit weight training. *RQES*. 1985;56:345–351.
13. Muntzing U. *Strength Training: One Set to Failure and One Set to Failure Plus Two Repetitions Compared to an Orthodox Weight Training Program*. Salt Lake City, UT: Brigham Young University; 1978. Thesis.
14. Stiggins CF. *Nautilus and Free Weight Training Program: A Comparison of Strength Development at Four Angles in the Range of Motion*. Salt Lake City, UT: Brigham Young University; 1978. Thesis.
15. Terbizan D, Bartels RL. The effect of set-rep combinations on strength gain in females age 18–35. *Lab Work Phys*. Columbus, OH: The Ohio State University; 1978. Thesis.
16. American College of Sports Medicine. Position statement on the recommended quantity and quality of exercise for developing and maintaining fitness in healthy adults. *Med Sci Sports Exerc*. 1990;22:265–274.
17. Westcott W. How much exercise is necessary? *Am Fitness Q*. 1990;April: 38–47.
18. Berkowitz MS. *Effects of Varying Rest Intervals Between Sets on the Acquisition of Muscular Strength*. University Park, PA: The Pennsylvania State University; 1978. Thesis.
19. Weir JP, Wagner LL, Housh TJ. The effect of rest interval length on repeated maximal bench presses. *J Strength Conditioning Res*. 1994;8:58–60.

Chapter 5

Aerobic Exercise

Caren J. Werlinger

CHAPTER OUTLINE

I. Benefits
II. Metabolic Pathways
III. Training Intensity
IV. Determining Target Heart Rate
V. Duration of Exercise
VI. Weather Considerations
VII. Aerobic Activities
VIII. Longevity Factors
IX. Research Findings
X. Chapter Summary

All exercise is performed either aerobically or anaerobically. The difference is how high the heart rate elevates during a given exercise and, based on heart rate, whether the body is receiving sufficient oxygen to fuel the working muscles for an extended period of time. Within this context, even a weight workout could be aerobic if it were vigorous enough to elevate and sustain a given heart rate for the entire workout. This is the concept behind circuit training classes now offered in many clubs. In this chapter we will consider the health benefits of activities more traditionally thought of as aerobic.

BENEFITS

The need to include aerobic training in any comprehensive exercise program stems from its ability to enhance both cardiovascular conditioning and weight control. Numerous studies over the past 15 years have proven that benefits are gained by improving a number of cardiac parameters, including increased stroke volume as cardiac muscle responds to training, lowered resting heart rate as the heart becomes more efficient, lowered levels of LDL cholesterol (the cholesterol component that can contribute to arterial plaque formation), lowered blood pressure, and increased VO_2 max. In addition, the skeletal muscles performing the exercise experience increased capillary density, which enhances oxygen exchange, and increased mitochondrial formation, which increases the muscles' metabolic activity, even at rest.[1–4] Accompanying these changes are better venous return, improved density in the bones involved in weight-loading during exercise, and enhanced blood flow to viscera and skin. Other benefits generally attributed to aerobic exercise include decreased stress, enhanced self-concept, lessened depression, improved sleep, and less absenteeism due to illness, although studies have been less conclusive in their findings on these topics.[5–9]

METABOLIC PATHWAYS

In aerobic exercise, the body is working at a submaximal effort at which the heart is able to deliver oxygen to the working muscles and remove the metabolic byproducts of carbohydrate and fat oxidation. These oxidative systems do not provide large amounts of energy, but can be sustained for hours at a time once the body has been trained to do so. Protein is also available as a potential source of energy, but is inefficient and, therefore, the last source utilized. The primary byproduct of aerobic metabolism is CO_2, although small amounts of lactate are formed during submaximal exercise.[10,11]

There are two anaerobic metabolic processes that can deliver high amounts of energy, but only for short periods of time. The first is a breakdown of phosphagens, consisting of adenosine triphosphate (ATP) and creatine phosphate (CP), which are available in small amounts. The other system is anaerobic glycolosis, in which glucose is metabolized for quick bursts of energy, but at the expense of rapid lactate buildup, which limits the amount of time this system can be utilized. When speedwork is added to an aerobic training program, it often calls for anaerobic intervals or short (15 second to 2 minute) sprints at maximal or near-maximal speed.[10,11]

TRAINING INTENSITY

For the past 10 to 15 years, since the running boom of the late 1970s, proponents of aerobic exercise have advocated training programs geared toward long, slow distances with training heart rates of about 60 to 70% of predicted max. This advice is still wise for people starting to exercise who need to build an aerobic base from which to work.[12–14] Many recreational exercisers may never wish to progress beyond the ability to run for 5 miles or cycle for 20 without hurting, and for them, long, slow distance training 3 to 5 times a week will be sufficient. But many others, once they have experienced the accomplishment of achieving those initial goals, want to push themselves farther and add speed to endurance. To accomplish this, they need to train at intensities of 85 to 90% of their max, or just below their anaerobic threshold.[4,15] The anaerobic threshold is the level of exercise intensity at which the heart can no longer deliver oxygen fast enough to supply the working skeletal muscle and remove the waste products that are building up. It is also called the lactate threshold, and corresponds with an increase in the blood lactate level. The anaerobic threshold can be improved with endurance training. Trained muscle appears to be better able to remove lactate from the system, so that after a period of training, the same amount of work will result in less lactate accumulation.[16] There are sophisticated lab tests that can pinpoint anaerobic threshold, but for practical purposes, it is the highest average heart rate that can be sustained for 20 to 30 minutes of continuous effort such as a long, steady climb on a bicycle or a flat time trial course.[13] Above this level of intensity, the body requires a very rapid production of energy for working muscles, and the anaerobic metabolic pathways can only produce enough for a very short time.

Aerobic metabolism, as mentioned earlier, uses primarily carbohydrate and fat. The proportion of carbohydrate versus fat varies with exercise intensity. During aerobic activity at a relatively low (65% of maximum heart rate [max HR]) intensity, the fat utilized will provide an increasing percentage of the calories burned as the activity is prolonged, up to about 50%.[12] This is another reason for beginning exercisers to work at a low level of intensity as they build an aerobic base. Once a moderate level of fitness is achieved, however, many people may find their weight loss tapering off if they maintain that same 65% intensity. At this level of exercise intensity, the carbohydrate being used is most likely consumed carbohydrate, utilizing very little of the muscles' glycogen stores. So any post-exercise carbohydrate consumed will not be used to replenish muscle glycogen stores, because these were not depleted, but rather, the excess will be stored as fat. At this exercise plateau, calories expended probably equal calories consumed.

When exercise moves to higher (85% of max HR) levels of intensity, the total number of calories burned will be higher during the same length of time exercising. The absolute number of fat calories will change less than the percent of fat calories; this is an important distinction when reading literature on exercise metabolism. The percent of fat calories will decrease because, at this higher level of intensity, glycogen is providing more of the total calories burned. Glycogen depletion will allow for more of the carbohydrates from post-exercise eating to be used in replenishing the glycogen stores in the muscles, leaving less excess to be stored as fat. Aerobically-trained muscle is capable of storing both more fat and more carbohydrate, and utilizing both efficiently when needed during exercise.[12,16]

DETERMINING TARGET HEART RATE

To determine a level of exercise intensity, it is necessary to first find a max HR. The American College of Sports Medicine (ACSM) guidelines do not call for physician supervision for maximal testing or strenuous exercise (above 60% intensity) for apparently healthy women under age 50 and men under age 40 who are asymptomatic for coronary artery disease (CAD), and who have fewer than two risk factors for CAD. Risk factors include blood pressure (BP) above 160 systolic or 90 diastolic on two separate occasions (or diagnosed hypertension with or without medication), serum cholesterol greater than 240 mg/dL, diabetes mellitus, and family history of CAD.[17]

It is important for the exercise professional to remember that a detailed history is critical, especially in a setting in which emergency assistance may not be immediately available. A client may need to be asked very specific questions to determine the presence of CAD symptoms. The ACSM guidelines offer cardiospecific questionnaires to aid in getting the appropriate responses.[17]

For individuals who fall into the above category, the 220 minus age formula is too general to get a max HR from which to calculate training intensities. It would be preferable to have those individuals undergo a maximal stress test if such equipment is available. If a stress test is not feasible, max HR can be determined by placing the subject on a stationary bicycle and increasing the resistance every couple of minutes for 10 to 15 minutes until the maximum is evident. A heart rate monitor facilitates this process tremendously. Blood pressure should also be monitored at each increase in intensity during this test. It must be stressed that, even though ACSM guidelines do not call for physician supervision, physician approval is strongly recommended prior to initiating a maximal effort. Once a max HR is determined, exercise intensity can be determined as a percentage of that number.

For those subjects for whom it is not safe to actually exercise to max HR because of factors such as age, the presence of two or more CAD risk factors, or diagnosed CAD, a submaximal stress test can assist in determining a target heart range. If submaximal testing is not available, the Karvonen equation will permit a reasonable estimation of target heart range.

220 − age = age-predicted max HR (APMHR)
APMHR − resting HR (RR) = HR reserve
(HR reserve × .65) + RR = low target HR
(HR reserve × .85) + RR = high target HR[17]

Another method of determining exercise intensity is the rating of perceived exertion (RPE), shown in Exhibit 5–1. Although this is a subjective rating, it has been closely correlated with HR readings in studies. Clinical trials have indicated that at first subjects will tend to underestimate the RPE. By about the third trial, however, they become much more familiar with their responses and how to rate them.[10] The RPE scale can be used in conjunction with HR data to gauge someone's response to exercise. Many factors can influence HR: fatigue, diet, temperature, and sleep. Individual perception of effort is often an accurate indicator, especially once a person is well-acquainted with her or his body's response to training. This scale is especially useful for subjects whose HR is artificially controlled with medications and is, therefore, not an accurate gauge of effort.

In recording an exercise session afterward, either HR or RPE—or both—can be used (see Exhibit 5–2), along with any symptoms or other comments. As training progresses, the RPE for a given HR should be less. In the event that a subject is becoming ill or being overtrained from inadequate rest, it is likely that both the RPE and the resting HR will rise, indicating a possible need for either complete rest for a few days or a change in type of activity. The benefit of utilizing several different types of exercise, or crosstraining, when designing a program, is that the likelihood of injury or overtraining is decreased. A variety of activities also serves to maintain interest and enjoyment in an exercise program. In addition, the metabolic benefits are enhanced if a variety of muscle groups receive training from several different exercises.

DURATION OF EXERCISE

Besides HR intensity and RPE, the other major factor in an aerobic exercise program is the length of the session. For

Exhibit 5–1 Rating of Perceived Exertion (RPE) Scale

6
7 very, very light
8
9 very light
10
11 fairly light
12
13 somewhat hard
14
15 hard
16
17 very hard
18
19 very, very hard
20

Source: Reprinted with permission from G.A. Borg, RPE Scale, *Medicine and Science in Sports and Exercise*, Vol. 14, pp. 377–387, © 1982, Williams & Wilkins.

people desiring only improved cardiovascular function, 20 to 30 minutes 3 to 5 times a week has been sufficient to show improvement in several parameters of cardiac function.[2,4,18–20] Those individuals wishing to pursue greater goals of enhanced exercise performance and weight loss will obviously need to exercise longer, but the activity chosen plays a role in length of exercise; 45 to 60 minutes may be a long run, but for a cyclist, 1.5 to 2 hours may be needed for a good 20 to 25 mile ride.

As a subject begins an aerobic exercise session, she or he should spend the first 10 to 15 minutes warming up at an intensity lower than the target HR. This allows the body to move into aerobic metabolism without excessive lactate buildup early in the session. It also opens peripheral blood flow in the working muscles, and allows the body to begin regulating through sweat the excess heat produced. For beginning exercisers, this may mean walking for 10 to 15 minutes if the primary activity (eg, bicycling or jogging) cannot be performed at a low enough level of intensity. After the warm-up period, the intensity can be increased to the target range established for that exercise session. The goal may be a hard session at 80 to 85% of max HR, it may be an easy recovery day at 65%, or it may be interval training with sprints at 90 to 100%.

Exhibit 5–2 Sample Heart Rate Recording Sheet

Date		Date		Date	
Target HR		Target HR		Target HR	
Actual HR		Actual HR		Actual HR	
RPE		RPE		RPE	
Comments		Comments		Comments	

WEATHER CONSIDERATIONS

Many aerobic activities are performed outdoors. Athletes use treadmills, stationary bicycles, and stairclimbers when necesary, but the real joy of a good run, walk, or ride is getting outside and enjoying the scenery. Even summer and winter extremes in temperature can be enjoyed comfortably with a little care.

In the heat of summer, a period of acclimatization is needed to give the body time to adapt to the stresses of heat regulation. An athlete should begin taking in fluids about ½ hour prior to starting exercise, and continue drinking at least 16 ounces (one large water bottle) of fluid each hour. It is recommended that a 5 to 10% carbohydrate solution be used to replace electrolytes lost in sweat.[13] Many cyclists prefer to carry one bottle of carbo solution and one of water. Individuals will need to experiment to see which brands are best tolerated by their digestive systems.

Exercising during the cooler parts of the day is another way to avoid the negative effects of training in the heat. Dressing in loose, light-colored clothing that can allow perspiration to evaporate and reflect some of the sun's rays will also help keep an athlete more comfortable.

Cold weather can be handled as well, with a little preparation. The trunk is the source of most of the body's heat, and can begin sweating on even the coldest days. Clothing should be layered, with the layers next to the skin made from a wicking material to pull perspiration to the outer layers, leaving the skin dry. Layering also creates cushions of warmed air around the body to preserve warmth. Peripheral structures such as the face, hands, and feet often suffer the most. Wearing a polypropylene or silk balaclava will protect the neck and as much of the face as needed. Socks made of materials such as Gore-Tex will allow sweat to evaporate without allowing outside moisture in. Cycling shoes can be covered with neoprene booties to keep wind and wetness out. Mittens work better than gloves to keep fingers warm, although they hamper dexterity. A good compromise is the V-shaped gloves which put two fingers into each side and leave the thumb free. Adding silk or polypropylene glove liners increases the dryness and warmth.

AEROBIC ACTIVITIES

This section contains a brief discussion of the important principles of a variety of aerobic exercises. This is certainly not an all-inclusive list, but simply a sampling of some of the most common activities.

Walking is the easiest, most accessible form of exercise for most people. It requires no more than a good pair of supportive cushioned shoes. Because it involves less bouncing than jogging, it is less stressful on the hips, knees, and feet. If the upper extremities are involved with powerful swinging (without weights, which can throw off the natural stride) or by using walking poles (which resemble ski poles), the cardiovascular benefit can be enhanced. Race walking is the most energetic form of walking. It involves exaggerated rotation of the pelvis to lengthen the stride, along with powerful swinging of the upper extremities.

Jogging or running is a natural progression of walking for people who want to increase the speed and cardiovascular level of their exercise. The choice of shoes becomes a little more important with running as the vertical load on the body increases. Many shoe companies manufacture models specifically designed to compensate for excessive pronation or supination. A reputable athletic shoe store should be able to offer advice on models most appropriate, especially if a biomechanical evaluation has been performed to determine the specific needs of a given exerciser.

Because of the increased vertical load of running, more consideration should be given to the type of surface a subject will be running on. Roads tend to be crowned for drainage, and because runners are supposed to face traffic, this places the left foot constantly in inversion and the right foot constantly in eversion. Therefore, it is advisable for a variety of surfaces to be used. Running tracks are boring to many people, but they are usually cushioned and flat, especially useful for the beginning runner whose joints are becoming accustomed to a new activity. Trail-running through woods or on cross-country courses provides lots of stimulation and variety, but the uneven terrain can be problematic for the untrained runner. Another option, especially in bad weather, is the use of a treadmill. A motorized treadmill, once an individual has become accustomed to it, can allow a more natural stride than the type in which the belt must be pushed backward over rollers with each step.

Besides varying the terrain, runners may need to vary their direction and stride to avoid overuse injuries. In some people, the hip flexors tend to get irritated with constant forward running. By utilizing brief stretches of backward running, cariocas (moving sideways with the lagging foot crossing first in front of, then behind the leading foot), and skipping, the monotony of a regular pace can be relieved and different muscles will be used.

Bicycling can be done indoors on a stationary bicycle, or on a regular bicycle either outdoors or clipped into a wind trainer. If a stationary bike is to be used, usually the only option for adjustment is seat height. The subject's knee should be only slightly flexed at the bottom of the pedal stroke. If a regular bicycle is to be used, there are a variety of adjustments to obtain an optimal fit. Unless the health professional is well-acquainted with cycling biomechanics, these adjustments should be done by a reputable bicycle shop that offers individualized service. It goes without saying that a helmet should be worn—properly fitted over the frontal area—at all times when riding outdoors. The type of bicycle, road or mountain, is not as important as bicycle fit and type of terrain.

The best cardiovascular workout is obtained by riding on the road where effort can be kept at a more constant level. Off-road riding is acceptable if the trail allows fairly continuous pedalling, rather than technical riding with heavy grinding up hills followed by coasting downhill.

The gearing, or on a stationary bike the resistance, should be chosen to allow a pedalling cadence of about 90 rpm, while still keeping the HR within the specified parameters for that ride. A heart rate monitor and a cycle computer will be able to track these two variables easily, and are worth the investment for someone who intends to ride regularly.

Steppers are machines that simulate the action of climbing stairs. There are many pneumatic and hydraulic units sold for home use, but the best choices are the ones that are regulated by a computer. These allow smoother action and decrease the risk of injury to the knees because the pedals are being followed in their descent according to the speed set, rather than actually being pushed against. The cardiovascular workout, therefore, comes from supporting the weight of the body as the lower extremities shift positions. Frequently, individuals using these machines support their body weight on the upper extremities as they tire, but this negates the effects of the exercise. The level of intensity and hill profile should be chosen to achieve and maintain the desired target HR.

Aerobics classes have evolved into a wide array of styles and intensity levels. The first consideration when choosing an aerobics class is the level of impact, that is, how much jumping and hopping are involved. Beginning exercisers, or those with a predisposition toward joint problems, should opt for a low-impact class. For those who are ready for a more strenuous workout, there are a variety of danced-based classes as well as classes that use steps of varying heights to make the workout harder. Again, appropriate footwear should be worn, with shoes designed to absorb the impact of the movements along with providing firm support.

There are a couple of certifications available for aerobics instructors, but these certification courses do not provide a great deal of depth in terms of exercise physiology. The testing requirements for certification with ACSM are much more stringent, and fitness instructors who pass the test should be able to devise classes with minimal chance of injury to clients.

Most classes contain a warm-up period, followed by 30 to 45 minutes of higher intensity exercise during which each participant should be trying to stay within target HR ranges, and finishing with a cool-down period.

Cross-country skiing is another activity that can be enjoyed either indoors or outdoors. Outdoor skiing is a wonderful, low-impact method of maintaining aerobic fitness during the off-season when many other outdoor activities are hampered by snow. For those who live in northern climates, cross-country skiing may be the primary aerobic activity. Ski rentals are inexpensive for those who only occasionally visit locations with appropriate trails. Purchasing a set of skis doesn't have to be a large investment, but in the last few years, various types of cross-country skis have been developed. The traditional long, thin ski is best for open areas with long, straight stretches of trail. Shorter skis are now available for wooded trails with lots of turns. A reputable ski shop will be able to set up a package of skis, boots, and poles appropriate for the terrain an individual will mostly be skiing.

Indoor ski machines are also an excellent aerobic workout. The use of the arms in coordination with the legs involves more major muscle groups than running or walking, and thus raises the HR faster and burns more calories. Beginners may need to use just the skis first without involving the arms until cardiovascular fitness and balance catch up. It is important to use a machine with a smooth glide to the skis. A poorly built machine that catches and slips will have a greater tendency to injure the knees and hips.

Outdoor skiing in cold weather can be very comfortable if, as mentioned earlier in this chapter, clothing is worn in layers to trap warmed air as insulation around the body. With wicking layers next to the skin, sweat will be drawn to the outer layers and the skin will stay dry.

Aerobic riders are machines that work with a scissor-like motion while the individual sits on the seat and push/pulls on both the foot bar and the handle. In effect, body weight is the resistance. This activity uses several muscle groups, so HR tends to rise rapidly.

All of the exercises mentioned above have the added benefit of involving some degree of compression of bones, mostly the lower extremities and the spine. This compression will positively influence bone deposition to help ward off the effects of osteoporosis. If these aerobic activities are combined with some weight work for the upper extremities, then the arms will also receive some additional benefit in increased bone density.

Swimming, while an excellent aerobic exercise, contributes almost nothing to increased bone density due to the buoyant effects of the water. Any variety of strokes will accomplish the cardiovascular goal of a swim workout, and mixing strokes may help prevent overfatiguing certain muscles. There are also a wide array of items, such as kick boards, fins, or webbed gloves, that can make the workout more interesting and can help strengthen any weaknesses in technique.

LONGEVITY FACTORS

Because aerobic activities typically require at least 30 minutes to obtain a cardiovascular benefit, many people become bored with the monotony of performing the same movement repetitively. Indoor exercise can seem to go much more quickly if accompanied by the television or music. Music headsets are not a good idea for outdoor activities near traffic, and are illegal for bicyclists in most states.

Most people find training more enjoyable with the comaraderie and friendly competition of a club or team. Having a coach to help structure workouts and critique form can be a great benefit. Exercising with a group that has a set start time also helps provide motivation on those days when it would be very easy to talk oneself out of exercising.

Exercising aerobically will also be less stressful to the body over time if more than one activity is part of a person's training program. Repetitive motions involved in activities such as running and cycling can lead to overuse injuries. Mixing activities not only spares the body from repetitive stress, but can actually enhance cardiovascular fitness by constantly surprising the body and not allowing it to adapt to a routine that never varies.

With all exercises discussed here, there should be a warm-up, followed by a period of more intense exercise aiming for a target HR, followed by a cool-down period. Remember that the goal is to help people adopt exercise as part of their lifestyle, so they should become independent at monitoring their HR and RPE.

RESEARCH FINDINGS

There is a large mass of research that supports the benefits of aerobic exercise. Children seem to benefit cardiovascularly as well as psychologically from being active.[7,9] For the purpose of weight loss, research has supported the use of aerobic exercise with dietary restriction to enhance the benefits.[3] One study looking at overweight women participating in an aerobics class found greater cardiovascular improvement when the intensity was controlled at a lower level than in most commercial aerobics classes.[14] Older people who have previously been sedentary also demonstrate significant improvement in several cardiovascular variables with the implementation of an aerobic training program.[1,2,4,21,22] Older people with osteo- or rheumatoid arthritis had fewer joint-related symptoms with participation in an aerobic exercise program, as well as improved perceptions of general health. Interestingly, subjects' perceived benefit from exercise appeared to be related to having exercised in their youth, certainly an indication for encouraging exercise in young people.[18,23]

In considering those who could benefit from preventive exercise, we ought not overlook the benefits to those who have sustained previous injuries or other diagnoses for whom exercise as rehabilitation is not really indicated, but rather to prevent further problems or deterioration. One study showed significant improvements in cardiorespiratory fitness and physical work capacity in disabled subjects after participation in an aerobic exercise program.[24] Another demonstrated significant improvement for sufferers of migraines.[25] Yet another looked at quality of life indicators for women with breast cancer, and found significant improvement with aerobic exercise.[26]

In summary, aerobic exercise bestows many health benefits involving improved cardiovascular function and enhanced weight control, as well as less tangible benefits such as reduced stress, improved self-esteem, and reduced symptoms of some other disease processes. In combination with flexibility and strength exercises, aerobic exercise is part of a comprehensive approach to preventive exercise.

CHAPTER SUMMARY

Aerobic exercise is a key part of any comprehensive exercise program, and provides numerous physical and psychological benefits. This chapter reviews, in basic terms, the processes of aerobic and anaerobic metabolism. It goes on to offer guidelines for intensity and duration of exercise. Aerobic exercise need not stop during the temperature extremes of summer or winter; the chapter suggests ways of continuing to exercise comfortably. Various forms of aerobic exercise are then covered, along with suggestions for maximizing the safety and enjoyment of each. Lastly, this chapter offers research that supports the benefits of aerobic exercise as prevention of further problems in people who have other diagnoses not specifically requiring rehabilitation.

REFERENCES

1. Blumenthal JA, Emery CF, Madden DJ, George LK, et al. Cardiovascular and behavioral effects of aerobic exercise training in healthy older men and women. *J Gerontol.* 1989;44:M147–M157.
2. Samitz G, Bachl N. Physical training programs and their effects on aerobic capacity and coronary risk profile in sedentary individuals. *J Sports Med Phys Fitness.* 1991;31:283–293.
3. Shinkai S, Watanabe S, Kurokawa Y, Torii J, et al. Effects of 12 weeks of aerobic exercise plus dietary restriction on body composition, resting energy expenditure and aerobic fitness in mildly obese middle-aged women. *Eur J Appl Physiol.* 1994;68:258–265.
4. Takeshima N, Tanaka K, Kobayashi F, Watanabe T, et al. Effects of aerobic exercise conditioning at intensities corresponding to lactate threshold in the elderly. *Eur J Appl Physiol.* 1993;67:138–143.
5. Cooper KH, Gallman JS, McDonald JL, Jr. Role of aerobic exercise in reducing stress. *Dent Clin North Am.* 1986;30:S133–S142.
6. Deshamais R, Jobin J, Cote C, Levesque L, et al. Aerobic exercise and the placebo effect: a controlled study. *Psychosom Med.* 1993;55:149–154.
7. MacMahon JR, Gross RT. Physical and psychological effects of aerobic exercise in boys with learning disabilities. *J Dev Behav Pediatr.* 1987;8:274–277.
8. Holmes DS, Roth DL. Effects of aerobic exercise training and relaxation training on cardiovascular activity during psychological stress. *J Psychosom Res.* 1988;32:469–474.
9. Tuckman BW, Hinkle JS. An experimental study of the physical and psychological effects of aerobic exercise on schoolchildren. *Health Psychol.* 1986;5:197–207.
10. Pate RR, Blair SN, Durstine JL, Eddy DO, et al. *ACSM's Guidelines for Exercise Testing and Prescription.* 4th ed. Philadelphia: Lea & Febiger; 1991.
11. Powers SK. Fundamentals of exercise metabolism. In: Durstine JL, King AC, Painter PL, Roitman JL, et al, eds. *ACSM's Resource Manual for Guidelines for Exercise Testing and Prescription.* 2nd ed. Philadelphia: Lea & Febiger; 1993.
12. Burke ER. The lose-weight debate. *Bicycling.* 1995;14:56–57.
13. Burke ER. *Serious Cycling.* Champaign, IL: Human Kinetics; 1995.
14. Gillett PA, Eisenman PA. The effect of intensity controlled aerobic dance exercise on aerobic capacity of middle-aged, overweight women. *Res Nurs Health.* 1987;10:383–390.
15. Spunway NC. Aerobic exercise, anaerobic exercise and the lactate thresold. *Br Med Bull.* 1992;48:569–591.
16. Wilmore JH, Costill DL. *Physiology of Sport and Exercise.* Champaign, IL: Human Kinetics; 1994.
17. Gordon NF, Mitchell BS. Health appraisal in the nonmedical setting. In: Durstine JL, King AC, Painter PL, Roitman JL, et al, eds. *ACSM's Resource Manual for Guidelines for Exercise Testing and Prescription.* 2nd ed. Philadelphia: Lea & Febiger; 1993.
18. Perlman SG, Connell KJ, Clark A, Robinson MS, et al. Dance-based aerobic exercise for rheumatoid arthritis. *Arthritis Care Res.* 1990;3:29–35.
19. Scordo KA. Effects of aerobic exercise training on symptomatic women with mitral valve prolapse. *Am J Cardiol.* 1991;67:863–868.
20. South-Paul JE, Rajagopal KR, Tenhilder MF. The effect of participation in a regular exercise program upon aerobic capacity during pregnancy. *Obstet Gynecol.* 1988;71:175–179.
21. Bruce RA. Exercise, functional aerobic capacity, and aging—another viewpoint. *Med Sci Sports Exerc.* 1984;16:8–13.
22. Elward K, Larson E, Wagner E. Factors associated with regular aerobic exercise in an elderly population. *J Am Board Fam Pract.* 1992;5:467–474.
23. Neuberger GB, Kasal S, Smith KV, Hassanein R, et al. Determinants of exercise and aerobic fitness in outpatients with arthritis. *Nurs Res.* 1994;43:11–17.
24. Santiago MC, Coyle CP, Kinney WB. Aerobic exercise effect on individuals with physical disabilities. *Arch Phys Med Rehabil.* 1993;74:1192–1198.
25. Labbe EE, Welsh MC, Delaney D. Effects of consistent aerobic exercise of the psychological functioning of women. *Percept Mot Skills.* 1988;67:919–925.
26. Young-McCaughan S, Sexton DL. A retrospective investigation of the relationship between aerobic exercise and quality of life in women with breast cancer. *Oncol Nurs Forum.* 1991;18:751–757.

CHAPTER 6

Flexibility

Caren J. Werlinger

CHAPTER OUTLINE

I. Physiology of Stretch
II. Specific Stretches
III. Research Findings
IV. Chapter Summary

An appropriate level of flexibility is required for the safe performance of any exercise activity, whether it be strength training or aerobic. If there is an asymmetry in flexibility, then there also exists an imbalance that predisposes a joint or soft tissues to injury. Even without the existence of a specific imbalance, muscles that have been properly warmed up and stretched are less likely to sustain injury during an exercise session.[1-5]

PHYSIOLOGY OF STRETCH

As soft tissue is stretched, the wavy configuration of the collagen fibers will become taut with very little force. As more stretch is applied, the tissue enters the elastic range of its stress-strain curve. It is within this range that the principle of *creep* can be used to advantage. If a low-intensity load is applied long enough, a change will take place in tissue length that will be maintained after the stretch force is removed. Time is the critical element, assuming the intensity of the force was low enough not to have caused tissue failure resulting in a sprain or strain. Most stretches should be held for at least 30 seconds. In the case of significantly shortened, tight muscles, longer stretches of 15 to 30 minutes may be needed. Any increased length gained will only be maintained if it is used; otherwise the tissue will slowly revert to its former length. The presence of heat facilitates the process of creep, so it is advisable for the athlete to undergo at least five minutes of easy warm-up exercise (eg, walking or cycling) prior to stretching, especially in cold weather. It is also advisable to stretch briefly after an exercise session as muscles are cooling down.[6,7]

Equally important is the type of stretch. A static, slowly applied stretch will usually be more beneficial than a ballistic type of stretch. If a ballistic or bouncing stretch is used, it will activate a reflex contraction of any muscle spindles caught in a stretched muscle. The resulting contraction of the muscle combined with the ballistic stretch force going in the opposite direction creates a high probability of micro- or macrotrauma to the muscle. Realize, though, that there are times when a ballistic stretch is required, usually when an activity requires a quick change in direction such as playing tennis or racquetball, or winding up for a throw. Muscles required to undergo these types of abrupt changes should be prepared for them gradually and in combination with strengthening exercises.

Static, maintained stretches can be applied using a variety of techniques. Passive stretches should be taken only to the point of discomfort; more force than that often results in involuntary muscle guarding. Active inhibition techniques utilize the nervous system's built-in inhibition mechanisms. Contract-relax stretches utilize the principle of autogenic inhibition in which a strong isometric contraction is followed by a heightened state of inhibition within that muscle, which allows greater passive stretch. Contract-relax-contract stretches utilize both autogenic inhibition and reciprocal inhibition by following the isometric contraction with a contraction of the antagonistic muscle, resulting in greater length of the agonist.[6,7]

How much length is normal is more difficult to determine. Textbooks offer charts of norms for most motion segments of the body, but that does not mean that that number is normal for a given individual. Athletes such as dancers, gymnasts, and swimmers obviously need much more range of motion (ROM) at certain joints to be able to perform their best. It will be up to the health professional and the client together to determine what normal range of motion should be. Caution should be used in providing stretch to any muscles or soft tissues lax enough to permit joint instability.

It is also very important that the stretch be applied to the intended tissue. Often, if there is a muscle or joint that has become tight, the body will have learned to substitute with excess motion at an adjoining motion segment. It would be easier for the stretch force to be diverted to the substituting segment that offers less resistance, than to the tight segment. Therefore, the subject must be taught stretches that control for any substitution, either by positioning or with the assistance of external restraints. The stretches presented in this chapter attempt to offer positions of isolation for the targeted tissues, but these may need to be altered for subjects with special needs.

In designing a flexibility program, special attention should be given to the spine, because it is the central base of support for all other movements. Remember that except for the upper cervical segments responsible for rotation, the other spinal motion segments each have limited movement in any given plane.[8] The position of the sacrum and pelvis influences the alignment of the rest of the spine. Attention should be paid, therefore, to stretches for the hamstrings and the hip flexors, iliopsoas, and rectus femoris.

SPECIFIC STRETCHES

The stretch program provided in Chapter 16 of this text is designed to cover most of the major muscle groups of the body. Most sports activities require a general approach to stretching, with perhaps some additional emphasis on certain muscle groups specific to that activity. The following are some sports-specific stretches.

1. *Cycling*—Most of the muscle groups used during cycling are covered in the stretches described: back extensors, quads, hamstrings, gastrocnemius/soleus. One of the areas most often complained about by cyclists is the cervical spine. With the weight of the upper body supported by the arms, the cervical spine is usually in extension for long periods of time, often with the shoulders shrugging up about the ears. Before and during the ride, stretch the neck, especially into flexion and into a chin tuck to target the upper cervical spine. Periodically depress and protract the scapulae to pull the shoulders back down into position.
2. *Ball sports*—This category includes baseball, football, tennis, racquetball, volleyball, or any other sport in which the upper extremities must be used, especially in overhead positions requiring combined abduction and external rotation. This is the shoulder's most vulnerable position for rotator cuff strains. The shoulder should be stretched carefully into external rotation, perhaps more than that provided by the corner or wall stretches explained in Part II. In addition, internal rotation can be performed by reaching each arm behind the back, trying to get the fingers to the opposite scapula. Normally the dominant shoulder will be tighter than the nondominant side.

    These sports often require a rapid deceleration from the triceps as a throw or serve is completed, so attention should also be paid to stretching the triceps by reaching overhead with the elbow flexed and pulling the stretch side into end range shoulder flexion.
3. *Golf*—Because of the strong rotational component of a golf swing, the spine is at particular risk of a strain. To stretch the spine, perform the flexion and extension stretches outlined in Part II. In addition, lie supine with the knees bent. Keeping the shoulders flat on the floor, roll the knees to one side, allowing them to fall gently toward the floor. Repeat on the other side. It must be stressed that stretching alone will not protect the spine from the strong forces caused by a full golf swing; the abdominal and back extensor muscles must also be strengthened with exercises such as those outlined in Part II.

RESEARCH FINDINGS

Although research has been less than unanimous in substantiating the role of flexibility exercises in preventing injuries, our knowledge of muscle physiology and a common sense approach to exercise would indicate the advisability of a regular stretching program. Research has demonstrated consistent improvement in tissue length with stretching, but because the incidence of actual injuries cannot be manipulated in a research design, there is little control of all possible variables. Agre has published a significant body of work on the role of stretching for athletes. One of the studies, looking at the musculoskeletal profiles of male college soccer players, found significant musculoskeletal abnormalities in 52% of the subjects. Yet even with this large number of asymmetries of flexibility and strength, no players sustained hamstring or groin strains in the two years of the study. Agre and Baxter concluded that this was attributable to the addition of a 15-minute warm-up and stretching program prior to each practice and match.[3]

With regard to the best time to perform stretches, a study by Cornelius et al indicated no significant difference in increased range of motion in subjects who did their stretches before, after, or before and after the activity of interest.[9] The researchers concluded that it may not be worth the time to stretch both before and after an exercise session if increased range of motion is the goal. However, a brief series of stretches after exercise may help eliminate post-exercise soreness.

A consistent stretching program prior to beginning an exercise session takes only about 15 minutes. A concise stretch routine that can be adapted or altered to fit the special requirements of any individual is presented in Part II.

CHAPTER SUMMARY

Flexibility adequate to allow the efficient performance of athletic activities is the goal of the stretches presented in this text. In this chapter, the physiology of effective stretch was addressed along with a discussion of static versus ballistic stretch. Normal range of motion varies with individual pursuits and needs despite the textbook lists of norms, and should therefore be tailored to meet each individual's requirements. A description of 10 flexibility exercises is found in Part II, selected to provide a general flexibility program for the major muscles of the body. Some sport-specific stretch suggestions are offered for muscle groups not covered in the general program. Research findings supporting the use of a flexibility program are discussed.

REFERENCES

1. Agre JC. Hamstring injuries: proposed aetiological factors, prevention, and treatment. *Sports Med.* 1985;2:21–33.
2. Agre JC. Static stretching for athletes. *Arch Phys Med Rehabil.* 1981;59:561.
3. Agre JC, Baxter TL. Musculoskeletal profile of male collegiate soccer players. *Arch Phys Med Rehabil.* 1987;68:147–150.
4. Agre JC, Baxter TL. Strength and flexibility characteristics of collegiate soccer players. *Arch Phys Med Rehabil.* 1980;62:539.
5. Bixler B, Jones RL. High school football injuries: effects of a post-halftime warm-up and stretching routine. *Fam Pract Res J.* 1992;12:131–139.
6. Kisner C, Colby LA. *Therapeutic Exercise: Foundations and Techniques.* 2nd ed. Philadelphia: Davis; 1990.
7. Liemohn W. Flexibility/range of motion. In: Durstine JL, King AC, Painter PL, Roitman JL, Zwiren LD, eds. *ACSM's Resource Manual for Guidelines for Exercise Testing and Prescription.* 2nd ed. Philadelphia: Lea & Febiger; 1993.
8. Nordin M, Frankel VH. *Basic Biomechanics of the Musculoskeletal System.* 2nd ed. Philadelphia: Lea & Febiger; 1989:189.
9. Cornelius WL, Hagemann RW, Jackson AW. A study on placement of stretching within a workout. *J Sports Med Phys Fit.* 1988;28(3):234–236.

CHAPTER 7

Posture

Caren J. Werlinger

CHAPTER OUTLINE

I. Postural Muscles
II. A Postural Base for Exercise
III. Postural Changes with Exercise Equipment
IV. Dynamic Posture Control
V. Posture and Aging
VI. Postural Exercises
VII. Chapter Summary

Postural considerations must be part of instructing a client in an exercise program. Just as therapeutic exercises cannot be properly performed with poor posture, neither can fitness exercises. A subject's posture is the "composite of the positions of all the joints of the body at any given moment."[1] If postural alignment is faulty, then energy cannot be safely transferred to the activity at hand.

Good posture, in general terms, will keep the muscle forces that are acting on the body as balanced as possible. In standing, this means a vertical plumb line would intersect right and left halves of the body equally in the sagittal plane. In the frontal plane, it would intersect the earlobe, the point of the shoulder, the midline of the trunk, the greater trochanter, just anterior to the midline of the knee, and just anterior to the lateral malleolus.[1] In this way there is a great deal of skeletal support, requiring only enough muscular effort to remain upright.

Trying to maintain good posture in dynamic situations is more difficult, because portions of the body's mass are always moving, changing the center of gravity and altering the muscular effort needed to maintain balance. In contrast to a static stance in which balance will be maintained as long as the line of gravity falls between the feet, many dynamic activities are a constant loss and recovery of balance. If a runner were suddenly arrested at any point in mid-run, the line of gravity would probably be outside the base of support (which at best would only be one foot), and that person would most likely fall over. Postural mechanisms in dynamic situations, therefore, are devoted to catching up with the body's hopefully controlled momentum.

POSTURAL MUSCLES

Muscles involved in postural control should be assessed when prescribing a preventive exercise program. Typically, these muscles have a higher concentration of Type I tonic muscle fibers, enabling them to maintain low levels of activity for prolonged periods of time without fatiguing. With habitual faulty posture, postural muscles can become weakened through disuse or by being in a constantly lengthened position.

Posteriorly, the muscles that are used to maintain an upright posture are the gastrocnemius/soleus, the hamstrings, gluteus maximus, erector spinae, trapezius, and cervical extensors. Anteriorly, the anterior tibialis, iliopsoas, rectus abdominus, internal and external obliques, pectoralis minor, and longus colli and longus capitus all offer balance to the posterior muscles. Part II offers a number of exercises to isolate and strengthen any of these muscles.

A POSTURAL BASE FOR EXERCISE

In exercise activities performed in standing, the client should try to maintain a neutral pelvis, without either an anterior or a posterior tilt. This will allow the lumbar spine to stay close to neutral lordosis and, combined with taut abdominals, will provide a fairly solid base of support from which to move. The habit of maintaining some tension in the abdominals during most activities is a difficult thing to teach, but helps to stabilize the spine with slightly increased intra-abdominal pressure and enhanced pelvic control.

The same principle of a neutral pelvis applies to activities performed in sitting, whether exercise or sedentary work. Keeping the hips and knees flexed at 90 degrees with a neutral lordosis gives the upper body a stable base from which to work.

The cervical lordosis is also an important postural component. A proper cervical lordosis cannot be maintained if the lumbar lordosis is absent, but good lumbar control does not guarantee good cervical position. Subjects must be taught to throw out the chest somewhat, allowing the upper extremities to hang properly from their muscular attachments. This technique is much more effective than trying to teach people to retract their scapulae, which does not really correct the problem. If the cervical and lumbar positions are correct, then usually the thoracic kyphosis will also fall within normal range.

POSTURAL CHANGES WITH EXERCISE EQUIPMENT

The situation changes once the subject is exercising with objects that become, in effect, part of the body mass. Holding weights and riding a bicycle are two examples of equipment that change the position of the body's center of gravity. The object's mass must be countered by the body's postural mechanisms. Balance will be altered, as will the speed of movement and the muscle force required for movement. Imagine someone standing with her back against a wall. If she were to lift two 3-lb dumbbells into 90 degrees of shoulder flexion, muscle force alone would probably enable her to accomplish the motion. However, if she tried to lift two 10-lb dumbbells, without the ability to counter the weight by swaying slightly backward, she most likely would fall forward. The physics involved are beyond the scope of this text, but it is important to grasp the concept that the extra mass of exercise equipment must be taken into consideration when a subject's form is being critiqued.

When riding a bicycle, a cyclist has to learn to adapt his responses to accommodate the bicycle's handling characteristics. Some bikes respond sluggishly, requiring more time to make adjustments to unexpected situations. High-performance bikes, though, are designed to respond almost immediately to the slightest shift in weight or body lean. In either case, the bicycle's mass becomes part of the total mass the rider must handle. Inexperienced cyclists will learn about these characteristics—either by instruction or by crashing.

DYNAMIC POSTURE CONTROL

The principle of a neutral lordosis is also applied to many dynamic exercises. Squats and lunges, for example, should be performed with muscle effort from the buttocks and thighs, not with the back extensors. If the lumbar lordosis is maintained, there will be minimal stress placed upon the spine with these movements. Any time weights are being lifted overhead, the lifter must be very careful to control lumbar position. An observer in any weight room will see a lifter attempting to perform an overhead lift with inadequate latissimus length, and compensating with excessive arch in the spine to bring his shoulders under the weight. Adequate flexibility is essential to proper posture.

In bicycling, the back should be kept relatively flat, the majority of the force coming, again, from the buttocks and lower extremities. The common complaint of neck ache while cycling will be minimized, if not eliminated, by keeping the scapulae protracted and keeping the neck long, as opposed to hanging from the scapulae with excessive cervical extension while hunched over the handlebars.

Runners often develop a tendency to tilt the pelvis anteriorly, especially as they try to lengthen their stride with inadequate length of the hip flexors. This results in frequent complaints of low back pain. Balancing the length of hip flexors and back extensors with the necessary strength of abdominals and hip extensors evens the forces acting on the spine.

POSTURE AND AGING

Learning the habits of good posture early in life can help prevent many of the skeletal problems associated with aging. Forward head posture is the cause of numerous musculoskeletal complaints including cervical pain syndromes, cervical facet joint irritation, problems in the thoracic outlet, impingement of the brachial plexus, temporomandibular joint disorders, and chronic headaches, just to name a few.[2] By providing the body with more balanced muscular support and good alignment, it would stand to reason that there would be less degeneration in some of the joints. And it has been proven that appropriately balanced weight-bearing exercise can increase bone density, therefore decreasing the likelihood of osteoporotic fractures.[3]

Even for those subjects who are beginning exercise later in life, postural exercises can help correct faulty posture. In a study by Itoi and Sinaki,[4] older women who performed back extensor strengthening exercises were able to decrease their thoracic kyphosis. Because this is a frequent site of compression fractures in elderly women, this study's findings are encouraging for a possible prevention of kyphotic deformities and fractures with the use of exercise.

POSTURAL EXERCISES

As stated in Chapter 6, adequate flexibility is essential to good posture. All the general stretches covered in Part II are recommended. For strengthening specifically of postural muscles, the movements in Exhibit 7–1 are suggested (see Part II for illustrations).

Exhibit 7–1 Resistive Exercise Movements That Emphasize Postural Muscles

• Abdominal curl	• Latissimus pulldown
• Trunk extension	• Posterior deltoid raises
• Hip extension	• Calf raises

CHAPTER SUMMARY

This chapter provided a discussion of the importance of proper posture in exercise, both static and dynamic. It covered basic principles of postural alignment and postural muscle fiber makeup, along with a general list of anterior and posterior postural muscles. The chapter then provided examples of postural considerations for various exercises, including how responses change with the addition of objects such as weights or a bicycle. The role of good posture in the aging process was discussed, and postural flexibility and strengthening exercises were suggested.

REFERENCES

1. Kendall FP, McCreary EK, Provance PG. *Muscles: Testing and Function.* 4th ed. Baltimore: Williams & Wilkins; 1993.
2. Kisner C, Colby LA. *Therapeutic Exercise: Foundations and Techniques.* 2nd ed. Philadelphia: Davis; 1990.
3. Heath GW. Exercise programming for the older adult. In: Durstine JL, King AC, Painter PL, Roitman JL, et al, eds. *ACSM's Resource Manual for Guidelines for Exercise Testing and Prescription.* 2nd ed. Philadelphia: Lea & Febiger; 1993.
4. Itoi E, Sinaki M. Effect of back-strengthening exercise on posture in healthy women 49 to 65 years of age. *Mayo Clin Prac.* 1994;69:1054–1059.

Chapter 8

Safety

Caren J. Werlinger

CHAPTER OUTLINE

I. Guidelines
II. Chapter Summary

Whether an exercise program is for general health, prevention of disease or injury, or rehabilitation of an existing injury, it will be nothing more than an exercise in futility if it is not designed and performed safely. If training injuries do occur, they almost always require the cessation of that particular activity until the injury heals.[1,2] The probability of this happening can be diminished with proper education and supervision.

When an individual is being instructed in an exercise program, the exercise professional should make a determination as to how much detail to impart regarding anatomy and biomechanics. Some people are not interested in more than a superficial explanation; but others are interested in pursuing more advanced training. Charts and illustrations can help with their understanding of the material.

The professional must also teach each technique or exercise with as much attention to detail as the client can comprehend. Many exercises require fine-tuning for each person (eg, how wide a grip to use with a barbell, how wide a stance to take for squats), and if the subject is taught to take the same preparatory steps each time a specific exercise is approached, the likelihood of injury due to faulty mechanics will be diminished. Written instructions with diagrams, such as those included in this text, should accompany any exercise prescription. This hard copy ensures that the subject will have an accurate reference should the details of the verbal instructions be forgotten. Any specific precautions or limitations can be spelled out for the protection of both the client and the exercise professional.

After the client has been instructed in an exercise program, the professional may need to give instruction at least two or three more times to correct errors in form or bad habits. If there is a single most common error in judgment made by health and fitness professionals, it is probably assuming that one instruction session is sufficient for people to perform their exercises correctly. Even small slips in technique should be corrected because, with time and repetition, they may cause overuse injuries. If an individual is to adopt an exercise program as a permanent lifestyle change, then at some point it will be performed without an instructor's supervision, and it hopefully will have become habit to perform the exercises correctly.

In the event that an injury does occur, it is possible and advisable to substitute other forms of training while the injured body part heals. If someone sustains a lower extremity running injury, activities such as cycling, swimming, or arm ergometry can be used to maintain cardiovascular fitness. If possible, strength training for the upper body and the uninjured leg should be continued. If a shoulder were injured doing a bench press, after an appropriate period of rest and rehabilitation (if needed), training could probably be resumed using light dumbbells to allow a more open-chained action and thereby avoid causing a chronic overuse injury. This is the reason that such a wide variety of exercises have been offered in this text; varying exercises not only provides more well-rounded conditioning, it also offers alternatives to alleviate stress on overworked tissues or joints.

In a study by Almekinders and Almekinders[3] that took a retrospective look at chronic overuse injuries, it was found that at an average of 27 months post-injury, 35% were unchanged. This would clearly indicate the advisability of preventing injuries in the first place, and treating them promptly when they do occur.

GUIDELINES

A brief warm-up should precede each exercise session. Stretches should be performed at low intensity to avoid triggering the muscle spindles, allowing sufficient time for muscle lengthening to take place.[4]

In resistance training, technique should always be emphasized over extra weight. Weights should never be used to try and force extra range of motion. The lift should be performed carefully within the available range, and should be at an intensity that can be controlled throughout the movement without the assistance of momentum or substitution.

Aerobic exercise should always be based on a target heart range that is a percentage of maximum heart range; usually 65 to 85% of maximum. Remember to include a warm-up period and a cool-down period after the main target heart range portion. Because aerobic exercise sessions tend to use the same repetitive motions for long periods of time, it is wise to vary the type of exercise and provide the muscles with different stimulation from time to time.

If subjects are to be exercising either at home or at another facility, it is wise for health professionals to acquaint themselves with any exercise facilities in their area. Exercise clubs vary widely in terms of the qualifications of their exercise instructors and the level of supervision provided to members. It would be most unfortunate for an enthusiastic novice to sustain an injury that might have been prevented under the watchful eye of more qualified staff.

Safe exercise also depends on safe equipment. Club equipment should be well-maintained and clean. It need not be new or shiny, but it should not have frayed cables, ripped upholstery, or broken weight plates. Any equipment in a public facility will need constant maintenance. An inspection of a facility that will be recommended to clients ought to go beyond the cosmetics.

The responsibility for safe equipment must also be shared by the exercising person. Running shoes will wear out biomechanically sooner than their appearance would indicate, so a serious runner must be prepared to replace them when necessary. A bicycle will need periodic tune-ups to grease the bearings in the hubs and bottom bracket. The headset, brake cables, pads, and drivetrain will all need maintenance. A bicycle should be checked by a bike mechanic at least once a year, and possibly more frequently if the bike has been ridden in wet, muddy weather.

Because the average person expects all health professionals to be exercise experts, it is our professional responsibility to stay abreast of current research. As more is learned about the body's response to training and its ability to adapt to exercise, we should be capable of interpreting that information for use with clients. This will also allow an exercise prescription to be based on scientific data rather than locker room advice or misconception. Only in this way can exercise programs be developed that help people accomplish their goals without endangering them.

CHAPTER SUMMARY

It is imperative that exercises be pursued safely if they are to be of any use in improving health. This chapter presents an overview of safety guidelines detailed in other chapters. It also covers the principles of alternative training in the event of an injury, and stresses the need to avoid overuse injuries. In addition to physiological principles of safety, there are practical safety needs in terms of equipment upkeep, both personal equipment and club equipment. Finally, the need for prescribers of exercise to stay abreast of current research was emphasized.

REFERENCES

1. Holmich P, Christensen SW, Darre E, Jahnsen F, et al. Non-elite marathon runners: health, training and injuries. *Br J Sprts Med*. 1980; 23:177–178.
2. Van Mechelen W. Running injuries. A review of the epidemiological literature. *Sports Med*. 1992;14:320–335.
3. Almekinders LC, Almekinders SV. Outcome in the treatment of chronic overuse sports injuries: a retrospective study. *J Orthop Sports Phys Ther*. 1994;19:157–161.
4. Kisner C, Colby LA. *Therapeutic Exercise: Foundations and Techniques*. 2nd ed. Philadelphia: Davis; 1990.

Chapter 9

Recovery and Overtraining

David Ash

CHAPTER OUTLINE

I. Signs and Symptoms of Overtraining
II. Resistive Exercise: How Many Sets and Repetitions?
III. Overtraining and Recovery in Aerobic Activities
IV. Chapter Summary

One of the most important and frequently overlooked components of a successful exercise program is sufficient recovery. Overtraining is simply the lack of recovery. These interrelated concepts, alluded to in Chapter 2, warrant further discussion.

Our society generally values hard work, self-sacrifice, and dedication. While these are indeed admirable traits, any desirable quality or activity when pursued to extremes may cause unfavorable imbalances. Problems may develop if exercise becomes excessive. When one exceeds a given amount of exercise, the health benefits begin to diminish. A simple analogy from the career/occupational realm involves the workaholic. As time at the office increases past some critical threshold, productivity declines.

Overtraining does not happen to the unmotivated. Rather, it is the highly motivated exerciser who must be wary of overtraining. If the highly motivated exerciser is not progressing with results every month (whether his or her goals are change in body composition, increase in repetitions on a particular resistive exercise movement, or mileage biked), one of two phenomena has occurred. Either the client has reached his or her genetic limit regarding that particular activity, or he or she is overtraining. Frequently the latter case is true. While certainly the vast majority of the population does need to exercise more, the small percentage that is highly motivated, and therefore susceptible to overtraining, may guide their exercise by the rule: Do not exercise more, exercise *more productively*.

SIGNS AND SYMPTOMS OF OVERTRAINING

Signs and symptoms of overtraining are many and variable. Signs may include increased resting heart rate, increased resting blood pressure, increased salivary cortisol, altered eating patterns, and decreased performance. Symptoms may include insomnia, lethargy, irritability, depression, and/or decreased ability to concentrate.

Prevention, rather than remediation, should be emphasized by the exercise professional. Education about productive and time-efficient exercise, recovery, and the common signs and symptoms of overtraining may help prevent this problem.

Raglin and Morgan[1] conducted an investigation of collegiate swimmers to determine whether psychological monitoring by use of the Profile of Mood States (POMS)[2] could provide sport coaches with a valid marker of overreaching. The value of such a marker is that exercise variables could be manipulated (eg, by introducing short periods of reduced training or rest) to prevent progression to the more serious state of overtraining.

Terminology was operationalized in the study as is shown in Table 9–1. The researchers then applied the seven-item training distress scale to track and field athletes and found it to be equally effective in identification of overreaching.

In addition to the signs and symptoms characteristic of overtraining as presented in Table 9–1, a review by Lehman et al[3] further contrasts overreaching and the more serious overtraining by adding loss of body weight, bradycardia, and tachycardia to the list of possible characteristics of over-

Table 9–1 Terminology Used in Overreaching and Overtraining

	Overreaching	Overtraining
Definition	Decrease by less than 5% or transient decrease or maintenance of performance only with increased difficulty and perception of effort.	Performance decrease of 5% with ongoing decrease in performance.
Synonym	Distress	Staleness
Signs/Symptoms	The following seven POMS items were the best predictors of overreaching: (1) worthlessness, (2) miserable, (3) bad-tempered, (4) guilty, (5) unworthy, (6) peeved, and (7) sad.	Clinical depression is frequently noted and behavioral problems such as sleep disturbances and appetite loss are also common.
Intervention	Manipulation of exercise variables (eg, introduction of short periods of reduced training or rest).	The athlete may have to stop training for a period of weeks or months to fully recover.

training. The *1995 American Heart Association Guidelines for Cardiovascular Exercise in Apparently Healthy Individuals*[4] cautions exercise professionals to watch for the following signs of overexercising:

1. inability to finish training session
2. inability to converse during the activity
3. faintness or nausea after exercise
4. chronic fatigue
5. sleeplessness
6. aches and pains in the joints

RESISTIVE EXERCISE: HOW MANY SETS AND REPETITIONS?

In research literature and particularly in advertising literature one can find resistive exercise programs that recommend one set per exercise movement, to as many as six to eight sets per movement. Perhaps the most common set/repetition protocol described is 3 × 10 (3 sets of 10 repetitions). What is the basis of performing 3 sets of 10 repetitions of a given exercise movement?

DeLorme, a Boston physician working with poliomyelitis patients, originally described the 10 repetition maximum (RM) in 1945.[5] In 1948, DeLorme and Watkins discussed their 3 sets of 10 repetitions protocol,

Set 1 = 10 repetitions with 50% of 10 RM
Set 2 = 10 repetitions with 75% of 10 RM
Set 3 = 10 repetitions with 10 RM

stating, "By use of small muscle loads initially, and then increasing them after each set of 10 repetitions, the muscle is 'warmed up' preparatory to exerting its maximum power for 10 repetitions."[6] In DeLorme and Watkins' own words, the initial 2 sets are warm-up sets.

Berger[7] "compared all possible combinations of 1, 2, and 3 sets and 2, 6, and 10 repetitions. Loads were always intended to elicit maximum effort for a given number of repetitions." This study indicated that 3 sets of 6 repetitions were more effective in increasing strength than the other set/repetition combinations.

Research by Reid et al[8] used each of the following protocols:

2 × 15 RM three times per week
1 × 10 RM twice per week, 1 × 3 RM once per week
3 × 6 RM three times per week

The researchers concluded that all three formats resulted in strength increases, but that the increases were not significantly different. The researchers commented that the conclusion of their study "fails to support Berger's findings." Other research comparing various set/repetition schemes with 3 sets of 6 repetitions also failed to support the superiority of 3 sets of 6 repetitions.[9–13]

Graves et al[14] conducted a 12-week study to assess the effect of decreased (1 to 2 days per week) resistive exercise. The study indicated that strength was maintained with decreased frequency of resistive exercise.

In 1989, Westcott[15] conducted a study in which the treatment group performed 20 minutes of exercise on each of 3 nonsuccessive days for 8 weeks. The 20-minute session consisted of 15 minutes of aerobic activity followed by 1 set of 8 to 12 bar dips and 1 set of 8 to 12 chin ups. At the conclusion of the study, the control group recorded small increases in cardiovascular endurance (3%), leg strength (3%), and upper body strength (3%). In contrast, the experimental group increased cardiovascular endurance by 11%, leg strength by 23%, and upper body strength by 24%. In addition, the experimental group improved body composition by

4%, as a result of an average loss of 3 lbs in fat and an average 2-lb increase in lean body mass. A post-study questionnaire revealed that 100% of the exercisers had a better attitude about exercise, with 95% committing to continue an exercise program. Westcott then repeated the study with a different group of subjects. In the second experiment, the exercise session consisted of 16 minutes of aerobic activity followed by 1 set of each of 3 different resistive exercise movements. The results of the second study were very similar to those of the first.

In a study conducted by Stone and Coulter,[16] 3 groups trained on the same resistive exercises for 9 weeks at 3 sets of 6 to 8 RM, 2 sets of 15 to 20 RM, and 1 set of 30 to 40 RM, respectively. The perception that heavy weights with low repetitions produce much greater increases in strength than medium repetitions (15 to 20) or high repetitions (30 to 40) was not supported in the study. The research database appears to be replete with studies supporting the idea that training can be productive regardless of the set and repetition scheme as long as the principles of overload and progression are utilized.

OVERTRAINING AND RECOVERY IN AEROBIC ACTIVITIES

Houmard et al[17] investigated the effects of 10 days of reduced training in collegiate distance runners. During this period, the runners decreased their mileage per week to 36% of pretaper volume (110 km/week to 40 km/week). The 10-day taper period consisted of 5 days of running and 5 rest days. No changes were identified between pretaper and posttaper measurements of maximal oxygen consumption, maximal heart rate, work time to exhaustion, body weight, percent body fat, submaximal treadmill runs (265 and 298 meters/minute), rating of perceived exertion, and 2-minute postrun lactate levels. Heart rate during a 6-minute run was elevated with respect to pretaper levels, as was heart rate at 1 and 2 minutes following the 6-minute run.

A study investigated the effects of 3 to 5 weeks of physical rest on selected physical, physiological, and psychological parameters of 12 Olympic athletes with recent underperformance. The data show that resting for 3 to 5 weeks helped these under-performing elite athletes improve their aerobic performance.[18]

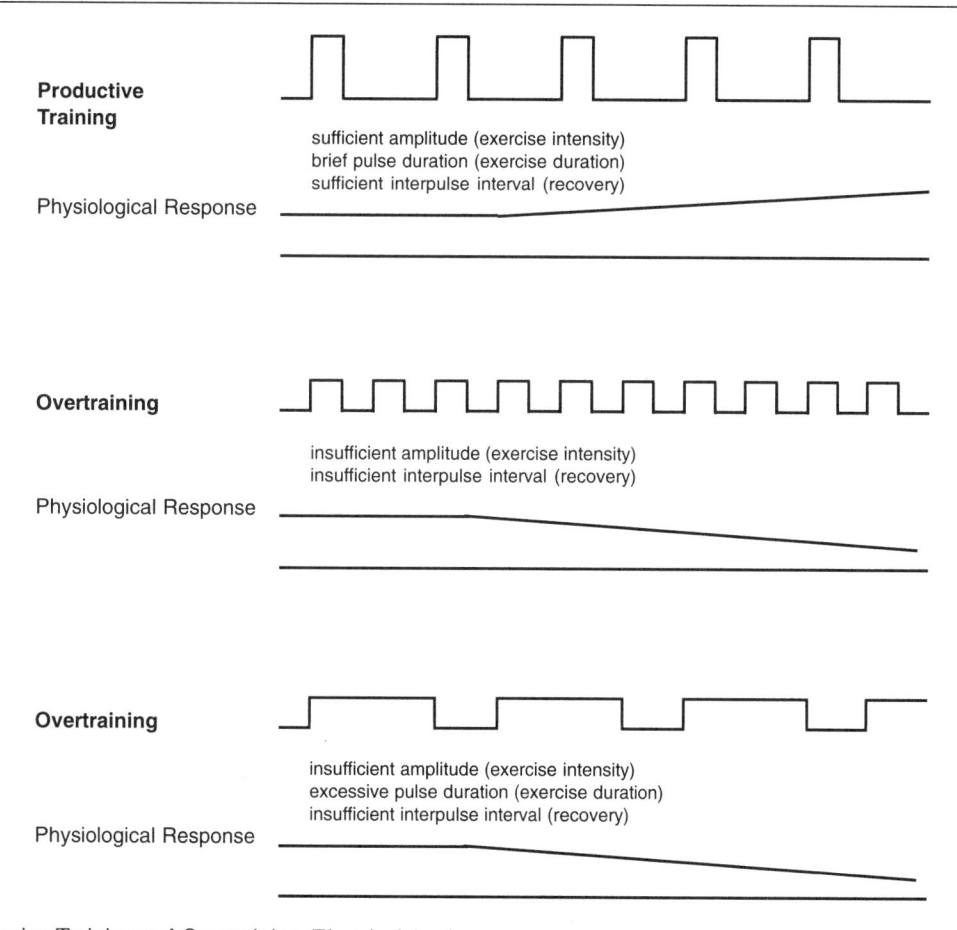

Figure 9–1 Productive Training and Overtraining: Electrical Analogy

A study conducted with competitive swimmers indicated that reduced training frequency improved swim power.[9]

Research appears to support the notion that quality rather than quantity of exercise may be the crucial variable with regard to physiological adaptation. An electrical analogy illustrates this concept in Figure 9–1. A general guideline recommended to help prevent the occurrence of overtraining is that one week of every month be scheduled as a recovery week. This recommendation applies to both aerobic and anaerobic emphasis activities and to exercisers from the novice to the professional athlete.

CHAPTER SUMMARY

Recovery is an integral, yet often overlooked, component to any successful exercise program. Overtraining is the absence of sufficient recovery. Highly motivated individuals are most vulnerable to overtraining. Signs and symptoms of overtraining have been identified. A literature review regarding the various set-repetition schemes proposed for resistive exercise was presented. It is recommended that the exercise consumer base exercise decisions on soundly designed, peer-reviewed research studies as opposed to advertising literature. Research regarding overtraining in aerobic activities was addressed.

REFERENCES

1. Raglin JS, Morgan WP. Development of a scale for use in monitoring training-induced distress in athletes. *Int J Sports Med*. 1994;15:84–88.
2. McNair DN, Lorr M, Droppleman LF. *Profile of Mood States Manual*. San Diego: Educational and Testing Service; 1991.
3. Lehman M, Foster C, Keul J. Overtraining in endurance athletes: a brief review. *Med Sci Sports Exerc*. 1993;25:854–862.
4. Fletcher GF, Balady G, Froelicher VF, Hartley LH, et al. Exercise standards: a statement for healthcare professionals from the American Heart Association. *Circ*. 1995;603–604.
5. DeLorme TL. Restoration of muscle power by heavy resistance exercises. *J Bone Joint Surg*. 1945;26:645.
6. DeLorme TL, Watkins AL. Techniques of progressive resistance exercise. *Arch Phys Med*. 1948;29:263–273.
7. Berger RA. Effects of varied weight training programs on strength. *Res Q*. 1962;33:168–181.
8. Reid CM, Yeater RA, Ullrich IH. Weight training and strength, cardiorespiratory functioning, and body composition of men. *Br J Sports Med*. 1987;21:40–44.
9. Johns RA, Houmard JA, Kobe RW, Hortobagyi T, et al. Effects of taper on swim power, stroke distance, and performance. *Med Sci Sports Exerc*. 1992;24:1141–1146.
10. Messier SP, Dill ME. Alterations in strength and maximal oxygen uptake consequent to Nautilus circuit weight training. *RQES*. 1985;56:345–351.
11. O'Shea P. Effects of selected weight training programs and the development of strength and muscle hypertrophy. *Res Q*. 1966;37:95–102.
12. Stiggins CF. *Nautilus and Free Weight Training Program: A Comparison of Strength Development at Four Angles in the Range of Motion*. Salt Lake City, UT: Brigham Young University; 1978. Thesis.
13. Withers RT. Effect of varied weight-training loads on the strength of university freshmen. *Res Q*. 1970;41:110–114.
14. Graves JE, Pollock ML, Leggett SH, Braith RW, et al. Effect of reduced training frequency on muscular strength. *Int J Sports Med*. 1988;9:316–319.
15. Westcott W. How much exercise is necessary? *Am Fitness Q*. 1990; April:38–47.
16. Stone WJ, Coulter SP. Strength/endurance effects from three training protocols with women. *J Strength Conditioning Res*. 1994;8:231–234.
17. Houmard JA, Kirwan JP, Flynn MG, Mitchell JB. Effects of reduced training on submaximal and maximal running responses. *Int J Sports Med*. 1989;10:30–33.
18. Koutedakis Y, Budgett R, Faulmann L. Rest in underperforming elite competitors. *Br J Sports Med*. 1990;24:248.

Chapter 10

Exercise Dependence

David Ash

CHAPTER OUTLINE

I. Exercise Dependence Defined
II. Intervention
III. Chapter Summary

Lambrinides[1] recalls he once knew an individual who purchased full memberships at two separate exercise facilities. When asked why, the individual responded that each of the facilities was closed one day of the year. The first facility was closed on Christmas Day, the second facility was closed on New Year's Day.

EXERCISE DEPENDENCE DEFINED

Exercise dependence as defined by Veale[2] is "a process that compels an individual to exercise in spite of obstacles, and results in physical and psychological symptoms when exercise is withdrawn." Exercise dependence is distinguished from overtraining in that overtraining is a physical action, whereas exercise dependence is a psychological construct. Exercise dependence can result in overtraining. Also called exercise addiction, dependence occurs when an individual exercises not for optimal physiological adaptations, but rather for psychological reasons or emotional needs.

Sachs[3] proposed an exercise continuum in which exercise dependence occurs when habitual exercise "has progressed from an important aspect of the individual's life to a controlling factor which dominates other choices" (see Exhibit 10–1).

Veale[2] proposed the following diagnostic criteria to assist in the identification of exercise dependence:

- Narrowing of repertoire leading to a stereotyped pattern of exercise with a regular schedule once or more daily
- Giving increasing priority to exercise over other activities to maintain the pattern of exercise
- Increased tolerance to the amount of exercise performed over the years
- Withdrawal symptoms related to a disorder of mood following the cessation of the exercise schedule
- Relief or avoidance of withdrawal symptoms by further exercise
- Subjective awareness of a compulsion to exercise
- Rapid reinstatement of the previous pattern of exercise and withdrawal symptoms after a period of abstinence

Identified withdrawal symptoms[2] resulting from cessation of exercise in individuals with this dependence include:

- depression
- anger
- tension
- frustration
- malaise
- guilt
- increased sexual tension
- anxiety
- irritability
- apprehension
- increased need for social interaction
- confusion
- decreased self-esteem
- relief
- impaired concentration
- muscle soreness
- sleep disturbance
- fatigue

Exhibit 10–1 Exercise Continuum

Habitual Exercise	Overtraining
exercise is positive	exercise is negative
an important component of the individual's life	a controlling factor that dominates other choices
the individual maintains control over the activity	the individual is controlled by the activity

- increased galvanic skin response
- gastrointestinal problems

INTERVENTION

The exercise professional's goal is to intervene prior to problem development. The intervention should include educating the exerciser about optimal amounts of exercise and the signs and symptoms of exercise dependence. If the exerciser reaches the point of dependence, it is questionable whether he or she will be responsive to the exercise professional. In all likelihood, the dependent individual has long been aware of recommended recovery guidelines, and signs and symptoms of dependence. If a professional is approached by an exercise-dependent client, the recommended course of action is to refer the client to professionals skilled in the psychological component of dependence.

CHAPTER SUMMARY

When exercise is performed not for optimal physiological adaptations, but rather to satisfy emotional or psychological needs, exercise dependence has developed. Exercise can be located anywhere along a continuum between the two extremes of being a positive addition to one's lifestyle, or at the other extreme, a negative and controlling factor. Diagnostic criteria for exercise dependence and common withdrawal symptoms were presented. Intervention was addressed.

REFERENCES

1. Lambrinides T. 1989. Personal communication.
2. Veale DC. Exercise dependence. *Br J Addict*. 1987;82:735–740.
3. Sachs ML. Compliance and addiction to exercise. In: Cantu RC, ed. *The Exercising Adult*. Boston: Collamore Press; 1982:19–27.

CHAPTER 11

Exercise for Children

David Ash

CHAPTER OUTLINE

I. Introduction
II. Benefits of Youth Exercise
III. Specific Activities and Injury Trends
IV. Recommendations
V. Prevention of Patellofemoral Dysfunction
VI. Chapter Summary

INTRODUCTION

Prepubescence is the time from childhood to onset of secondary sex characteristics. *Adolescence* begins with the onset of secondary sex characteristics and continues until physical and skeletal maturity. These are crucial periods during which physical activity patterns that may have long-term health implications are formed. Cunnane[1] states that low exercise level is a contributing factor to childhood obesity and hypertension and predisposes the individual to premature death from coronary heart disease. Fortunately, through intervention in children and adolescents in the form of education and motivation, exercise level may be increased.

BENEFITS OF YOUTH EXERCISE

The benefits of youth physical activity include fitness, weight control, and the development of habits having the potential to span a lifetime. A study was conducted to systematically determine the amount of moderate to vigorous physical activity students obtain during elementary and middle-school physical education classes (time spent performing moderate to vigorous physical activity/total class time). The researchers concluded that the amount of physical activity observed (elementary schools, 8.6%; middle schools, 16.1%) was significantly less than the estimated national average of 27% and far below the national recommendation of a minimum of 50%.[2] A review of current youth fitness data indicates that children in the United States are fatter, slower, and weaker than children in other developed nations. Also, children in the United States appear to be developing a sedentary lifestyle at earlier ages. Recommendations for improvement must involve programs that increase physical activity both in school and at home. Parental education is recommended to address the importance of parent participation in physical activity with their children. A balance between sedentary activity and physical activity is optimal. To facilitate improvement in youth fitness, involvement of communities, state and federal governments, health professionals, and the media are necessary.[3]

Several research studies elucidate the criticality of exercise habit formation at early ages. Efforts early in life to promote cardiovascular health may have a dramatic effect beyond the pediatric age. Focus should not be limited to traditional childhood diseases but should include adult diseases that have their origins in childhood. Five major target areas for cardiovascular health promotion in childhood are obesity, cardiovascular fitness, hypertension, hypercholesterolemia, and smoking prevention.[4] Cardiovascular risk factors tend to track from childhood to adulthood. Therefore, programs to increase consistent physical activity in youths have potential for reducing adult cardiovascular diseases.[5] A 16-year cohort study was conducted with 115,195 registered nurses serving as subjects. Both weight gain of greater than 10 kg after age 18 years and a body mass index of greater than 22.0 at age 18 years were predictors of overall mortality and death from cardiovascular disease in middle adulthood.[6] With respect to developing youth interest in exercise/physical activity and ongoing compliance, education and skill development of entire families about the prevention of cardiovascular disease can be emphasized. The targeting of the entire family system—rather than one individual—for behavioral change enhances social support, self-confidence, and the probability of behavioral skill maintenance.[7]

Participation in physical activity throughout one's entire life span has benefits that supercede participation only during selected parts of the life cycle. Shephard[8,9] has maintained that the school setting is an ideal intervention site to expose children to exercise on a regularly scheduled basis. He states, "The allocation of one hour for physical education per academic day does not negatively influence learning at the elementary school level. Indeed, any enhancement of self-image and relief of boredom may enhance classroom performance." Budgeting time for physical education and other physical activities should be included when planning school curriculums. Summaries of additional studies are presented in Table 11–1.

SPECIFIC ACTIVITIES AND INJURY TRENDS

In 1993, Mazur et al[27] reviewed types and causes of injuries to preadolescents and adolescents resulting from

Table 11–1 Additional Studies Regarding Benefits of Youth Exercise

Summary	Researchers/Authors
Strength training is associated with strength gains in adolescents and is safe when supervised by knowledgeable adults.	Purcell and Hergenroeder[10]
"The main conclusion of this study is that the derived measurement of body fatness is correlated with risk factors for coronary heart disease and non–insulin-dependent diabetes mellitis."	Gutin, Islam, Manos, and Cucuzzo[11]
"The results of this study indicate that the encouragement of heart healthy dietary intake patterns and participation in physical activity can decrease accelerated weight gain and obesity, even in preschool children."	Klesges, Klesges, Eck, and Shelton[12]
This study examined the effects of a 14-week resistive exercise program on prepubescent males. Exercisers achieved significant increases in strength and flexibility. Musculoskeletal scintigraphy indicated no damage to epiphyses, bone, or muscles. The program should be individualized based on the young exerciser's developmental status, ability, and special needs.	Weltman et al[13]; Weltman[14]
The developing musculoskeletal structures of the immature athlete are uniquely susceptible to injury, particularly at the physes. While early literature suggested that weight training might be inappropriate for these athletes, recent evidence suggests that, properly done, strength/resistance training may not only be safe, it may also help reduce the risk of injury for the young athlete.	Metcalf and Roberts[15]
Early gains in muscular strength resulting from resistance training in prepubescent children may be attributed to increased muscle activation.	Ozmun, Mikesky, and Surburg[16]
The results of a seven-year cohort study of adolescents in two communities, one of which had school-based intervention for cardiovascular health promotion, revealed that physical appearance was the most valued characteristic of adolescents in both communities. Students in the intervention community tended to retain positive values about physical exercise while the reference community demonstrated gradual reductions.	Prokhorov, Perry, Kelder, and Klepp[17]
"High-intensity resistance training appears to be effective in increasing strength in preadolescents. Children make similar relative, but smaller absolute strength gains when compared with adolescents and young adults. Resistance training appears to have little if any hypertrophic effect, rather being associated with increased levels of neuromuscular activation. The risk of injury from prudently prescribed and closely supervised resistance training appears to be low during preadolescence."	Blimke[18]

continues

Table 11-1 continued

Summary	Researchers/Authors
"Strength training stimulates predictable cardiovascular and neuromuscular responses. The cardiovascular responses result in nonpathologic concentric left ventricular hypertrophy with preservation of ejection fraction and no diastolic dysfunction. Resting heart rates and blood pressures in strength trained individuals remain unchanged or decrease slightly. Strength gains occur from enhanced neuromuscular activation over the initial eight weeks and from increased muscle fiber density and hypertrophy during subsequent weeks. Significant strength gains are possible in all populations, including children, women, and the elderly, when exposed to an adequate strength training program."	Lillegard and Terrio[19]
Salminen et al conducted a prospective three-year study of low back pain in the young. The researchers comment, "The high prevalence of low back pain (LBP) in the adult population and its impact on individuals and society suggest there is a need for studies on the early stages of the problem. However, LBP in adolescents has been under-investigated (despite the fact that) school-based surveys have shown a very high prevalence of backache and particularly LBP among children and teenagers." The researchers concluded that nearly 8% of the subjects "recognize LBP as a recurring problem after the age of rapid physical growth. At this age, and for a couple years to follow, these persons are characterized by a low frequency of leisure time physical activity and decreased spinal function, and increasing bodyweight. . . ."	Salminen, Erkintalo, Laine, and Pentti[20]
Motivation of adolescents to exercise may be facilitated by joining physical activity to the adolescent's personal interests or activities the entire family can integrate into the family lifestyle.	Telama[21]
Studies show no increased risk of injury when prepubescents participate in resistive exercise.	Sewall and Micheli[22]
"A risk that must be considered in the immature skeleton is the susceptibility of the growth cartilage of the epiphyseal plate. Weight training in a submaximal controlled, supervised situation is beneficial to bone deposition. Strength training can be a valuable and safe mode of exercise provided (1) instructors are properly educated, (2) participants are properly instructed, and (3) the absolute necessity of avoiding maximal lifts is reinforced."	Schafer[23]
In-season strength was maintained with performance of resistive exercise one day per week in pubescent male baseball players.	DeRenne, Hetzler, Buxton, and Ho[24]
Neither Olympic-style lifting nor powerlifting are indicated for prepubescents or adolescents due to the high injury risk associated with these activities.	Kuland, Dewey, and Brubaker[25]; Cahill[26]
"Although injuries can occur during the use of weight machines, most apparently happen during the aggressive use of free weights. Prepubescent and older athletes who are well-trained and supervised appear to have low injury rates in strength training programs. Good coaching, proper lifting techniques, and other injury prevention methods are likely to minimize the number of musculoskeletal problems caused by weight training."	Mazur, Yetman, and Risser[27]

weight lifting/training. The researchers concluded that "prepubescent and older athletes who are well-trained and supervised appear to have low injury rates in strength training programs." The information in Tables 11-2 through 11-4 is reprinted from that report. Trends regarding types of movements resulting in injury may be noted by the reader.

RECOMMENDATIONS

In addition to the resistive exercise guidelines discussed in Chapter 4, the exercise professional should be cognizant of the following regarding resistive exercise for prepubescents and adolescents. See Table 11-5 for recommended exercise variables.

Table 11-2 Injuries in Case Reports

Injury	Reference	Cause	Age, Sex
Lumbar ring apophyseal fracture	Browne, Yost, and McCarron[28]	Power lifts	16, M
Distal radioulnar joint dislocation	Francobandiera, Maffuli, and Lepore[29]	Squat lift	23, F
Cardiac rupture leading to death	George, Stakin, and Wright[30]	Barbell fell on chest from rack above bench	9, M
Transchondral fracture of the dome of the talus	Mannis[31]	Squat lift	17, M

Source: Reprinted with permission from L.J. Mazur, R.J. Yetman, and W.L. Risser, Weight-Training Injuries: Common Injuries and Preventative Methods, *Sports Medicine*, Vol. 16, No. 1, pp. 57-63, © 1993.

1. The physically immature individual should exercise at a lower intensity and duration than the mature adult.
2. As mentioned previously, intensity level is determined by the physician, specified in the physician's permission to exercise, and is based on the physician's physical examination.
3. Repetition maximums should not be attempted under any circumstances.
4. Competition should be discouraged.
5. Olympic lifting should not be attempted under any circumstances.
6. Exercises that require a great deal of practice before they can be performed safely (eg, squats, deadlifts) should be discouraged.
7. Antagonistic muscle groups should be addressed to prevent imbalance.
8. Body weight exercises should be used.
9. The exercise session is an excellent environment to encourage communication and socialization skill development.
10. Variety should be employed.
11. Exercise should be fun.

PREVENTION OF PATELLOFEMORAL DYSFUNCTION

A dysfunction for which the exercise professional should remain constantly observant in all exercisers—but particularly prepubescents and adolescents—is patellofemoral disease. Misaligned tracking of the patella in the groove of the distal femur may eventually result in this pathology. Steinkamp et al[42] presented a discussion of joint stresses occurring in open chain and closed chain resistive exercises (see Figures 11-1, 11-2, and 11-3). Patellofemoral joint stress in closed chain movements increases with increasing

Table 11-3 Injuries in Case Series

Injury	Reference	Cause	Number of Patients (Age and Range in Years)
Spondylolysis	Kotani et al[32]; Rossi and Dragoni[33]	Major lifts; weightlifting	8; 22 (18-24)
25 lumbar strains requiring bedrest and/or traction; 2 ruptured lumbar discs; 2 spondylolisthesis; 6 avulsions-anterior iliac spine; 4 meniscus tears of knee; 4 cervical sprains	Brady, Cahill, and Bodnar[34]	8 deadlift; 4 Universal gym; 2 leg machine	43 (13-19)
Osteolysis of distal clavicle	Cahill[35]	Bench press	43 (mean 23.3)
Fractures of radius and/or ulna	Gumbs, Segal, Halligan, and Lower[36]; Ryan and Salciccioli[37]	Clean and jerk; overhead press	5; 2 (12-17)

Source: Reprinted with permission from L.J. Mazur, R.J. Yetman, and W.L. Risser, Weight-Training Injuries: Common Injuries and Preventative Methods, *Sports Medicine*, Vol. 16, No. 1, pp. 57-63, © 1993.

Table 11–4 Injuries in Cohort Studies (Presented by Number and by Percent of Total)

Injuries	71 Powerlifters[38]	354 American Football Players[39]	10,908 American Football Players[40]
Injury Type			
Muscle strains	59 (61.2)	20 (74.1)	15 (44)
Tendonitis	12 (12.2)	1 (3.4)	2 (6)
Muscle cramps	10 (10.2)		1 (3)
Sprains	4 (4.1)	3 (11.1)	7 (20)
Abrasions/contusions	4 (4.1)		1 (3)
Nerve injuries	3 (3.1)	1 (3.7)	
Fractures	2 (2.0)	2 (7.4)	1 (3)
Dislocations	1 (1.0)		1 (3)
Lumbar disc injuries			2 (6)
Patellar subluxation			2 (6)
Hernia			1 (3)
Torn cartilage (knee)			1 (3)
Injury Site			
Lower back	49 (50.0)	13 (48.1)	15 (44)
Upper back	4 (4.1)	3 (11.1)	6 (18)
Chest	7 (7.1)		1 (3)
Abdomen	3 (3.1)		1 (3)
Neck		1 (3.7)	3 (9)
Shoulder	6 (6.1)	4 (14.8)	5 (15)
Elbow	6 (6.1)		
Hand	4 (4.1)	2 (7.4)	
Wrist	2 (2.0)	1 (3.4)	
Knee	8 (8.2)	2 (7.4)	3 (9)
Groin	4 (4.1)		
Thigh	3 (3.1)		
Leg			2 (6)
Ankle	2 (2.0)	1 (3.4)	1 (3)

Source: Reprinted with permission from L.J. Mazur, R.J. Yetman, and W. L. Risser, Weight-Training Injuries: Common Injuries and Preventative Methods, *Sports Medicine,* Vol. 16, No. 1, pp. 57–63, © 1993.

---

knee flexion. However, during the open chain knee extension movement, this joint stress increases with increasing knee extension.

In related research, Doucette and Child[43] conducted a study to investigate patellar tracking at various joint angles during open and closed chain resistive exercise in subjects with lateral patellar compression syndrome. Computed tomography was utilized for evaluation of congruence angle, the dependent variable.[44] Results of the Doucette and Child study are as follows:

1. From 0 to 40 degrees of knee flexion, patellofemoral congruence progressively increased (therefore lateral patellar tracking *decreased)* for both open chain and closed chain conditions.
2. Significantly more lateral tracking was identified for the open chain movement than the closed chain movement from full extension (0 degrees) to 20 degrees of knee flexion.
3. At 30 and 40 degrees of knee flexion, differences in lateral patellar tracking as indicated by congruence angle became insignificant (see Figure 11–4).
4. Doucette and Child cite the work of van Kampen and Huiskes[45] in suggesting that the differences in tibial rotation in open and closed chain movements may contribute to the differences in patellar tracking identified, particularly in the early range of knee flexion, 0 degrees to 25 degrees.

In additional research, Brownstein et al[46] have identified VMO EMG activity as highest between 60 and 90 degrees of knee flexion and lowest between 0 and 30 degrees of knee flexion. Grabiner et al[47] also state that short arc quadriceps

Table 11–5 Recommended Exercise Variables

	Prepubescent	Adolescent
Aerobic	American College of Sports Medicine guidelines,[41] however, not to exceed moderate intensity.	American College of Sports Medicine guidelines.[41]
Flexibility	Agonist and antagonist, 60 second static, alternating days.	Agonist and antagonist, 60 second static, alternating days.
Resistive	Resistance not to exceed 25 rM, perceived intensity is light, 2 sessions of 15 to 20 minutes per week.	Resistance not to exceed 20 rM, perceived intensity is moderate, 2 sessions of 20 to 30 minutes per week.

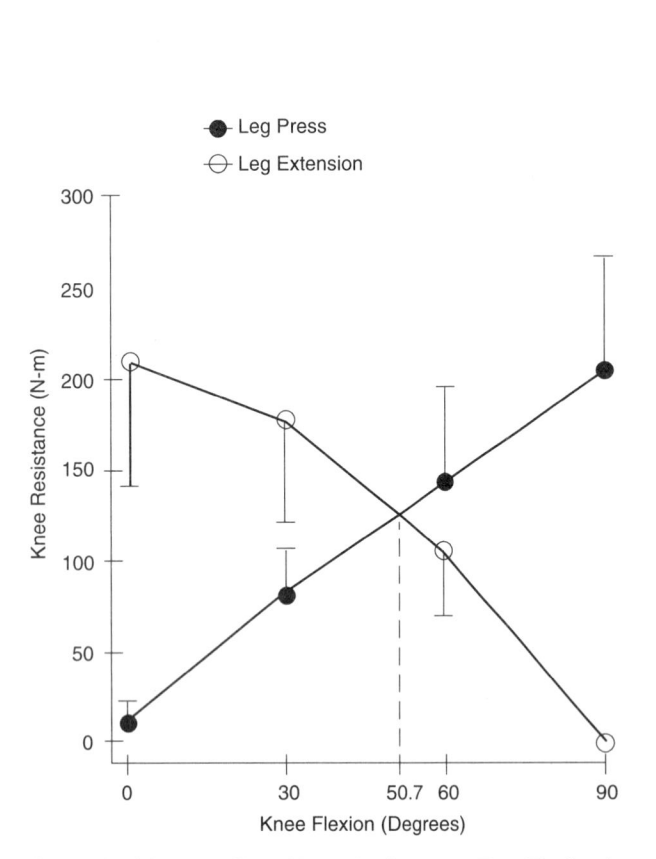

Figure 11–1 Mean (+ SD) of Knee Resistance at Four Flexion Angles. *Source:* Reprinted with permission from L.A. Steinkamp et al, Biomechanical Considerations in Patellofemoral Joint Rehabilitation, *The American Journal of Sports Medicine*, Vol. 21, No. 3, pp. 438–444, © 1993, The American Orthopaedic Society for Sports Medicine.

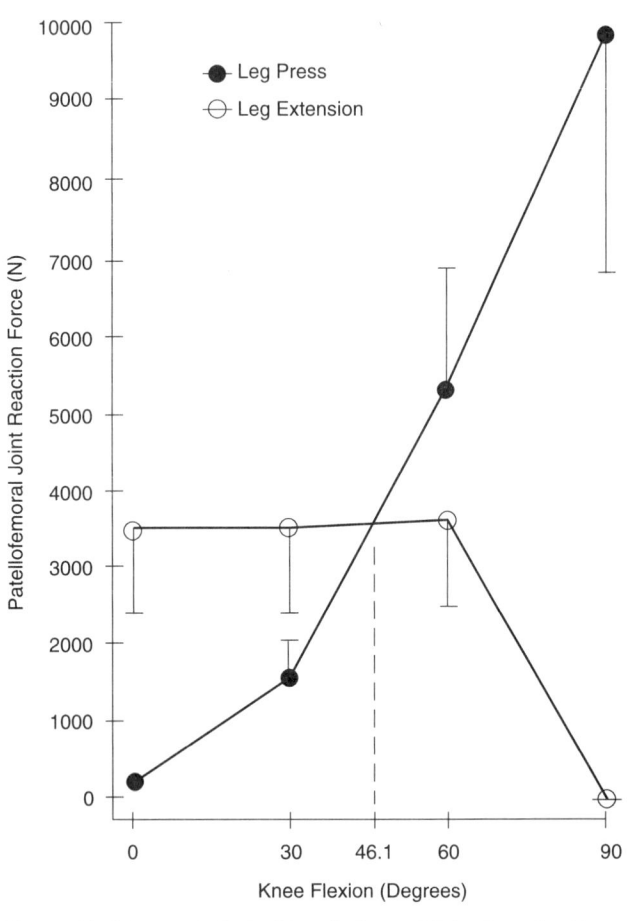

Figure 11–2 Mean (+ SD) of Patellofemoral Joint Reaction Force at Four Flexion Angles. *Source:* Reprinted with permission from L.A. Steinkamp et al, Biomechanical Considerations in Patellofemoral Joint Rehabilitation, *The American Journal of Sports Medicine*, Vol. 21, No. 3, pp. 438–444, © 1993, The American Orthopaedic Society for Sports Medicine.

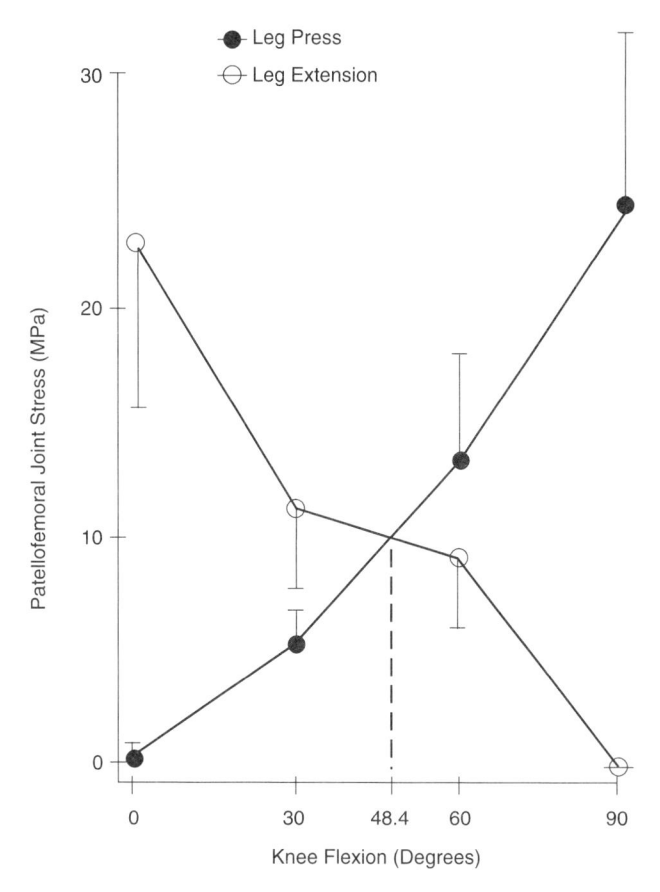

Figure 11–3 Mean (+ SD) of Patellofemoral Joint Stress at Four Flexion Angles. *Source:* Reprinted with permission from L.A. Steinkamp et al, Biomechanical Considerations in Patellofemoral Joint Rehabilitation, *The American Journal of Sports Medicine*, Vol. 21, No. 3, pp. 438–444, © 1993, The American Orthopaedic Society for Sports Medicine.

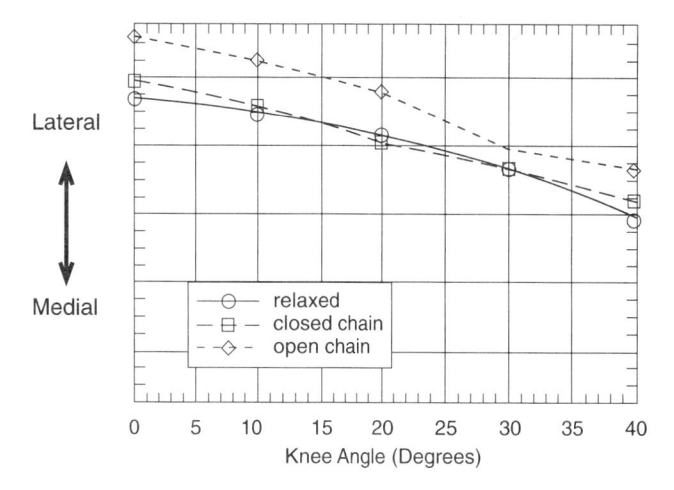

Figure 11–4 The Relationship between Muscle Condition and Knee Joint Angle as Measured by Congruence Angle. *Source:* S.A. Doucette and D. Child, The Effect of Open and Closed Chain Exercise and Knee Joint Position on Patellar Tracking in Lateral Patellar Compression Syndrome, *Journal of Orthopaedic and Sports Physical Therapy*, Vol. 23, No. 2, pp. 104–110, © 1996, Williams & Wilkins.

movements (terminal knee extensions) have not been identified to selectively recruit VMO fibers.

It is recommended that the open chain resisted knee extension movement be performed within the range of 90 to 60 degrees or 90 to 45 degrees of knee flexion. It is recommended that the leg press movement be contained to the 0 to 30 or 0 to 45 degree ranges. By utilizing the two movements in a complementary manner, the full range of knee extension is addressed without excessive joint stress.

CHAPTER SUMMARY

Prepubescence is the time from childhood to onset of secondary sex characteristics. Adolescence is the period after onset of secondary sex characteristics until physical and skeletal maturity. These are crucial periods in which physical activity habits are developed. These exercise patterns may have long-term health implications. Research is reviewed that addresses the benefits of safe exercise supervised by qualified individuals. Powerlifting and Olympic lifting differ from resistive exercise (strength training) in their emphasis on single repetition maximums and/or explosive movements. Powerlifting and Olympic lifting are contraindicated in the prepubescent and adolescent. A study reviewing types and causes of injuries is presented to allow the reader to examine the data for trends regarding injurious activities. Recommendations are made for prepubescent and adolescent comprehensive exercise. Open and closed chain knee extension movements are discussed for effects at the patellofemoral joint.

REFERENCES

1. Cunnane SC. Childhood origins of lifestyle-related risk factors for coronary heart disease in adulthood. *Nutr Health.* 1993;9:107–115.
2. Simons-Morton BG, Taylor WC, Snider SA, Huang IW, et al. Observed levels of elementary and middle school children's physical activity during physical education classes. *Prev Med.* 1994;23:437–441.
3. DiNubile NA. Youth fitness—problems and solutions. *Prev Med.* 1993;22:589–594.
4. Bronfin DR, Urbina EM. The role of the pediatrician in the promotion of cardiovascular health. *Am J Med Sci.* 1995;310.
5. Harsha DW. The benefits of physical activity in childhood. *Am J Med Sci.* 1995;310 Suppl:S109–S113, S42–S47.

6. Manson JE, Willett WC, Stampfer MF, et al. Body weight and mortality among women. *N Engl J Med.* 1995;333:677–685.
7. Johnson CC, Nicklas TA. Health ahead—the Heart Smart Family approach to prevention of cardiovascular disease. *Am J Med Sci.* 1995; 310 Suppl:S27–S32.
8. Shephard RJ. Physical activity, health, and well-being at different life stages. *RQES.* 1996;66:298–302.
9. Shephard R, Lavallee H, Volle M, LaBarre R, et al. Academic skills and required physical education: the Trois Rivieres experience. *CAHPER Res Suppl.* 1994;1:1–12.
10. Purcell JS, Hergenroeder AC. Physical conditioning in adolescents. *Curr Opin Pediatr.* 1994;6:373–378.
11. Gutin B, Islam S, Manos T, Cucuzzo N. Relation of percentage of body fat and maximal aerobic capacity to risk factors for atherosclerosis and diabetes in black and white seven to eleven-year-old children. *J Pediat.* 1994;125:847–852.
12. Klesges RC, Klesges LM, Eck LH, Shelton ML. A longitudinal analysis of accelerated weight gain in preschool children. *Pediatr.* 1995; 95:126.
13. Weltman A, et al. The effects of hydraulic resistance strength training in prepubescent males. *Med Sci Sports Exerc.* 1986;18:638.
14. Weltman A. 1993. Personal communication.
15. Metcalf JA, Roberts SQ. Strength training and the immature athlete: an overview. *Pediatr Nurs.* 1993;19:325–332.
16. Ozmun JC, Mikesky AE, Surburg PR. Neuromuscular adaptations following prepubescent strength training. *Med Sci Sports Exerc.* 1994; 26:510.
17. Prokhorov AV, Perry CL, Kelder SH, Klepp KI. Lifestyle values of adolescents: results from Minnesota Heart Health Youth Program. *Adoles.* 1993;28:637–647.
18. Blimke CJ. Resistance training during preadolescence: issues and controversies. *Sports Med.* 1993;15:389–407.
19. Lillegard WA, Terrio JD. Appropriate strength training. *Med Clin North Am.* 1994;78:457–477.
20. Salminen JJ, Erkintalo M, Laine M, Pentti J. Low back pain in the young: a prospective three-year follow-up study of subjects with and without low back pain. *Spine.* 1995;20:2101–2108.
21. Telama R. Nature as motivation for physical activity. In: Oja P, Telama R, eds. *Sport for All.* Amsterdam: Elsevier; 1991:607–616.
22. Sewall L, Micheli LH. Strength training for children. *J Pediatr Orthop.* 1986;6:146.
23. Schafer J. Prepubescent and adolescent weight training: is it safe? Is it beneficial? *Natl Strength Conditioning Assoc J.* 1991;13:39–45.
24. DeRenne C, Hetzler RK, Buxton BP, Ho KW. Effects of training frequency on strength maintenance in pubescent baseball players. *J Strength Conditioning Res.* 1996;10:8–14.
25. Kuland DN, Dewey JB, Brubaker CE, et al. Olympic weightlifting injuries. *Physician Sports Med.* 1978;6:111.
26. Cahill BR. *Proceedings of the Conference on Strength Training and the Prepubescent.* Chicago: American Orthopedic Society of Sports Medicine; 1988.
27. Mazur LJ, Yetman RJ, Risser WL. Weight-training injuries: common injuries and preventative methods. *Sports Med.* 1993;16:57–63.
28. Browne TD, Yost RP, McCarron RF. Lumbar ring apophyseal fracture in an adolescent weight lifter. *Am J Sports Med.* 1990;18:533–535.
29. Francobandiera C, Maffulli N, Leopore L. Distal radio-ulnar joint dislocation, ulnar volar in a female body builder. *Med Sci Sports Exerc.* 1990;22:155–158.
30. George DH, Stakin K, Wright CJ. Fatal accident with weightlifting equipment: implications for safety standards. *Can Med Assoc J.* 1989; 140:925–926.
31. Mannis CI. Transchondral fracture of the dome of the talus sustained during weight training. *Am J Sports Med.* 1983;11:354–356.
32. Kotani PT, Ichikawa N, Wakabayashi W, et al. Studies of spondylolysis found among weight lifters. *Brit J Sports Med.* 1971;6:4–7.
33. Rossi F, Dragoni S. Lumbar spondylolysis: occurrence in competitive athletes: updates, achievements in a series of 390 cases. *J Sports Med Phys Fit.* 1990;30:450–452.
34. Brady TA, Cahill BR, Bodnar IM. Weight training-related injuries in high school athletes. *Am J Sports Med.* 1982;101:1–5.
35. Cahill BR. Osteolysis in the distal part of the clavicle in male athletes. *J Bone Joint Surg.* 1982;64:1053–1058.
36. Gumbs VL, Segal D, Halligan JB, Lower G. Bilateral distal radius and ulnar fractures in adolescent weight lifters. *Am J Sports Med.* 1982; 10:375–379.
37. Ryan JR, Salciccioli GG. Fractures of the distal radial epiphysis in adolescent weight lifters. *Am J Sports Med.* 1976;4:26–27.
38. Brown EW, Kimball RG. Medical history associated with adolescent powerlifting. *Pediatr.* 1983;72:636–644.
39. Risser WL, Risser JM, Preston D. Weight training injuries in adolescents. *Am J Disease Child.* 1990;144:1015–1017.
40. Zemper ED. Four-year study of weightroom injuries in a national sample of college football teams. *Natl Strength Conditioning Assoc J.* 1990; 12:32–34.
41. American College of Sports Medicine. Position statement on the recommended quantity and quality of exercise for developing and maintaining fitness in healthy adults. *Med Sci Sports Exerc.* 1990;22: 265–274.
42. Steinkamp LA, Dillingham MF, Markel MD, Hill JA, et al. Biomechanical considerations in patellofemoral joint rehabilitation. *Am J Sports Med.* 1993;21:438–444.
43. Doucette SA, Child D. The effect of open and closed chain exercise and knee joint position on patellar tracking in lateral patellar compression syndrome. *JOSPT.* 1996;23:104–110.
44. Merchant AC, Mercer RL, Jacobson RH, Cool CR. Roentgenographic analysis of patellofemoral congruence angles. *J Bone Joint Surg.* 1974; 56A:1391–1396.
45. van Kampen A, Huiskes R. The three dimensional tracking pattern of the human patella. *J Orthop Res.* 1990;8:372–382.
46. Brownstein BA, Lamb RL, Mangine RE. Quadriceps torque and integrated electromyography. *J Orthop Sports Phys Ther.* 1985;6:309–314.
47. Grabiner M, Koh T, Miller G. Fatigue rates of vastus medialis obliquous and vastus lateralis during static and dynamic knee extension. *J Orthop Res.* 1991;9:391–397.

CHAPTER 12

Exercise for Older Persons

David Ash

CHAPTER OUTLINE

I. Introduction
II. Research
III. Functional Benefits
IV. Falling in Older Persons: Exercise as Prevention
V. Exercise and Self-Efficacy
VI. Exercise Programming for Older Persons
VII. Chapter Summary

INTRODUCTION

Judge[1] stated that the "major goal of prevention from a geriatric perspective is to prolong functional independence. Physical exercise and activity may be the most effective strategy health care professionals can recommend to middle-aged and older persons who wish to maintain their independence into their ninth and tenth decades."

Judge's *functional independence* may be expanded to the construct *quality independence*. Quality independence is operationally defined as the physical ability to perform desired leisure, recreational, social, and exercise activities, as well as activities of daily and occupational living.

While the percentage of older persons participating in regular physical activity is increasing,[2] a 1992 study[3] indicated that almost 50% of this population participates in no regular physical activity. It is expected that exercise participation will increase as a result of health care cost containment measures.

A decline in many physiological functions formerly attributed to aging is increasingly considered more a function of sedentary lifestyle. Bokovy and Blair[4] indicate that lifestyle interventions (eg, nutrition, cessation of smoking, exercise) may modify many age-related changes. Lowenthal and colleagues concur, stating, "It appears that many of the diseases associated with age, as well as aging itself, can be either treated or blunted by an active lifestyle. Cardiac, pulmonary, musculoskeletal and metabolic-endocrine changes associated with age and/or disease can show a change in progression (being forestalled or rectified) as a result of physical activity."[5] The International Society and Federation of Cardiology[6] recommends that physical inactivity be viewed as a significant factor in coronary heart disease, and that physical activity be encouraged in preventive programs.

RESEARCH

Given demographic trends, research regarding the effects of various types of exercise on older persons is of great interest. Older persons, defined here as individuals 65 years of age or older, can realize substantial health benefits from exercise. Table 12–1 illustrates a sampling of the research base regarding exercise for older persons.

FUNCTIONAL BENEFITS

Ades et al,[27] in a study designed to examine the effects of a 12-week resistive exercise program, selected walking endurance, a functional activity, as the dependent variable. The researchers concluded that "resistance training for 3 months improves both leg strength and walking endurance in healthy, community-dwelling elderly persons. This finding is relevant to older persons at risk for disability, because walking endurance and leg strength are important components of physical functioning."[27] Results of the Ades et al study are displayed graphically in Figure 12–1.

Table 12–1 Research Regarding Exercise for Older Persons

Summary	Researchers/Authors
"The highly conditioned elderly women in this study had superior NK and T-cell function when compared with their sedentary counterparts."	Nieman et al[7]
"These results demonstrate that strength training increases insulin action and lowers plasma insulin levels in middle-aged and older men."	Miller et al[8]
"Increasing the back extensor strength in healthy estrogen-deficient women helps decrease thoracic kyphosis."	Itoi and Sinaki[9]
"Correlations between exercise behaviors and perceptions of internal and external competence were positively related."	Mobily et al[10]
Significant reductions in intra-abdominal adipose tissue and an increase in strength and muscle area were observed after a strength training program in healthy older women. These changes may be important in preventing the negative health outcomes associated with the age-related increase in intra-abdominal obesity.	Treuth et al[11]
"High-intensity strength training exercises are an effective and feasible means to preserve bone density while improving muscle mass, strength, and balance in post-menopausal women."	Nelson et al[12]
"Possible benefits to exercise participants include increased longevity, decreased risk of cardiovascular disease, improved psychological well-being and greater fitness. The few controlled studies that exist (regarding the effect of exercise on arthritis) may be interpreted to suggest that reasonable recreational exercise carried out within limits of comfort, putting joints through normal motions, and without underlying joint abnormality, need not inevitably lead to joint injury, even over many years."	Panush and Holtz[13]
"The results demonstrate that the skeletal muscles of elderly individuals can adapt to heavy resistance exercise and do so by increases in both muscle size and strength."	Roman, Fleckenstein, Stray-Gunderson, and Alway[14]
"The data demonstrate a graded inverse relationship between total physical activity and mortality. Furthermore, vigorous activities, but not non-vigorous activities were associated with longevity. These findings pertain to only all cause mortality; non-vigorous exercise has been shown to benefit other aspects of health."	Lee, Hsieh, and Paffenbarger[15]
"Men who maintained or improved adequate physical fitness were less likely to die from: (1) all causes and (2) from cardiovascular disease during follow up than persistently unfit men. Physicians should encourage unfit men to improve their fitness by starting a physical activity program."	Blair et al[16]
"Evidence from well-conducted, large prospective studies indicated that exercise reduces the risk of cardiovascular disease and that it reduces total mortality in men. Beginning exercise late in life is beneficial, whereas stopping exercise is harmful. Exercise may reduce the risk of malignancy (particularly colon cancer)."	Thompson[17]
"The study results suggest that prolonged moderate to high intensity resistance training may be carried out by older adults with reasonable compliance, and that such training leads to sustained increases in muscle strength. These improvements are rapidly achieved and accompanied by hypertrophy of both type I and type II muscle fibers."	Pyka, Lindenberger, Charette, and Marcus[18]
Increased bone density and increased muscle strength were realized by a treatment group of women in their 60s as a result of resistive exercise performed twice per week.	Hartard, Haber, Ilieva, and Preisinger[19]

continues

Table 12–1 continued

Summary	Researchers/Authors
"Recent studies show a 50% reduction in the risk of dying from cardiovascular disease in men who increase physical activity and improve physical fitness, a magnitude of risk reduction comparable to smoking cessation."	Physical activity, health, and well-being: An international scientific consensus conference consensus statement[20]
"Walking more than four hours/week may reduce the risk of hospitalization for cardiovascular disease events. The association of walking more than four hours/week with reduced risk of death may be mediated by effects of walking on other risk factors."	La Croix et al[21]
This study was designed to investigate the relationships between aerobic exercise, quality of sleep, and daytime sleepiness. The exercise group (n = 46) reported greater sleep quality as determined by (1) greater sleep duration, (2) less time to fall asleep, and (3) less daytime sleepiness, when compared to the nonexercising controls (n = 33).	Brassington and Hicks[22]
"Exercise is becoming more widely used to prevent and treat the diseases that are most prevalent in the United States: coronary artery disease, stroke, hypertension, diabetes, arthritis, osteoporosis, dyslipidemia, obesity, depression, cancer, and chronic obstructive pulmonary disease."	Elrick[23]
A study conducted with 851 women aged 45 to 64 indicated that leisure time physical activity has a beneficial effect on HDL cholesterol, fibrinogen, and insulin levels in postmenopausal women.	Greendale, Bodin-Dunn, Ingles, and Itaile[24]
"Older adults who engage in weight lifting with heavy submaximal loads are exposed to no more peak circulatory stress than that created during a few minutes of inclined walking."	Benn, McCartney, and McKelvie[25]
This study attempted to integrate social cognitive and impression management perspectives regarding anxiety related to exercise. Exercise participation resulted in significantly increased self-efficacy. Increased self-efficacy was determined to be a significant predictor of reductions in physique anxiety, even when controlled for the influence of gender, body fat reductions, body weight, and girth measurements. Emphasizing health and fitness outcomes associated with exercise rather than appearance outcomes may help reduce negative body image.	McAuley, Bane, and Mihalko[26]

Figure 12–2 is adapted from Shephard[28, 29] and presents a logical argument that "the most common basis for loss of independence is simple deterioration of physical condition."[28]

Table 12–2 summarizes the results of several studies that have investigated the effects of exercise on specific functional variables.

FALLING IN OLDER PERSONS: EXERCISE AS PREVENTION

A literature review identifies the following facts about falls in older persons.

- Approximately one-fourth of all individuals aged 65 to 74 report having fallen. Of these falls, about 15% require medical care. Approximately 50% of those able to walk independently prior to a fall resulting in hip fracture, subsequently require ambulatory assistance.[46]
- It is probable that the rate of falling in elderly is underestimated, as falls may not be reported if they do not warrant medical attention.[47]
- The incidence of falls increases to one person in three with respect to those older than 74 years of age.[48]
- Approximately two-thirds of older persons who fall incur another fall within the next six months.[49]
- A fall may leave the individual with a fear of falling of sufficient intensity to decrease mobility and independence. Up to 50% of those who have fallen avoid activities due to fear of fall recurrence.[50]
- Muscle weakness is associated with injuries resulting from falls.[46]

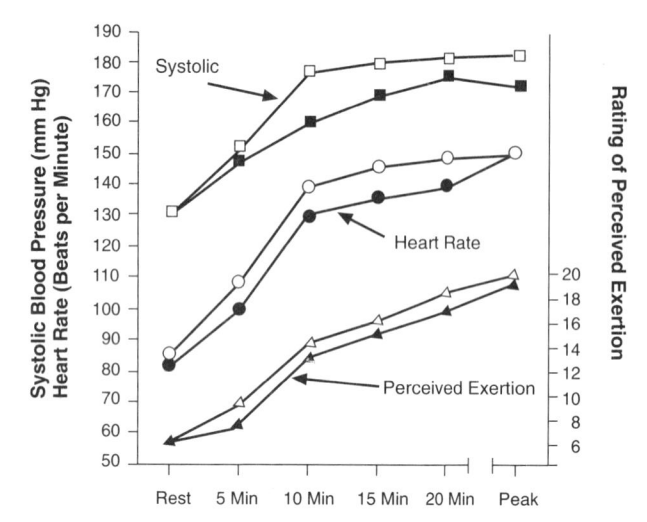

Figure 12–1 Conditioning Data in the Resistance-Training Group. *Source:* Reprinted with permission from P.A. Ades et al, Weight Training Improves Walking Endurance in Healthy Elderly Persons, *Annals of Internal Medicine*, Vol. 124, p. 568, © 1996, American College of Physicians.

Note: Open symbols indicate values before conditioning; closed symbols indicate values after conditioning.

- "Accidental falls are the primary cause of femoral neck fractures. Preventive actions should be directed toward intrinsic (e.g., oxygen tension), as well as extrinsic risk factors for falls. Hypoxemia might be a risk factor for falls, especially those falls that occur at night."[51]
- Exercise participation can result in improved sensorimotor function in women aged 60 to 85 years. High compliance with an exercise program may reduce the frequency of falls.[52]

- "After adjusting for fall risk factors, Tai Chi was found to reduce the risk of multiple falls by 47.5%. A moderate Tai Chi intervention can have favorable effects upon the occurrence of falls."[53]
- "Treatments including exercise for elderly adults reduce the risk of falls."[54]
- A study with 112 women (mean age 71.2, SD = 5.4) serving as subjects, was conducted by Lord, Ward, and Williams to analyze the effects of a 12-month exercise program. The frequency and duration of the exercise program were 2 sessions per week of approximately 60 minutes, which included warm-up and cool-down. The exercise activities included aerobic exercises, balance activities, hand/foot-eye coordination, and strengthening exercises. At the conclusion of the study, the exercise group demonstrated significant performance improvement in the maximal balance range test and the coordinated stability test. The control group demonstrated no improvement in these tests. The treatment group also demonstrated improved hip flexion strength, hip extension range, and dorsiflexion range, not seen in the control group. The researchers concluded that "exercise can significantly improve dynamic postural stability in older persons."[55]
- Risk factors to falling in the elderly population may be categorized as resulting from the individual (intrinsic) or from the environment (extrinsic).[56] Muscular weakness would be an example of an intrinsic factor, with an icy sidewalk being classified as extrinsic. Several authors suggest that falls are oftentimes a result of factors of both categories.[57,58]
- Lower extremity weakness has been significantly associated with repeated falls in the elderly population.[59,60]

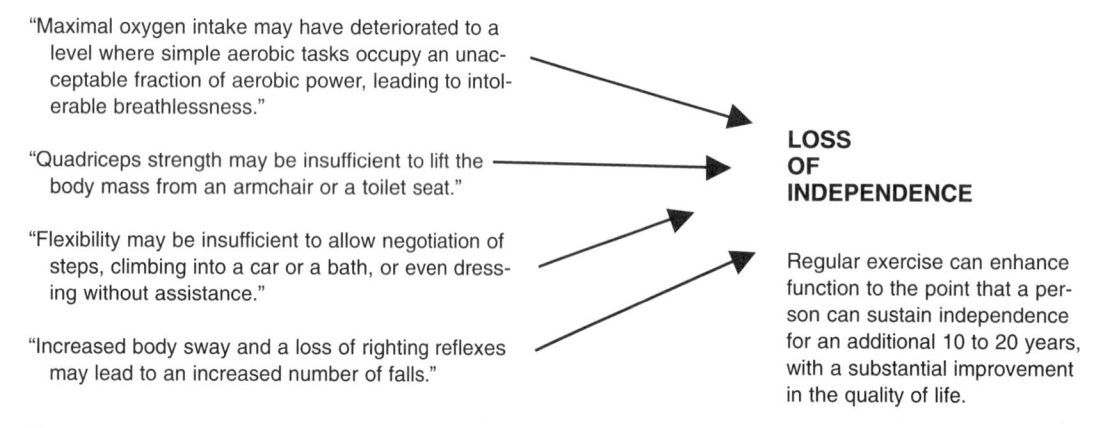

"Maximal oxygen intake may have deteriorated to a level where simple aerobic tasks occupy an unacceptable fraction of aerobic power, leading to intolerable breathlessness."

"Quadriceps strength may be insufficient to lift the body mass from an armchair or a toilet seat."

"Flexibility may be insufficient to allow negotiation of steps, climbing into a car or a bath, or even dressing without assistance."

"Increased body sway and a loss of righting reflexes may lead to an increased number of falls."

→ **LOSS OF INDEPENDENCE**

Regular exercise can enhance function to the point that a person can sustain independence for an additional 10 to 20 years, with a substantial improvement in the quality of life.

Figure 12–2 Loss of Independence. *Source:* Data from R.J. Shephard, Fitness and Aging, *Aging Into the Twenty-First Century*, pp. 22–35, © 1991, Captus Publications; and R.J. Shephard, Physical Activity, Health, and Well-Being at Different Life Stages, *Research Quarterly for Exercise and Sport*, Vol. 66, pp. 298–302, © 1995.

Table 12-2 Effects of Exercise on Specific Functional Variables

Summary	Researchers/Authors
"Exercise may play a role in improving a number of sensorimotor systems that contribute to stability in older persons."	Lord and Castell[30]
"The intervention (which included an exercise component) resulted in a significant reduction in the risk of falling in the subjects."	Tinetti et al[31]
"Exercise emphasizing strength and balance achieved improvement in gait velocity."	Judge, Underwood, and Gennosa[32]
"Long-term resistance training in older people is feasible and results in increases in dynamic muscle strength, muscle size and functional capacity."	McCartney, Hicks, Martin, and Webber[33]
"This study demonstrated improvements in single stance postural sway in older women with exercise (resistive exercise, brisk walking, and postural exercises) training."	Judge, Lindsey, Underwood, and Winsemius[34]
"After strength conditioning, healthy older women showed not only substantially increased strength but also improvements in walking velocity and the ability to carry out daily tasks such as rising from a chair and carrying a box of groceries."	Hunter[35]
"Increased habitual activity patterns are likely to be indicative of improvements in functional ability, lifestyle, and independence."	Hamdorf, Withers, Penhall, and Haslam[36]
"Increased neural activation accompanies an increase in muscle strength at least during eccentric action in already rather active elderly men and muscle endurance may also be improved with training."	Grimby et al[37]
"The study suggests that physical activity offers benefits to physically capable older adults, primarily in reducing the risk of functional decline and mortality."	Simonstick et al[38]
"In a US Agricultural Research Service study, 100 volunteers in their 80s and 90s doubled their leg muscle strength in 10 weeks and became more physically active in general."	Agricultural Research Service[39]
"Weight training leads to significant gains in muscle strength, size, and functional mobility among frail residents of nursing homes up to 96 years of age."	Fiatarone et al[40]
Joint impairment and quadriceps strength contribute significantly to walking velocity in older persons.	Gibbs et al[41]
"Twelve weeks of daily walking at a self-selected walking pace by ambulatory nursing home residents produced significant improvements in walk endurance capacity."	MacRae et al[42]
"Gait speed is a useful indicator of activities of daily living function in geriatric patients."	Potter, Evans, and Duncan[43]
A randomly assigned program of resistive exercise, implemented within a population of 100 nursing home residents, resulted in significant improvements in strength and functional status.	Evans[44]
A study was designed to examine the relationship between recreational physical activity among physically capable older persons and functional status, incidence of particular chronic conditions, and mortality over three and six years. Data suggest that physical activity offers benefits to physically capable older individuals, primarily in decreased risk of functional decline and mortality.	Simonsick et al[38]
Enhanced physiological and psychological function helps to maintain independence and lessens the need for acute and chronic care services. From an economic standpoint, the costs of well-designed exercise programs could likely be offset by savings in medical expenses. Primary care physicians can assist older patients to realize these benefits through encouragement to increase physical activity and by prescribing appropriate exercise.	Shephard[45]

EXERCISE AND SELF-EFFICACY

Self-efficacy is the power to produce intended results by one's self. A literature review identifies the following information about exercise and self-efficacy in older persons.

- Range of motion (ROM) exercise is a simple activity that can have significant results. ROM exercise can enhance an elderly person's quality of life by increasing self-efficacy, independence, and self-esteem.[61]
- "Acute and long-term exercise were associated with enhanced perceptions of personal efficacy in previously sedentary middle-aged adults."[62]
- In a review of literature regarding the determinants of physical activity, factors are commonly grouped into the following three divisions: (1) personal characteristics (ie, education level, age), (2) psychological variables (ie, self-efficacy, goal setting skills), and (3) environmental factors (ie, family support, proximity of exercise facility).[63]
- A study attempted to integrate social, cognitive, and impression management perspectives regarding anxiety related to exercise. Exercise participation resulted in significantly increased self-efficacy. Increased self-efficacy was determined to be a significant predictor of reductions in physique anxiety, even when controlled for the influence of gender, body fat reductions, body weight, and girth measurements. Emphasizing health and fitness outcomes associated with exercise rather than appearance outcomes may help reduce negative body image.[26]

EXERCISE PROGRAMMING FOR OLDER PERSONS

In general, the American College of Sports Medicine guidelines for exercise programming for healthy adults (see Appendix A) apply to older persons as well. The only exception is that the intensity level will be slightly decreased in favor of slight increases in duration and frequency. Pollock and colleagues comment as follows:[64]

> The basic guidelines of frequency, intensity, and duration of training and the mode of activity recommended by the American College of Sports Medicine for healthy adults are also appropriate for the elderly. The difference in the exercise prescription for the elderly participant is the manner in which it is applied. Given that the elderly person is more fragile and has more physical-medical limitations than the middle-aged participant, the intensity of the program is usually lower while the training frequency and duration are increased. The prescribed training heart rate for the elderly at 40 to 80% of maximal heart rate reserve is slightly lower than the 50 to 85% recommended for young and middle-aged participants, but its relationship to relative metabolic work and rating of perceived exertion are similar to those found for younger participants. Because of the importance of maintaining muscle mass and bone in middle and old age, a well-rounded program including strength/resistance exercise of the major muscle groups is recommended.

Judge[1] lists the following as exercise principles for older persons, which appear to be applicable to all age groups: (1) program goals should be client-centered, (2) the program must account for any existing limitations of the client, (3) the program should be progressed slowly, and (4) to decrease the likelihood of musculoskeletal injury, new activities are introduced only after mastery of prerequisite activities.

With regard to specific exercise components (frequency, intensity, duration, and mode), Judge appears to support the American College of Sports Medicine guidelines for maintaining fitness in healthy adults, with addition of a functional component. Judge includes a "functional training/balance" subcomponent within the flexibility component. Classified as functional training/balance activities are: (1) transfers from sit to stand, (2) picking up objects from the floor (with correct body mechanics), (3) transfer from standing to prone-supine (rolling on a floor mat) and (4) forward leaning, backward leaning, lateral leaning, and rotation.[1]

Dishman's[65] recommendations for improving fitness after the age of 65 also appear to reinforce American College of Sports Medicine guidelines, with the adjustment of decreased intensity. Dishman's guidelines are as follows:[65]

1. The types of activities should emphasize movement, flexibility, and some resistive exercise.
2. Exercise intensity is moderate.
3. Overloading should be done with gradual progression.
4. Duration of exercise is individualized and may be accumulated in multiple sessions per day.
5. Exercise sessions can be performed on most days, with lower intensity activity, such as walking, being performed every day.

Shephard[29] insightfully suggests an important topic for exercise researchers to consider: "Despite substantial information on the physiological benefits of physical activity for the middle-old and very old, there remains an urgent need to determine the most effective methods of *encouraging* exercise in those who are over 65 years of age."

CHAPTER SUMMARY

The increasing proportion of the United States population over the age of 50 years has prompted researchers to focus on the effects of exercise within this population. Almost 50% of older persons do not participate in a regular exercise program. The growth of preventive exercise participation due to health care cost containment measures is expected. A sampling of the research literature was provided. In general, the American College of Sports Medicine guidelines for development and maintenance of fitness in healthy adults apply to older persons, though intensity is decreased.

REFERENCES

1. Judge JO. Exercise programs for older persons: writing an exercise prescription. *Conn Med.* 1993;57:269–275.
2. Stephans T. Secular trends in physical activity: fitness boom or bust. *Res Q Exerc Sport.* 1987;58:94–108.
3. Wagner EH, et al. Effects of physical activity on health status in older adults 1: observational studies. *Annu Rev Publ Health.* 1992;13:451–468.
4. Bokovy JL, Blair SN. Aging and exercise: a health perspective. *J Aging Phys Activity.* 1994;2:243–260.
5. Lowenthal DT, Kirschner DA, Scarpace NT, Pollock M, et al. Effects of age on disease. *South Med J.* 1994;87:5.
6. Bijnen FC, Mosterd WL, Caspersen CJ. *Physical inactivity: a risk factor for coronary heart disease. A position statement for the World Health Organization, governments, heart foundations, societies of cardiology, and other health professionals.* Geneva: International Society for the World Health Organization; 1992:2–6.
7. Nieman DC, Henson DA, Gusewitch G, Warren BJ, et al. Physical activity and immune function in elderly women. *Med Sci Sport Exerc.* 1993;25:823–831.
8. Miller JP, Pratley RE, Goldberg AP, Gordon P, et al. Strength training increases insulin action in healthy 50–65-year old men. *J Appl Physiol.* 1994;77:1122–1127.
9. Itoi E, Sinaki M. Effect of back strengthening exercise on posture in healthy women 49 to 65 years of age. *Mayo Clin Proc.* 1994;69:1054–1059.
10. Mobily, et al. Leisure repertoire in a sample of midwestern elderly: the case for exercise. *J Leisure Res.* 1993;25:84–99.
11. Treuth MS, Hunter GR, Kekes-Szabo T, Weinsier RL, et al. Reduction in intra-abdominal adipose tissue after strength training in older women. *J Appl Physiol.* 1995;78:1425–1431.
12. Nelson ME, Fiatarone MA, Morganti CM, Trice I, et al. Effects of high intensity strength training on multiple risk factors for osteoporotic fractures. A randomized controlled trial. *JAMA.* 1994;272:1909–1914.
13. Panush RS, Holtz HA. Is exercise good or bad for arthritis in the elderly? *South Med J.* 1994;87:74–77.
14. Roman WJ, Fleckenstein J, Stray-Gunderson J, Alway SE. Adaptations in the elbow flexors of elderly males after heavy resistance training. *J Appl Physiol.* 1993;74:750–754.
15. Lee IM, Hsieh C, Paffenbarger R. Exercise intensity and longevity in men: the Harvard Alumni Health Study. *JAMA.* 1995;273:1179–1184.
16. Blair SN, Kohl HW, Barlow CE, Paffenbarger RS, et al. Changes in physical fitness and all cause mortality: a prospective study of healthy and unhealthy men. *JAMA.* 1995;273:1093–1098.
17. Thompson WG. Exercise and health: fact or hype? *South Med J.* 1994;87:567.
18. Pyka G, Lindenberger E, Charette S, Marcus R. Muscle strength and fiber adaptations to a year-long resistance training program in elderly men and women. *J Gerontol.* 1994;49:M22–M27.
19. Hartard M, Haber P, Ilieva D, Preisinger D. Systematic strength training as a model of therapeutic intervention. *Am J Phys Med Rehabil.* 1996;75:21–28.
20. Physical activity, health, and well-being: an international scientific consensus conference consensus statement. *RQES.* 1996;66:v.
21. La Croix AZ, Leveille SG, Hecht JA, Grothaus LC, et al. Does walking decrease the risk of cardiovascular disease hospitalizations and death in older adults? *J Am Geriatr Soc.* 1996;44:113–120.
22. Brassington GS, Hicks RA. Aerobic exercise and self-reported sleep quality in elderly individuals. *J Aging Phys Activity.* 1995;3:120–134.
23. Elrick H. Exercise is medicine. *Physician Sports Med.* 1996;24:72–79.
24. Greendale GA, Bodin-Dunn L, Ingles S, Itaile R. Leisure, home, and occupational physical activity and cardiovascular risk factors in postmenopausal women. The Postmenopausal Estrogens/Progestins Intervention (PEPI) Study. *Arch Intern Med.* 1996;156:418–424.
25. Benn SJ, McCartney N, McKelvie RS. Circulatory responses to weight lifting, walking, and stair climbing in older males. *J Am Geriatr Soc.* 1996;44:121–125.
26. McAuley E, Bane SM, Mihalko SL. Exercise in middle-aged adults: self-efficacy and self-presentational outcomes. *Prev Med.* 1995;24:319–328.
27. Ades PA, Ballor DL, Ashikaga T, Utton JL. Weight training improves walking endurance in healthy elderly persons. *Ann Intern Med.* 1996;124:568.
28. Shephard RJ. Fitness and aging. In: Blais C, ed. *Aging Into the Twenty-First Century.* New York: Captus Publications; 1991:22–35.
29. Shephard RJ. Physical activity, health, and well-being at different life stages. *RQES.* 1995;66:298–302.
30. Lord SR, Castell S. Physical activity program for older persons; effect on balance, strength, neuromuscular control, and reaction time. *Arch Phys Med Rehabil.* 1994;75:648–652.
31. Tinetti ME, Baker DI, McAvay G, Claus EB, et al. A multifactorial intervention to reduce the risk of falling among elderly people living in the community. *New Engl J Med.* 1994;331:821–827.
32. Judge JO, Underwood M, Gennosa T. Exercise to improve gait velocity in older persons. *Arch Phys Med Rehabil.* 1993;74:400.
33. McCartney N, Hicks AL, Martin J, Webber CE. Long-term resistance training in the elderly: effects on dynamic strength, exercise capacity, muscle, and bone. *J Gerontol A Biol Sci Med Sci.* 1995;50: B97–B104.
34. Judge JO, Lindsey C, Underwood M, Winsemius D. Balance improvement in older women: effects of exercise training. *Phys Ther.* 1993;73(4).
35. Hunter GR, et al. The effects of strength conditioning on older women's ability to perform daily tasks. *J Am Geriatr Soc.* 1995;43:756–760.
36. Hamdorf PA, Withers RT, Penhall RK, Haslam MV. Physical training effects on the fitness and habitual activity patterns of elderly women. *Arch Phys Med Rehabil.* 1992;73:603.
37. Grimby G, Aniansson A, Hedberg M, Henning GB, et al. Training can improve muscle strength and endurance in 78–84 year old men. *J Appl Physiol.* 1992;73:2517–2523.
38. Simonstick EM, et al. Risk due to inactivity in physically incapable older adults. *Am J Publ Health.* 1993;83:1443–1450.
39. Agricultural Research, US Department of Agriculture. Agricultural Research Service. November 1994. 6303 Ivy Lane, Room 408, Greenbelt, MD 20770.

40. Fiatarone MA, Marks CE, Ryan ND, Meredith CN, et al. High-intensity strength training in nonagenarians—effects on skeletal muscle. *JAMA*. 1990;263:3029–3034.
41. Gibbs J, Hughes S, Dunlop D, Singer R, et al. Predictors of change in walking velocity in older adults. *J Am Geriatr Soc*. 1996;44:126–132.
42. MacRae PG, Asplund LA, Schnelle JF, Ouslander JG, et al. A walking program for nursing home residents: effects on walk endurance, phyical activity, mobility, and quality of life. *J Am Geriatr Soc*. 1996;44:175–180.
43. Potter JM, Evans AL, Duncan G. Gait speed and activities of daily living function in geriatric patients. *Arch Phys Med Rehabil*. 1995;76:997–999.
44. Evans WJ. Effects of exercise on body composition and functional capacity of the elderly. *J Gerontol A Biol Sci Med Sci*. 1995;50:147–150.
45. Shephard RJ. Exercise and aging: extending independence in older adults. *Geriatr*. 1993;48:61–64.
46. Tideiksaar R. Preventing falls: how to identify risk factors, reduce complications. *Geriatr*. 1996;51:43–53.
47. Nevitt MC. Falls in older persons: risk factors and prevention. In: Berg RL, Cassells JF, eds. *The Second Fifty Years: Promoting Health and Preventing Disability*. Washington DC: Institute of Medicine National Academy Press; 1990:263–290.
48. Tinetti ME, Speechley M, Ginter SF. Risk factors for falls among elderly persons. *N Engl J Med*. 1988;319:1701–1707.
49. Perry BC. Falls among the elderly. *J Am Geriatr Soc*. 1982;30:367–371.
50. Nevitt MC, Cummings SR, Kidd S, Black D. Risk factors for recurrent falls: a prospective study. *JAMA*. 1989;261:2663–2668.
51. Nyberg L, Gustafson Y, Berggren D, Brannstrom B, et al. Falls leading to femoral neck fractures in lucid older people. *J Am Geriatr Soc*. 1996;44:156–160.
52. Lord SR, Ward JA, Williams P, Strudwick M. The effect of a 12-month exercise trial on balance, strength, and falls in older women: a randomized controlled trial. *J Am Geriatr Soc*. 1995;43:1198–1206.
53. Wolf SL, Barnhart HX, Kutner NG, McNeeley E, et al. Reducing frailty and falls in older persons: an investigation of Tai Chi and Computerized Balance Training. *J Am Geriatr Soc*. 1996;44:489–497.
54. Province MA, Hadley EC, Hornbrook MC, Lipsitz LA, et al. The effects of exercise on falls in elderly patients: a pre-planned meta-analysis of the FICSIT trials. Frailty and injuries: cooperative studies of intervention techniques. *JAMA*. 1995;273:1341–1347.
55. Lord SR, Ward JA, Williams P. Exercise effect on dynamic stability in older women: a randomized controlled trial. *Arch Phys Med Rehabil*. 1996;77:232–236.
56. Robbins AS, Rubenstein LZ, Josephson DR, et al. Predictors of falls among elderly people: results of two population-based studies. *Arch Intern Med*. 1989;149:1628–1633.
57. Lipsitz LA, Johnson PV, Kelly MM, et al. Causes and correlates of recurrent falls in ambulatory frail elderly. *J Gerontol*. 1991;46:M114–M122.
58. Tideiksaar R. Geriatric falls in the home. *Home Health Nurs*. 1986;4:14–23.
59. Studenski SA, Duncan PW, Chandler JM. Postural responses and effector factors in persons with unexplained falls: results and methodological issues. *J Am Geriatr Soc*. 1991;39:229–234.
60. Whipple RH, Wolfson LI, Amerman P. The relationship of knee and ankle weakness to falls in nursing home residents: an isokinetic study. *J Am Geriatr Soc*. 1987;35:13–20.
61. Dawe D, Curran-Smith J. Going through the motions. *Can Nurs*. 1994;90:31–33.
62. Lianov L, et al. Referral outcomes from a community based preventive health care program for elderly people. *Gerontologist*. 1991;31:543–547.
63. Marcus BH. Exercise behavior and strategies for intervention. *Res Q Exerc Sport*. 1995;66:319–323.
64. Pollock ML, Graves JF, Swart DL, Lowenthal DT. Exercise training and prescription for the elderly. *South Med J*. 1994;87:88–95.
65. Dishman RK. Motivating older adults to exercize. *South Med J*. 1994;87:S79–S83.

CHAPTER 13

Home Exercise

Caren J. Werlinger

CHAPTER OUTLINE

I. Aerobic Exercise
II. Strength Training
III. Stretches
IV. Safety
V. Chapter Summary

Much of the information provided in this text assumes the availability of a commercial exercise facility. There will be many individuals who will not have access to such equipment either because of cost, lack of facilities near home or work, or lack of time to leave home to exercise. Many of the exercises presented in the various chapters in this text can be adapted for home programs.

AEROBIC EXERCISE

Activities such as walking, running, or cycling can be done near most peoples' homes without difficulty. Indoor equipment can be very convenient to allow combined exercise with supervision of children, preparation of meals, and other responsibilities. Cross-country ski machines, treadmills, stationary bicycles, aerobic riders, and home aerobic video tapes all can make home workouts stimulating and cardiovascularly challenging.

The same format of a 5 to 10 minute warm-up, followed by 30 to 45 minutes of intense exercise aimed at a target heart rate, then a cool-down ought to be used for home workouts.

There is a huge market for home exercise equipment at various prices. Experience has shown that there truly is a difference in the quality of inexpensive versus expensive machines. More expensive machines are built with better quality components that work more smoothly and last considerably longer than cheap ones. Longevity is definitely a factor when there is no club manager to maintain broken equipment. Well-built, smooth-running machines are also a pleasure to exercise on. It is no fun for anyone to fight against poorly machined parts that stick and grab. The frustration can be enough to raise a person's heart rate all by itself. As a general rule, the adage "you get what you pay for" really does apply to exercise equipment. Someone wanting to exercise conscientiously would be well-advised to get the best equipment the budget will realistically allow.

STRENGTH TRAINING

There are several home gyms on the market. They use various types of resistance ranging from weight stacks to rubberbands to hydraulic or pneumatic cylinders. Most of these can be adapted to perform a number of different exercises by moving a bar to different positions.

Every muscle group in the body also can be strengthened using either body weight as resistance or using common household items as weights. Several of the trunk exercises presented in Part II use body weight (eg, trunk extension and abdominal crunches) as the resistance. These exercises can be performed on a mattress or floor, and are illustrated with pillows as trunk support when needed.

Weights can be bought either for home use or can be made out of items such as soup cans or milk jugs partially filled with liquid or dirt. Most of the shoulder, chest, and back exercises in Part II can be adapted to weights such as these instead of dumbbells. A broomstick can be slid through the handle of a milk jug to provide a barbell-type resistance. Ankle weights are made easily by filling plastic sealable bags with dirt, gravel, or dried beans to the desired weight, and then fastening them to the ankles with a belt.

Surgical tubing is another option for elastic resistance. It is obtained easily at most medical supply stores.

STRETCHES

All of the stretches presented in Part II can be done easily at home without special equipment. Stretching should accompany each exercise session, whether it is a cardiovascular or strength session. The working muscles will be more fluid and efficient, with less chance of injury.

SAFETY

Any home exercise equipment should be set up according to the manufacturer's instructions. Many home gyms must be anchored to a wall for safety. Some cross-country ski machines need an extra two to three feet of clearance in the rear. Motorized treadmills must be placed where the cord will not become a hazard. Take space availability into consideration when deciding what equipment to purchase.

CHAPTER SUMMARY

Regular exercise is a difficult commitment for many people to make due to time or family constraints. This chapter outlines some ways to use home equipment or household items to provide an adequate workout without commercial facilities.

CHAPTER 14

Alternative Resistive Exercise Movements: Use of a Biomechanical Model

David Ash

CHAPTER OUTLINE

I. Purpose
II. Example Exercise Movements
III. The Future

PURPOSE

The purpose of presenting the following biomechanical model is to introduce a series of alternative resistive exercise movements and to stimulate resistive exercise research. Human motion rarely occurs purely around one of the three cardinal axes (the anteroposterior, superoinferior, and mediolateral axes).

Movement takes place around *various combinations* of these axes. However, for the purpose of illustrating the pattern by which the alternative movements are derived, the movements will be described with reference to the cardinal axes, movements, and planes. The derived movements begin with a resisted movement to place the body segment in position to perform a second movement. The second movement is performed while maintaining the resisted muscle action necessary to achieve the initial movement (see Table 14–1). For movements at multi-axial joints, two derived movements or "derivatives" exist. For bi-axial joints, a movement will have one derivative. Uni-axial joints do not mechanically allow a derived movement. Once the basic pattern is conceptualized, the model is very simple. Examples will help the reader begin to visualize the underlying concepts.

Axis	*Movement*	*Movement Plane*
anteroposterior	adduction, abduction	frontal (coronal) plane
superoinferior	rotation	transverse (horizontal) plane
mediolateral	flexion, extension	sagittal plane

Table 14–1 Resistance Exercise Movement Derivative Model

Resistance Key
TC = tubing or cable resistance
BW = body weight, cuff weights may be added to increase resistance
FW = free weight
MR = manual resistance
M = machine

Primary Movement	Axis	Derivative Axis	Osteokinematics	Resistance	Description/Points of Emphasis
hip extension	z	x	adduction/abduction	TC, BW	
		y	rotation	TC, BW	
hip flexion	z	x	adduction/abduction	TC, BW	Exerciser is upright. Tubing remains in position to resist flexion.
		y	rotation	TC, BW	Exerciser is upright. Tubing remains in position to resist flexion.
hip adduction	x	y	rotation	TC, BW	Resistance is directed against adduction throughout movement.
		z	flexion/extension	TC	Body weight resistance is not applicable because stabilization with contralateral foot would prevent clearance. Resistance is against adduction throughout.
hip abduction	x	y	rotation	TC, BW	BW is contralateral side-lying with resisted abduction throughout.
		z	flexion/extension	TC, BW	BW is contralateral side-lying with resisted abduction throughout.
hip medial rotation	y	x	adduction/abduction	MR	Exercise professional applies only a lateral rotation resistance. MR is indicated as other modes will not produce only rotatory resistance. Patient stands on contralateral leg.
		z	flexion/extension	MR	Exercise professional applies only a lateral rotation resistance. MR is indicated as other modes will not produce only rotatory resistance. Patient stands on contralateral leg.
hip lateral rotation	y	x	adduction/abduction	MR	As above with therapist now applying medial rotation resistance.
		z	flexion/extension	MR	As above with therapist now applying medial rotation resistance.
trunk flexion	z	x	lateral flexion	BW	
		y	rotation	BW	
trunk extension	z	x	lateral flexion	BW	
		y	rotation	BW	
trunk lateral flexion	x	y	rotation	BW	Contralateral side-lying
		z	flexion/extension	BW	Contralateral side-lying
trunk rotation	y	x	lateral flexion	TC	Resistance from contralateral side to outstretched arms to create a rotation resistance.
		z	flexion/extension	TC	Resistance from contralateral side to outstretched arms to create a rotation resistance.

continues

Copyright © 1997, Aspen Publishers, Inc.
Exercises for Health Promotion

Table 14–1 continued

Primary Movement	Axis	Derivative Axis	Osteokinematics	Resistance	Description/Points of Emphasis
shoulder abduction	x	y	rotation	TC, BW, FW	
		z	horizontal adduction/abduction	TC, BW, FW	
shoulder adduction	x	y	rotation	TC	Resistance is directed from ipsilateral side. BW, FW not applicable here because it is difficult to produce an abduction resistance.
		z	flexion/extension	TC	Resistance is directed from ipsilateral side. BW, FW not applicable here because it is difficult to produce an abduction resistance.
shoulder flexion	z	x	adduction/abduction	TC, FW, BW	
		y	rotation	TC, MR	
shoulder extension	z	x	adduction/abduction	TC, FW, BW	For FW and BW, prone position is required to produce shoulder flexion resistance.
		y	rotation	TC	For FW and BW, prone position is required to produce shoulder flexion resistance.
shoulder horizontal abduction (shoulder horizontal extension)	z	y	rotation	BW, FW	Prone on exercise table or bench
		x	adduction/abduction	TC, BW, FW	Prone on exercise table or bench
shoulder medial rotation	y	x	adduction/abduction	TC, BW, FW	Resistance positioned to create shoulder lateral rotation resistance throughout the derived movement. TC: standing with elbow flexed to 90 degrees, resistance from anterior. (Variation: While not a full contraction of the medial rotators, greater ad/ab range of motion will be available if resistance is positioned from anterior, with medial rotators stabilizing forearm in the yz [coronal] plane.) For FW, BW: prone with elbow flexed to 90 degrees and forearm maintained in horizontal plane.
		z	flexion/extension	TC	TC: elbow flexed to 90 degrees with forearm in xy (sagittal) plane for optimal sagittal plane motion. Tubing secured to ipsilateral side to create shoulder lateral rotation resistance. (Note: shoulder adductors will actively stabilize humerus in xy plane.) BW, FW: Not applicable because to maintain lateral rotation resistance with elbow at 90 degrees, the exerciser would have to be ipsilateral side-lying, which would prevent flexion and extension movements.

continues

Table 14-1 continued

Primary Movement	Axis	Derivative Axis	Osteokinematics	Resistance	Description/Points of Emphasis
shoulder lateral rotation	y	x	adduction/abduction	TC, BW, FW	Elbow flexed to 90 degrees, shoulder in full lateral rotation. Resistance from anterior to create medial rotation resistance. BW, FW can be used in prone position. Cocontraction of shoulder extensors will maintain humerus in frontal plane if TC, in horizontal plane if BW, FW.
		z	flexion/extension	MR	Exercise professional provides conjoint medial rotation resistance and flexion/extension resistance. Note: for flexion, the professional must apply a medial rotation resistance at the wrist and an extension resistance at the shoulder.
Medial rotation derivative of shoulder flexion not recommended due to impingement.					
cervical flexion	z	x	lateral flexion	BW, MR	Supine
		y	rotation	BW, MR	Supine
cervical extension	z	x	lateral flexion	BW, MR	Prone
		y	rotation	BW, MR	Prone
cervical lateral flexion	x	y	rotation	BW, MR	Contralateral side-lying
		z	flexion/extension	BW, MR	Contralateral side-lying
cervical rotation	y	x	lateral flexion	MR	Exercise professional provides resistance to + or − cervical rotation in addition to applying resistance to lateral flexion.
		z	flexion/extension	MR	Exercise professional provides resistance to + or − cervical rotation in addition to applying resistance to flexion/extension.
Bi-axial joints (one derivative available)					
elbow flexion	z	y	pronation/supination	TC, MR, FW	From prone position, fully flex elbow while keeping arm at side of thorax. Pronate, supinate.
elbow extension	z	y	pronation/supination	TC, FW	TC: standing; FW: prone. Stabilize humerus so pronation only at elbow rather than shoulder rotation occurs.
pronation	y	z	elbow flexion/extension	TC	Resistance from ipsilateral side. Grasp tubing in supinated position, then pronate to start position. Stabilize humerus against thorax.
supination	y	z	elbow flexion/extension	TC	Resistance from contralateral side. Grasp tubing in pronated position, then supinate to start position. Stabilize humerus.
plantarflexion	z	x	inversion/eversion	TC, MR	Maintain dorsiflexion resistance while providing inversion/eversion resistance.

continues

Table 14–1 continued

Primary Movement	Axis	Derivative Axis	Osteokinematics	Resistance	Description/Points of Emphasis
dorsiflexion	z	x	inversion/eversion	TC, MR	Maintain plantarflexion resistance.
inversion	x	z	plantar/dorsiflexion	TC, MR	Resistance to inversion throughout plantarflexion/dorsiflexion.
eversion	x	z	plantar/dorsiflexion	TC, MR	Maintain inversion resistance.
forefoot pronation	y	z	plantar/dorsiflexion	MR	Stabilize rear foot in neutral while providing resistance to forefoot supination and ankle plantarflexion/dorsiflexion.
forefoot supination	y	z	plantar/dorsiflexion	MR	Stabilize rear foot in neutral while providing resistance to forefoot supination and ankle plantarflexion/dorsiflexion.
wrist flexion	z	x	radial/ulnar deviation	MR, TC	If using TC, maintain forearm vertically.
wrist extension	z	x	radial/ulnar deviation	MR, TC	If using TC, mintain forearm vertically.
radial deviation	x	z	flexion/extension	MR, TC	If using TC, stabilize forearm horizontally.
ulnar deviation	x	z	flexion/extension	MR, TC	If using TC, stabilize forearm horizontally.

Note: No wrist movement about y axis. Pronation/supination occurs at the elbow.

Primary Movement	Axis	Derivative Axis	Osteokinematics	Resistance	Description/Points of Emphasis
knee flexion	z	y	medial/lateral tibial rotation	M, TC, MR	Fully flex knee against resistance. Stabilize thigh to prevent rotation at the hip. Exerciser fully rotates tibia as professional provides resistance to tibial rotation.
knee extension	z	y	tibial rotation	BW, MR	Fully extend knee against resistance. Stabilize thigh to prevent rotation at the hip. Exerciser fully rotates tibia as professional provides resistance.
medial tibial rotation	y	z	flexion/extension	MR, TC	Seated with ankle in neutral. Resistance placed around forefoot from ipsilateral side to create lateral rotation resistance. Stabilize thigh.
lateral tibial rotation	y	z	flexion/extension	MR, TC	Seated with ankle in neutral. Resistance placed around forefoot from contralateral side to create medial rotation resistance. Stabilize thigh as exerciser flexes and extends knee while holding leg in lateral rotation.

Example Exercise Movements

Axis Key

x axis = anteroposterior axis
y axis = superoinferior axis
z axis = mediolateral axis

Example 1

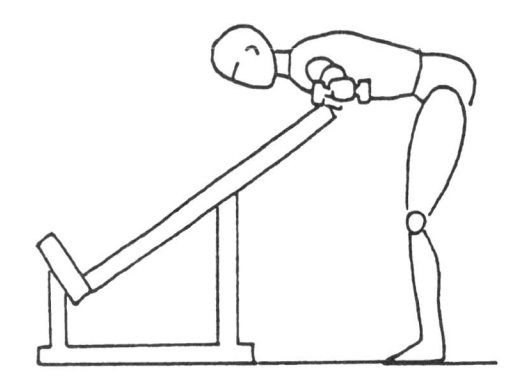

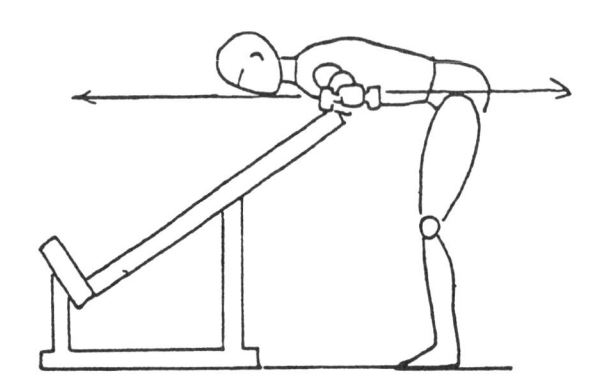

Start/Finish   Movement

Shoulder transverse abduction is a resistive exercise movement to strengthen posterior shoulder structures. The movement may prevent pathology resulting from an excessive anterior shoulder/posterior shoulder strength imbalance. In addition to standard shoulder transverse abduction, two additional supplementary options are adduction/abduction (as shown above) from a position of full shoulder transverse abduction and shoulder rotation from a position of shoulder transverse abduction.

Example 2

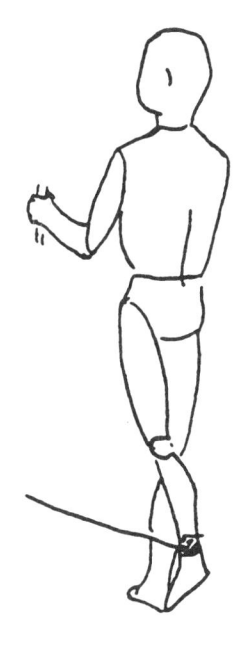

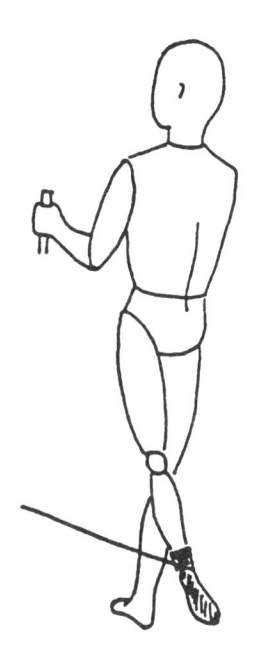

Start/Finish **Movement**

Resisted hip extension is a sagittal plane movement about the z axis. The two hip extension derivatives are rotation (transverse plane movement about the y axis), and adduction/abduction (coronal plane movement about the x axis). As a supplement to pure resistive hip extension movements (sagittal plane motion), resistive hip extension can be sustained while simultaneously performing hip mediolateral rotation (transverse plane motion) as shown above, hip adduction/abduction (coronal plane motion), or combinations of movements in both the transverse and coronal planes.

Copyright © 1997, Aspen Publishers, Inc.
Exercises for Health Promotion

Example 3

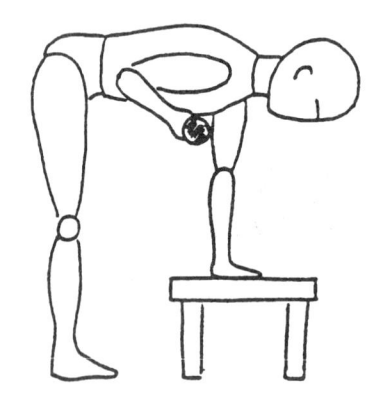

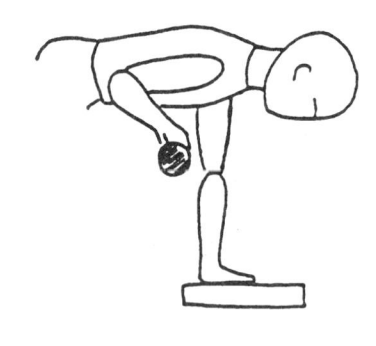

Start/Finish   **Movement**

At the elbow, flexion and extension occur in the sagittal plane about the z axis. The single derivative is forearm rotation, which normally occurs in the transverse plane about the y axis. The rotation is performed while holding the elbow in full flexion against resistance.

Example 4

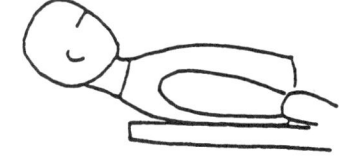

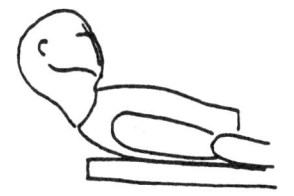

Start/Finish **Movement**

Resistive cervical flexion occurs in the sagittal plane. Because the cervical vertebrae also allow lateral flexion (coronal plane movement) and rotation (transverse plane movement), two derivatives are available. From a position of resisted full cervical flexion, the cervical spine may be rotated, laterally flexed, or simultaneously rotated and laterally flexed.

Example 5

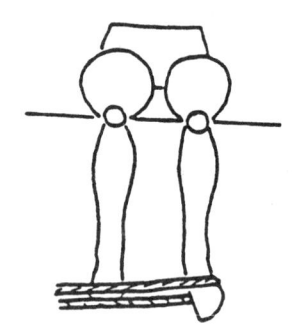

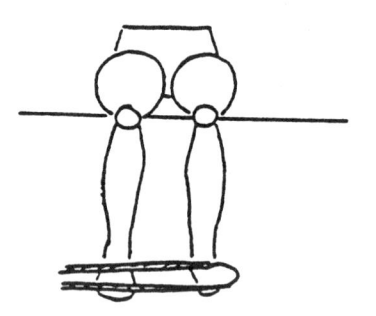

Start/Finish **Movement**

Resistive exercise targeted at the lateral structures of the leg may play a role in prevention of inversion injury. Movements available at the subtalor and midtarsal joints are supination and pronation. As an option to resisted pronation, the foot could be held in resisted pronation while simultaneously plantarflexing and dorsiflexing the talocrural joint. This combination of movements may strengthen the lateral structures of the leg through a greater range of functional positions than pure pronation alone.

THE FUTURE

Edward Cornish, current president of the World Future Society, succinctly wrote, "when we recognize that we, ourselves, create our future, we recognize our powers over the future. We inevitably begin to anticipate the consequences of what we do and to do those things that will improve our future; in short, we begin to act wisely."[1] What is the future of health care? What advances will we see? What will change? What role will preventive exercise play in health care? Coates hypothesizes, "All human diseases and disorders will have their linkages, if any, to the human genome identified. In several parts of the world the understanding of human genetics will lead to explicit programs to enhance people's overall physical and mental abilities—not just prevent diseases. More people in advanced countries will be living to their mid-80s while enjoying a healthier, fuller life."[2]

Throughout this period of flux, exercise professionals should be prepared not only to update continually their knowledge through consistent research literature review, but also to contribute actively to the preventive exercise research base. Exercise professionals may view the future not with apprehension, but rather as a grand opportunity to embark on an exciting adventure in which they will respond to unknown challenges and continually adapt to meet the health care needs of tomorrow.

REFERENCES

1. Cornish E. Responsibility for the future. *Futurist*. 1994;May–June:60.
2. Coates JF. The highly probable future: 83 assumptions about the year 2025. *Futurist*. 1994;28:29–35.

Part II

Exercises

Chapter 15

Resistive Exercise Movements

David Ash

RESISTIVE EXERCISE TERMINOLOGY

See Table 15–1 for a list of resistive exercise terms used in this chapter.

RESISTIVE EXERCISE MOVEMENTS

In this section, a variety of resistive exercise movements are presented. Movements that offer stimulation to the major muscle groups of the body are described. It is the responsibility of the exercise professional to include appropriate movements in the program after a detailed evaluation of each individual exerciser's needs and goals.

It is important to realize that an isolation movement for each muscle group need not be performed during each session. A dumbbell chest press movement, in addition to providing stimulation to the fibers of the pectoral and anterior deltoid muscles, concurrently stimulates the tricep group. Most upper extremity pulling movements, in addition to addressing the shoulder extensors and adductors, also recruit the elbow flexors. The point is that each of the body's major muscular structures can be provided with an overload during each session without a specific isolation movement for each muscle group being performed within each session. Refer to Appendix G for sample programs that illustrate this principle.

The resistive exercise movements are presented in groups based on osteokinematic motion (eg, knee flexion, shoulder extension), with each movement within that group listed by its generic name (eg, leg curl, lat rowing). The primary muscle groups recruited during performance of each movement are listed.

Start/Finish and Movement drawings for each movement are provided, accompanied by a description of correct performance of the movement. The sample movements use a variety of exercise equipment types. Emphasis is placed on using equipment to which the exerciser has access. The movements illustrated may be performed in commercial fitness, home, clinic, or travel settings. While reviewing the exercise movements, the reader should keep in mind that within any given exercise session, one or perhaps at most two exercises from a particular osteokinematic group are performed.

Table 15–1 Resistive Exercise Terminology

Term	Operational Definition
Resistive exercise	A type of exercise in which multiple repetitions of various movements are performed against some type of resistance. The objective is enhanced fitness and injury prevention. Resistive exercise is also called weight training.
Olympic weightlifting	A sport in which the goal of the participant is to demonstrate the ability to lift as much weight as possible in two movements: the snatch and the clean and jerk.
Powerlifting	A sport in which the goal of the participant is to demonstrate the ability to lift as much weight as possible in three movements: bench press, dead lift, and squat.

continues

Table 15–1 continued

Term	Operational Definition
Bodybuilding	A sport in which resistance is performed with the objective being to demonstrate hypertrophy and symmetry.
Concentric muscle action	Development of tension as muscles shorten.
Eccentric muscle action	Development of tension as muscles lengthen.
Isometric muscle action	Tension production without muscle lengthening or shortening.
Agonist	Muscle that causes movement by shortening.
Antagonist	Muscle which becomes lengthened as a result of a movement.
Torso	That part of the body from the waist to the neck, excluding the arms.
Thigh	The body segment between the hip and the knee.
Leg	The body segment between the knee and the ankle.
Arm	The body segment between the shoulder and the elbow.
Forearm	The body segment between the elbow and the wrist.

Exercise 1

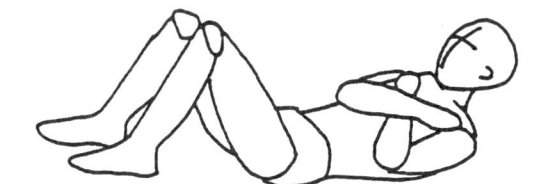

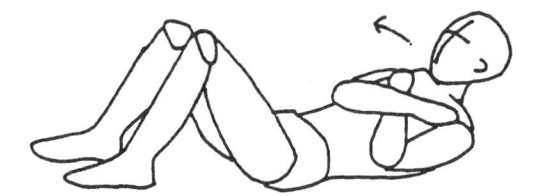

Start/Finish   **Movement**

Movement: Abdominal curl
Target Muscles: Abdominals, obliques
Instructions: With your knees bent and feet on the floor but *not* anchored, slowly raise your head and shoulder blades up from the floor by contracting your abdominal muscles. Your arms are crossed in front of your chest with hands on opposite shoulders throughout the movement.

Repetitions: _____
Goal: _____
Precautions/Comments: _____
_____
_____

Exercise 2

Start/Finish **Movement**

Movement: Heels up
Target Muscles: Abdominals, obliques
Instructions: Begin on your back with arms and legs upright. Attempt to raise your heels and fingertips straight upward by contracting your abdominal muscles.

Repetitions: _____
Goal: _____
Precautions/Comments: _____
_____
_____
_____

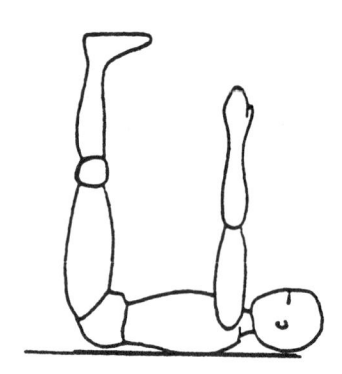

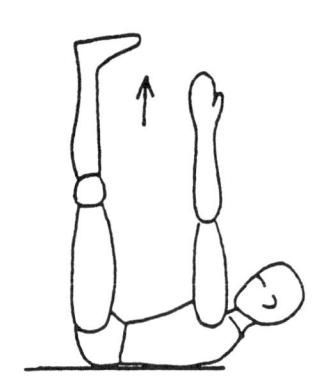

Copyright © 1997, Aspen Publishers, Inc.
Exercises for Health Promotion

Exercise 3

Start/Finish **Movement**

Movement: Standing side bends
Target Muscles: Obliques
Instructions: Position yourself with feet shoulder width apart. Begin the movement from the side-bending right position. Side bend fully to your left as you pull the resistance. Move only left and right. Do not let your trunk bend forward or backward. When finished, perform the movement from left to right.

Repetitions: _____
Goal: _____
Precautions/Comments: _____
_____
_____

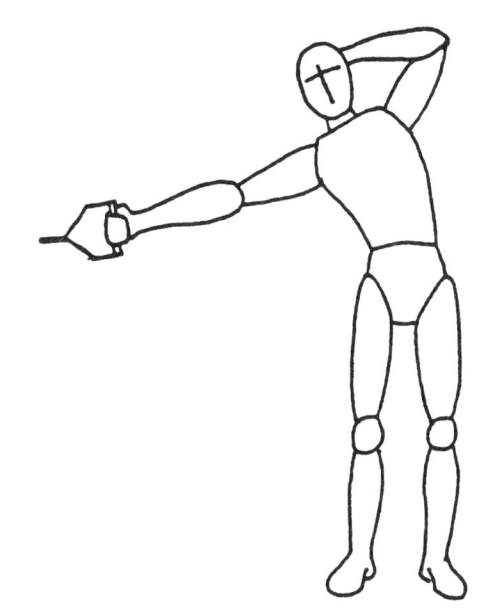

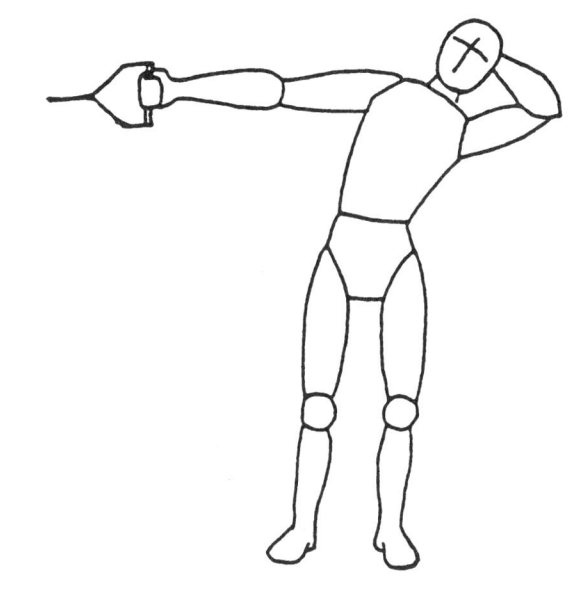

Exercise 4

Start/Finish **Movement**

Movement: Side-lying lateral curl
Target Muscles: Obliques
Instructions: Start from a side-lying position with your legs held in place by a partner. Bend to your side, making your "top" shoulder raise. Do not bend forward or backward, only to the side.

Repetitions: _____
Goal: _____
Precautions/Comments: _____
_____
_____

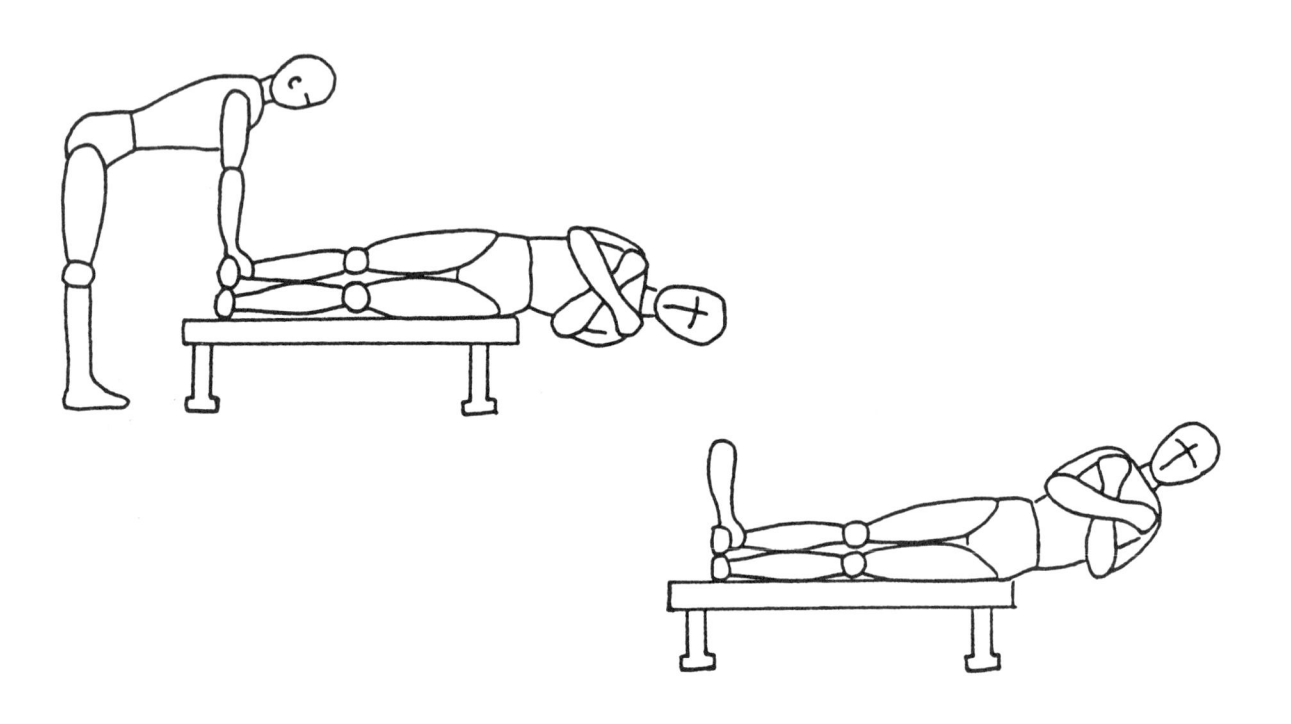

Exercise 5

Start/Finish **Movement**

Movement: Twisting abdominal curl
Target Muscles: Abdominals, obliques
Instructions: Start with your knees bent and feet on the floor but not anchored. As with the standard abdominal curl, use your stomach muscles to curl your upper body until your shoulder blades are off the floor. Add a gradual twist to either side throughout the upward curl. Lower slowly. Alternate the twisting motion to left and right.

Repetitions: _____
Goal: _____
Precautions/Comments: _____
_____
_____
_____

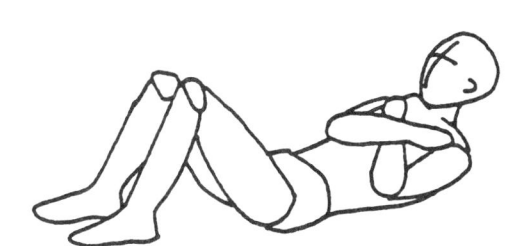

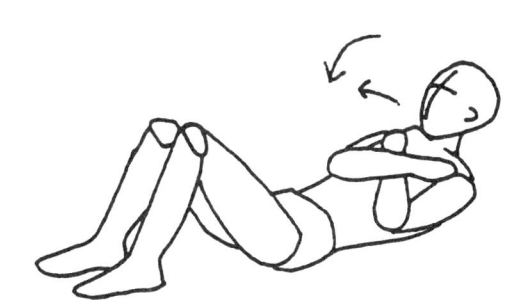

Exercise 6

Start/Finish   **Movement**

Movement: Trunk rotation on machine
Target Muscles: Obliques, rotational back muscles
Instructions: Begin this movement from the position of full rotation to either side. As you rotate to the opposite side, make sure that your entire upper body rotates (as opposed to keeping your torso stationary and only rotating your arms). When finished moving to the left, use the lever to rotate your seat. Repeat the movement twisting to the right.

Repetitions: _____
Goal: _____
Precautions/Comments: _____
_____
_____

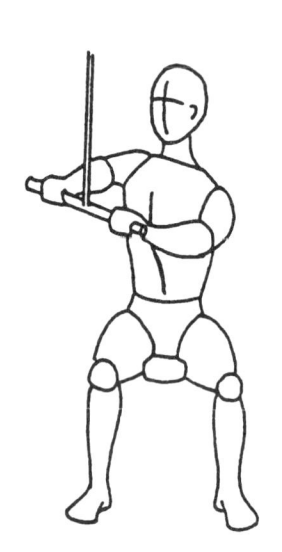

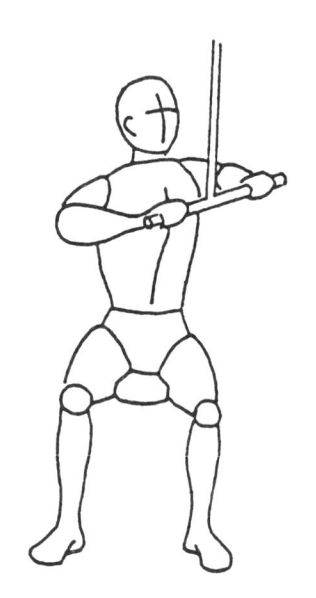

Copyright © 1997, Aspen Publishers, Inc.
Exercises for Health Promotion

Exercise 7

Start/Finish   **Movement**

Movement: Prone back extension
Target Muscles: Erector spinae
Instructions: Begin by lying on your stomach with a pad or pillow at waist level. Your arms and legs are outstretched. Maintain your thighs in contact with the floor. Raise your upper body until your thighs, hips, and shoulders are in a straight line. Do not hyperextend.

Repetitions: _____
Goal: _____
Precautions/Comments: _____
_____
_____
_____

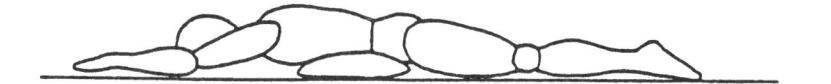

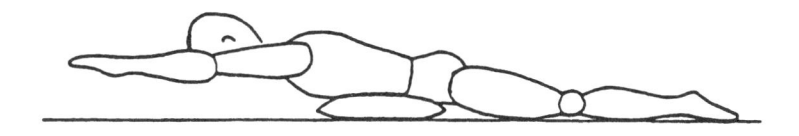

Exercise 8

Start/Finish **Movement**

Movement: Back extension on machine
Target Muscles: Erector spinae
Instructions: From the machine's starting position, extend backward. Do not hyperextend at either your low back or neck.

Repetitions: _____
Goal: _____
Precautions/Comments: _____
_____
_____

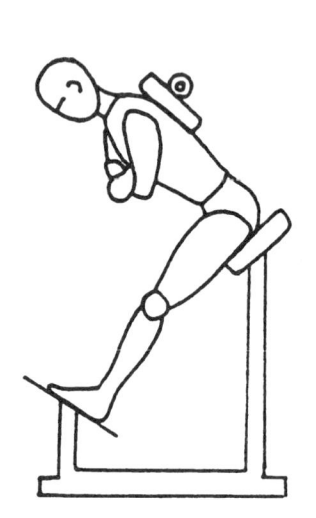

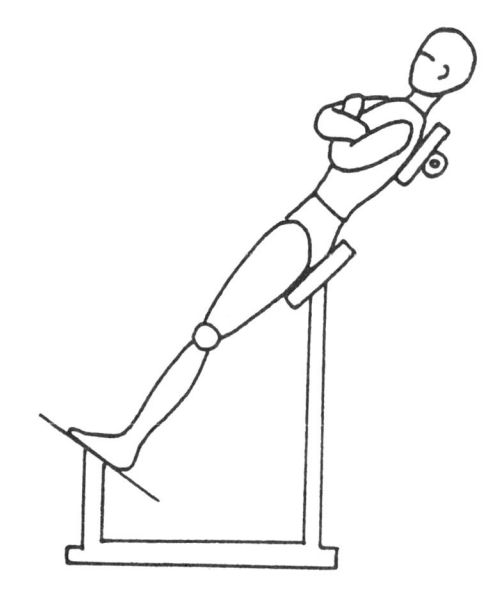

Exercise 9

Start/Finish **Movement**

Movement: Leg press
Target Muscles: Gluteus maximus, quadriceps, hamstrings
Instructions: Before you begin, adjust your seat so that in the Start/Finish position your knees are flexed no more than 30 to 45 degrees. As you press out, concentrate on pushing equally with both legs. Extend your knees fully as you move in a slow, controlled, continuous motion between lifting and lowering the weight. Do not lock your knees to take a rest as this results in a hyperextension stress to the knees.

Repetitions: _____
Goal: _____
Precautions/Comments: _____
_____
_____
_____

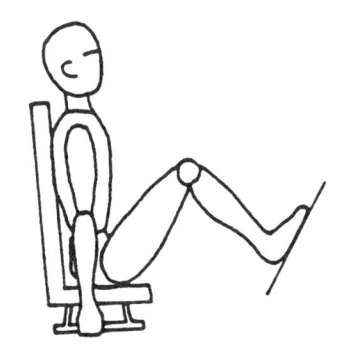

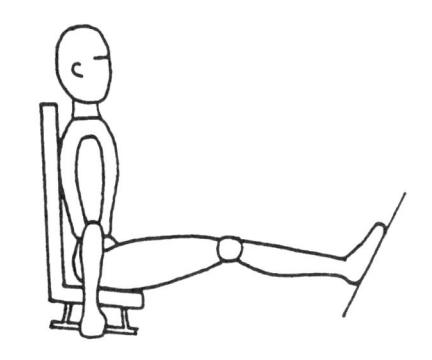

Exercise 10

Start/Finish   **Movement**

Movement: Dumbbell lunge
Target Muscles: Gluteus maximus, hamstrings, quadriceps
Instructions: Begin with dumbbells in your hands and your feet shoulder width apart. Slowly step forward with one leg, placing your foot so you maintain shoulder width between your feet. Slowly lower your body as you maintain your torso vertically. Lower your back knee *almost* to the point of touching the floor but do not allow it to touch the floor. Use the initial repetitions to adjust your step length so that at the lowest point of the movement, your front knee is at a 90 degree angle. To return to the Start/Finish position, emphasize a controlled push from the heel of your front foot. Do not allow the dumbbells to swing at any time throughout the movement. Alternate legs.

Repetitions: _____
Goal: _____
Precautions/Comments: _____
_____
_____

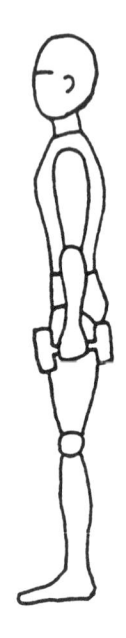

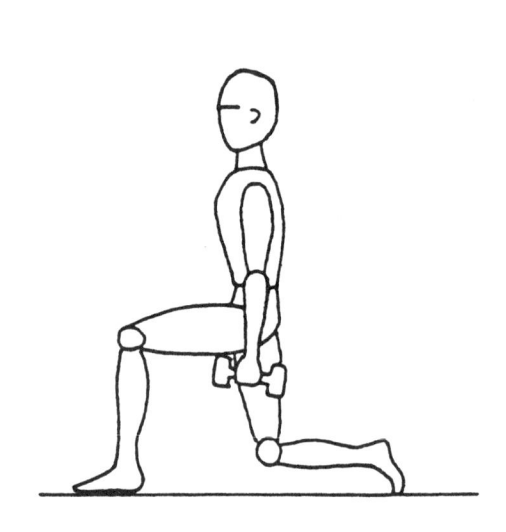

Exercise 11

Start/Finish **Movement**

Movement: Hip extension on multi-hip machine
Target Muscles: Gluteals, hamstrings
Instructions: Before you begin, adjust the resistance arm of the machine so that it is horizontal or angled slightly upward. The machine will have a bar or some type of handle for you to grasp for support. The key to correct performance of this movement is maintaining your support leg and your upper body vertically as you extend your moving thigh as far back as possible.

Repetitions: _____
Goal: _____
Precautions/Comments: _____
_____
_____

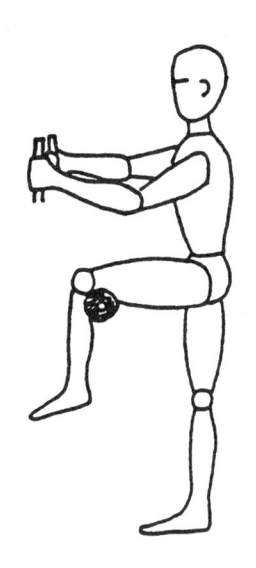

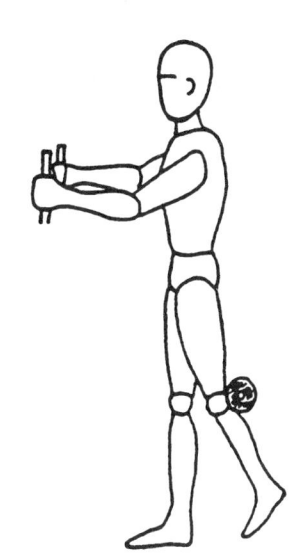

Exercise 12

Start/Finish   **Movement**

Movement: Squat
Target Muscles: Gluteals, quadriceps, hamstrings
Instructions: The squat movement can be a safe movement; however, extreme caution must be taken to ensure that the movement is performed and spotted correctly. If the squat is performed, it is recommended that you use light weight and emphasize correct body mechanics. Proper squat and spotting technique require multiple learning/practice sessions with a qualified exercise professional.

Repetitions: _____
Goal: _____
Precautions/Comments: _____
_____
_____

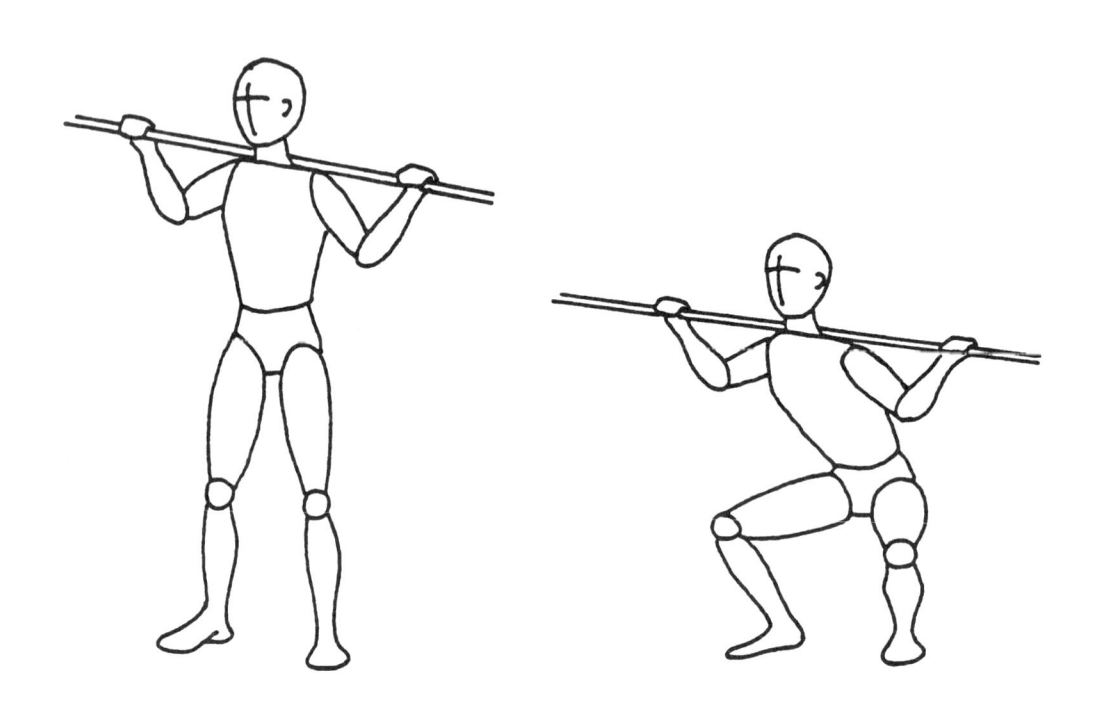

Exercise 13

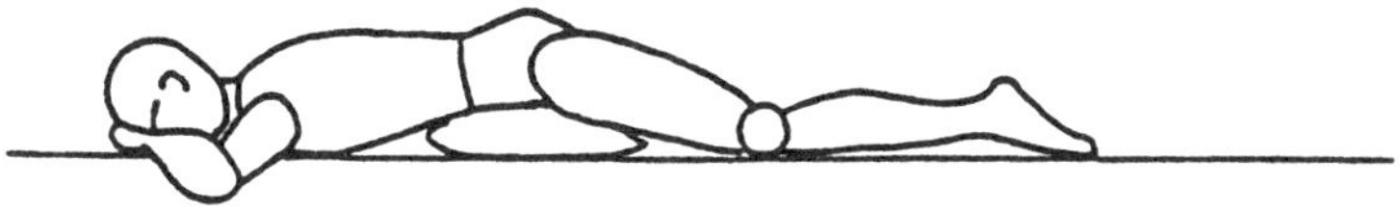

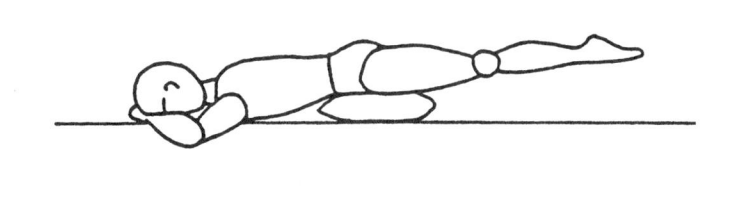

Start/Finish **Movement**

Movement: Prone hip extension
Target Muscles: Gluteals
Instructions: Begin by lying on your stomach on a weight bench (a bed works just as well). Position your hips at the edge of the bench to isolate movement at the hips. Hold your upper body against the bench with your arms. The movement is performed by extending your hips so your thighs move to a horizontal position.

Repetitions: _____
Goal: _____
Precautions/Comments: _____
_____
_____
_____

Exercise 14

Start/Finish **Movement**

Movement: Full body extension
Target Muscles: Gluteals, erector spinae
Instructions: Begin by lying on your stomach with a pad or pillow at waist level. Simultaneously raise your chest, arms, and legs from the floor until your body forms a straight line (180 degrees). Do not hyperextend.

Repetitions: _____
Goal: _____
Precautions/Comments: _____
_____
_____

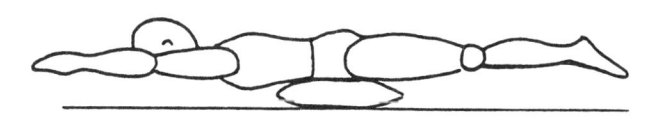

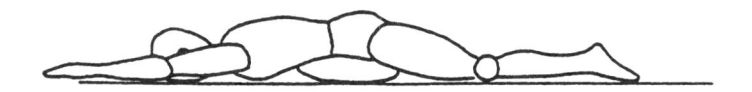

Exercise 15

Start/Finish **Movement**

Movement: Hip flexion on multi-hip machine
Target Muscles: Iliopsoas
Instructions: Before you begin, select your desired weight. Stand on the platform with erect posture. There will be a bar or handles for you to grasp for support. Adjust the resistance arm of the machine so that it places a comfortable stretch on the front of the leg to be exercised. Flex your thigh, raising your knee as high as you can, while keeping torso and stance leg aligned vertically. Slowly return to the Start/Finish position. To exercise the hip flexors of your opposite leg, reverse your position on the platform and reset the resistance arm.

Repetitions: _____
Goal: _____
Precautions/Comments: _____
_____
_____

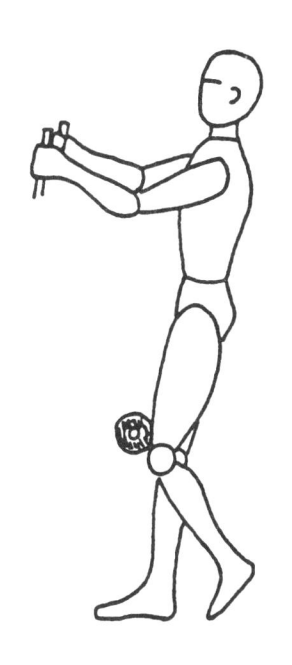

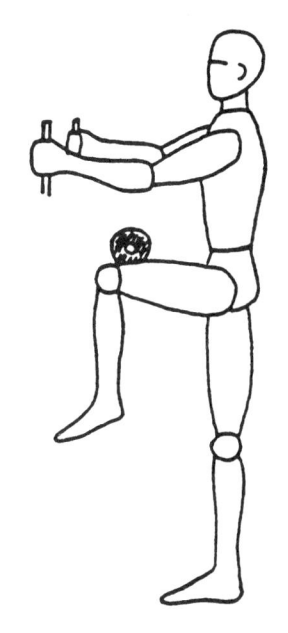

Exercise 16

Start/Finish   **Movement**

Movement: Hip adduction on adduction machine
Target Muscles: Adductor magnus, longus, and brevis
Instructions: To determine your correct starting position, spread your legs to a position of comfortable stretch. From that position, use the hand lever to set the thigh supports one setting inward. This will ensure that you do not overstretch. Move your thighs together. You will feel the machine's rubber bumpers when you have reached the end of the inward movement. Slowly return to the Start/Finish position.

Repetitions: _____
Goal: _____
Precautions/Comments: _____
_____
_____

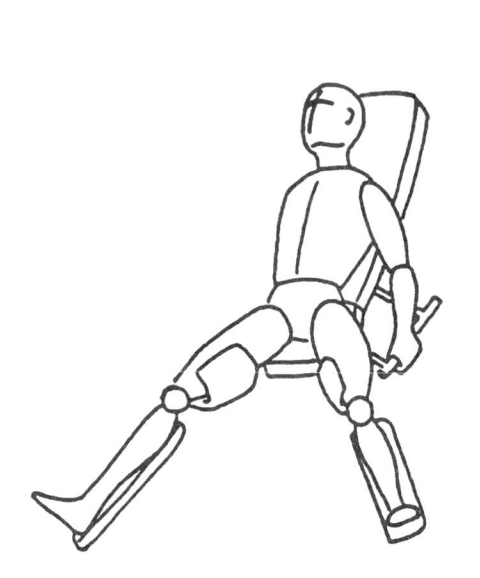

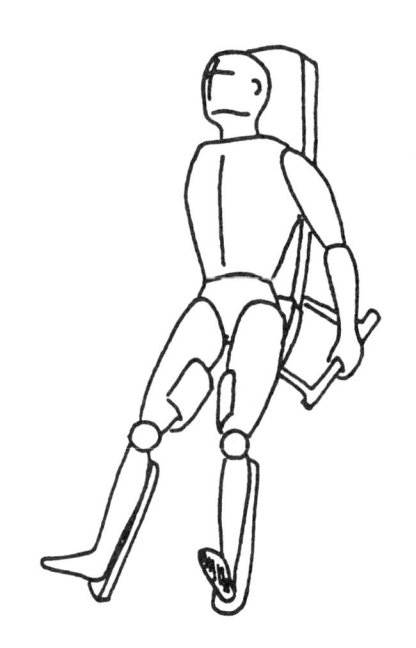

Exercise 17

Start/Finish **Movement**

Movement: Hip adduction on multi-hip machine
Target Muscles: Adductor magnus, longus, and brevis
Instructions: Before you begin, adjust the resistance arm of the machine so that it is angled slightly less than 90 degrees toward the leg to be exercised. Place your thigh so it contacts the outer side of the roller pad, thus putting the inner thigh muscles on a slight, comfortable stretch. This is your Start/Finish position. To exercise, move your leg to midline, then as far past midline as you can. Slowly return to the Start/Finish position. The machine will have a bar or some type of handles you can grasp for support. Maintain a vertical torso throughout the movement.

Repetitions: _____
Goal: _____
Precautions/Comments: _____
_____
_____
_____

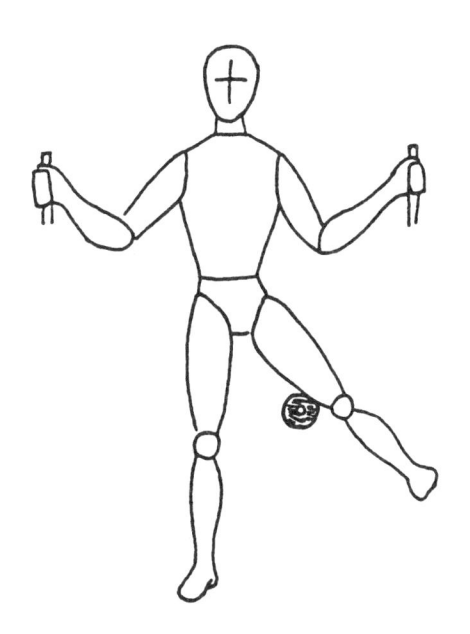

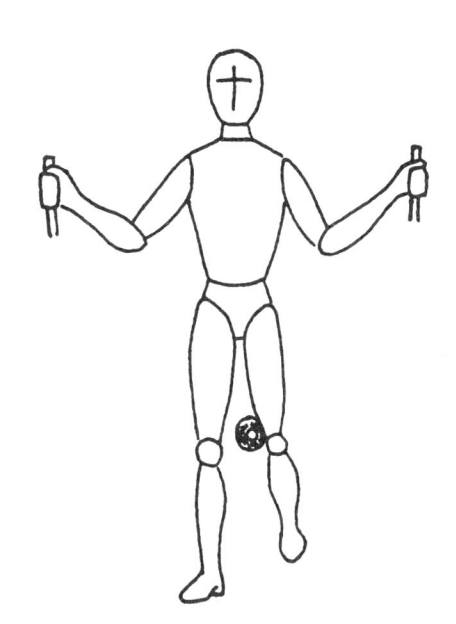

Exercise 18

Start/Finish **Movement**

Movement: Hip adduction with cuff weight
Target Muscles: Adductor magnus, longus, and brevis
Instructions: From a side-lying position on the floor, place the foot of your supporting leg either in front of or behind the distal thigh of your exercising leg. As you raise your leg straight upward (adduction) maintain your body in a straight line.

Repetitions: _____
Goal: _____
Precautions/Comments: _____
_____
_____
_____

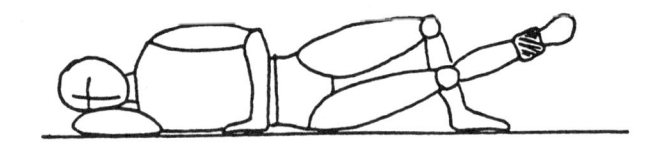

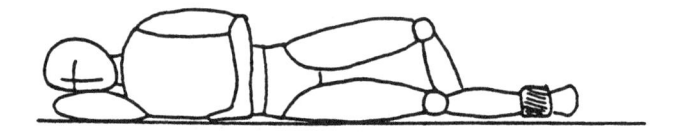

Exercise 19

Start/Finish **Movement**

Movement: Lateral lunge
Target Muscles: Hip abductors of stepping leg, hip adductors of other leg
Instructions: Begin with your feet slightly wider than shoulder width. Slowly step with your left leg to the left. As your body lowers, maintain your torso upright. Concentrate on using both legs equally as you step to the side. As you return to the Start/Finish position, concentrate on pushing with your left leg and pulling with your right leg. Alternate stepping to the left and right.

Repetitions: _____
Goal: _____
Precautions/Comments: _____
_____
_____

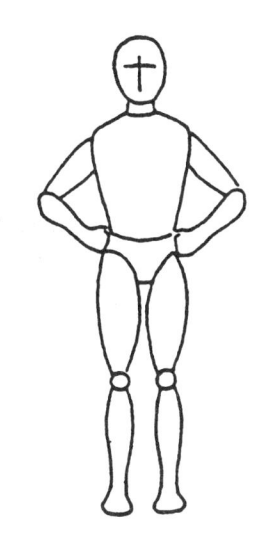

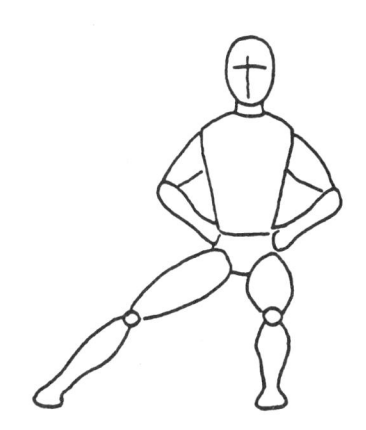

Exercise 20

Start/Finish **Movement**

Movement: Hip abduction on abduction machine
Target Muscles: Gluteals, tensor fasciae latae
Instructions: Use the hand lever to adjust the thigh supports so that they are as close together as possible. This is the Start/Finish position. To perform the movement, spread your legs apart against the resistance.

Repetitions: _____
Goal: _____
Precautions/Comments: _____
_____
_____

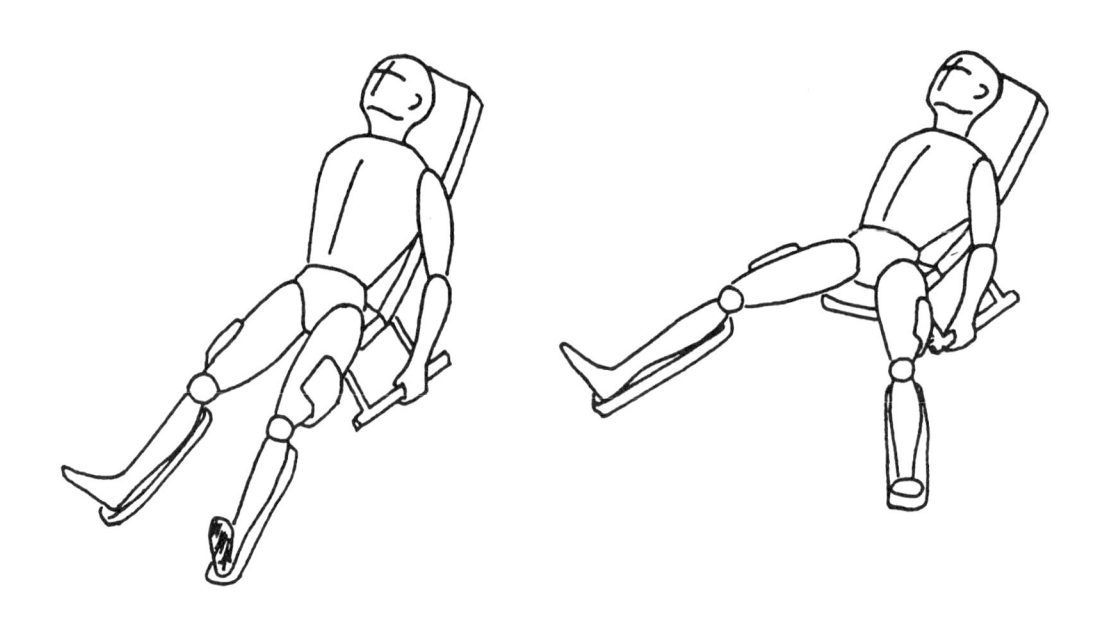

Exercise 21

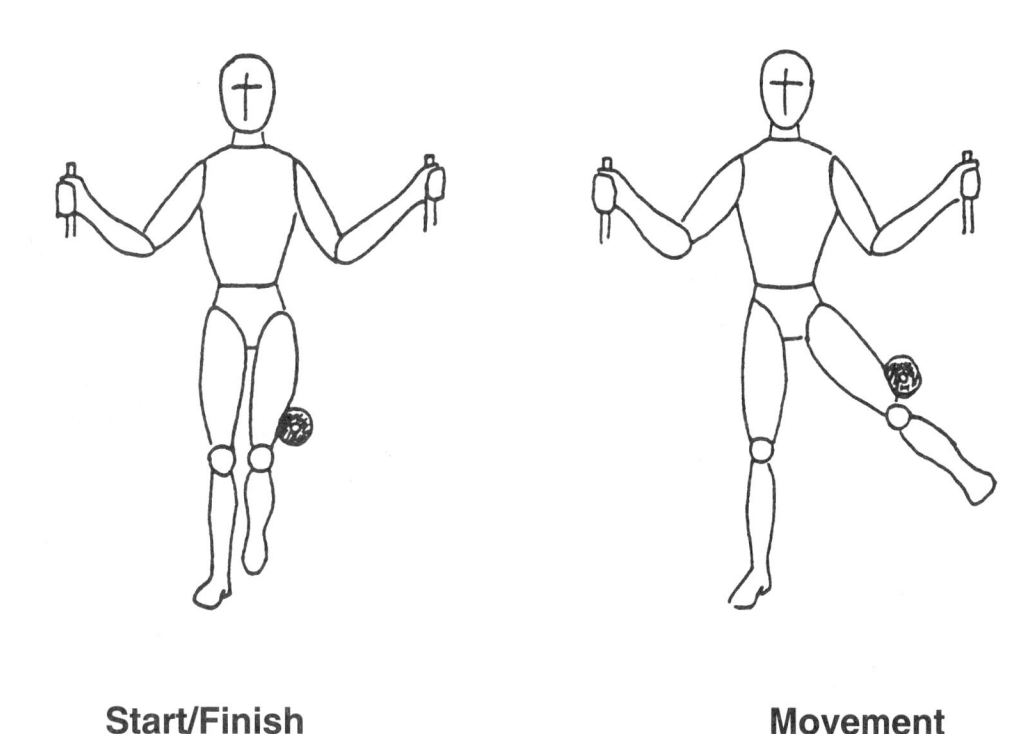

Start/Finish   **Movement**

Movement: Hip abduction with multi-hip machine
Target Muscles: Gluteals, tensor fasciae latae
Instructions: Maintain your body and your stance leg in a vertical position. The machine will have a bar or handles to grasp for support. Adjust the roller pad so that it contacts the outer side of the exercising thigh just proximal to the knee. Adjust the resistance arm so that it is vertical (or just slightly angled toward the stance leg for a little more stretch). This is the Start/Finish position. Move your thigh to the side against the resistance. Maintain your stance leg and torso in vertical alignment. You will feel that this movement utilizes the hip muscles of not only the moving thigh but the stance leg as well.

Repetitions: _____
Goal: _____
Precautions/Comments: _____
_____
_____
_____

Exercise 22

Start/Finish **Movement**

Movement: Hip abduction with cuff weight
Target Muscles: Gluteals, tensor fasciae latae
Instructions: Begin from a side-lying position with a cuff weight on the ankle of the upper leg. Concentrate on maintaining your legs and upper body in a straight line as you raise your leg vertically.

Repetitions: _____
Goal: _____
Precautions/Comments: _____
_____
_____

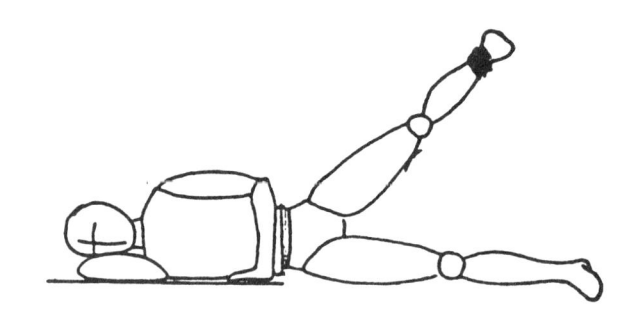

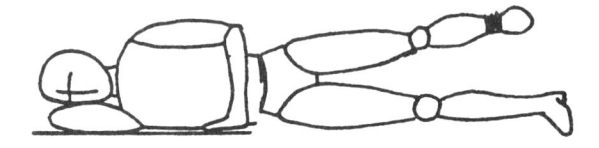

Exercise 23

Start/Finish **Movement**

Movement: Hip medial rotation in side-lying position with cuff weight
Target Muscles: Gluteus medius and minimus, tensor fasciae latae
Instructions: To exercise the medial rotators of your right hip, begin by lying on your left side on a weight bench. Your right hip and right knee begin from a position of 90 degrees of flexion. Grasp your hand to your wrist to maintain the right thigh horizontally. Slowly lower your right ankle toward the floor while maintaining the knee and hip in 90 degrees of flexion. This is the Start/Finish position. The movement is performed by rotating your right hip to raise your right ankle as high as possible. As with all movements, hold the maximally contracted position for a full second before slowly returning to the Start/Finish position. In addition to strengthening the medial rotators, this movement will help lengthen the frequently foreshortened lateral rotators. When finished, reverse body position to exercise the medial rotators of the left hip.

Repetitions: _____
Goal: _____
Precautions/Comments: _____
_____
_____

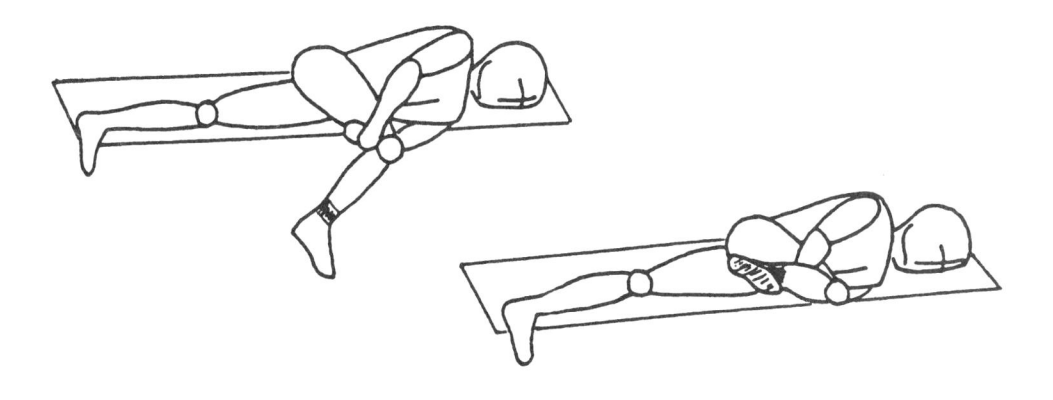

Exercise 24

Start/Finish   **Movement**

Movement: Standing hip medial rotation with elastic band or tubing
Target Muscles: Gluteus medius and minimus
Instructions: Begin from a standing position with arms extended to a wall for support. Your right hip will begin from a position of lateral rotation. The knee is maintained in 90 degrees of flexion. Rotate at the hip, concentrating on maintaining your right thigh vertically as your right ankle pulls the resistance across behind your body. Do not lean forward at the hips; maintain erect posture throughout. Reverse body position and line of pull of resistance to address the medial rotators of your left hip.

Repetitions: _____
Goal: _____
Precautions/Comments: _____
_____
_____
_____

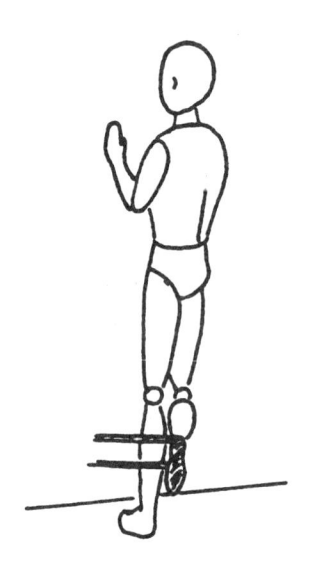

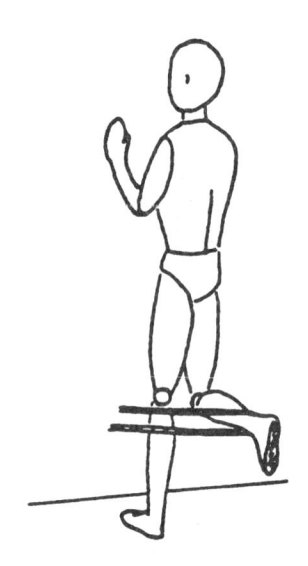

Exercise 25

Start/Finish **Movement**

Movement: Seated hip medial rotation with elastic band or tubing
Target Muscles: Gluteus medius and minimus
Instructions: Begin this movement from a seated position with your thighs together and your knees flexed to 90 degrees. To perform the movement, concentrate on rotating both your hips such that your thighs and knees do not change location, but your ankles move outward against the elastic resistance.

Repetitions: _____
Goal: _____
Precautions/Comments: _____
_____
_____
_____

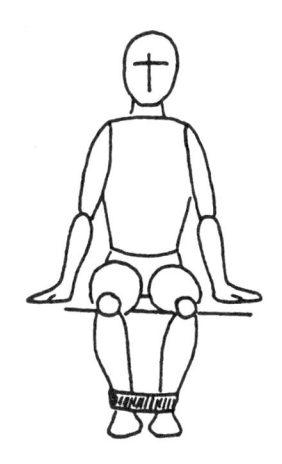

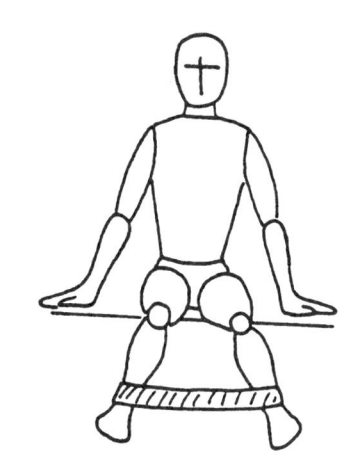

Exercise 26

Start/Finish **Movement**

Movement: Hip lateral rotation in side-lying position with cuff weight
Target Muscles: Gluteus maximus and medius
Instructions: To exercise the lateral rotators of your left hip, begin from a left side-lying position on a weight bench. Use your arms to support your hip in a position of 90 degrees of flexion and to maintain your thigh horizontally. Slowly lower your ankle by allowing your left hip to medially rotate. This is the Start/Finish position. Keep your hip and knee in 90 degrees of flexion and rotate at the left hip to raise the left ankle against the resistance provided by the cuff weight. Slowly lower to the Start/Finish position and repeat. Reverse body position to exercise the lateral rotators of the right hip.

Repetitions: _____
Goal: _____
Precautions/Comments: _____
_____
_____
_____

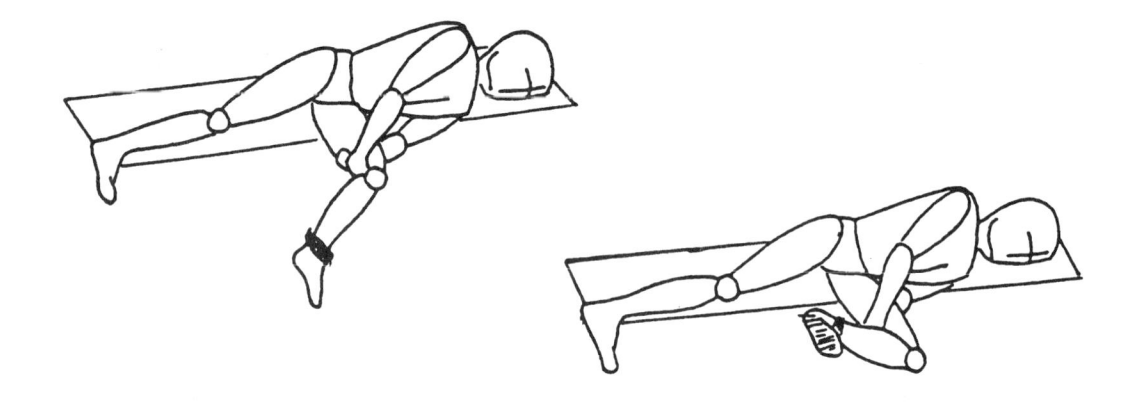

Exercise 27

Start/Finish **Movement**

Movement: Standing hip lateral rotation with elastic band or tubing
Target Muscles: Gluteus maximus and medius, piriformis
Instructions: Stand upright with your arms placed against a wall for support. This is your Start/Finish position. Your right knee is flexed to 90 degrees. To exercise the lateral rotators of the right hip, you will begin from a position of medial rotation. Rotate your right hip so that you pull the elastic resistance to the left. Note that your right thigh rotates, but it does not change location.

Repetitions: _____
Goal: _____
Precautions/Comments: _____
_____
_____

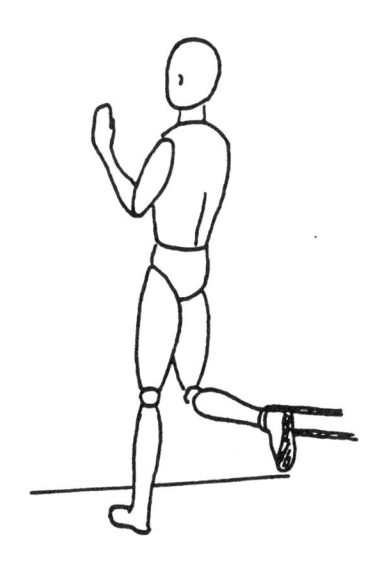

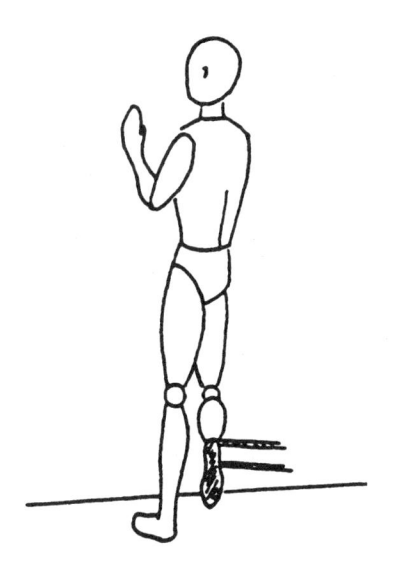

Exercise 28

Start/Finish **Movement**

Movement: Prone knee flexion
Target Muscles: Hamstrings
Instructions: Position yourself on the seat, lying on your stomach. Your kneecaps should not be in contact with the thigh pad. Slowly bend your knees, pulling the roller pad as close to your buttocks as possible. Concentrate on using both legs equally.

Repetitions: _____
Goal: _____
Precautions/Comments: _____

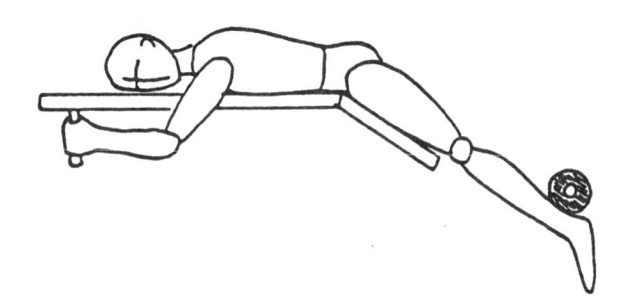

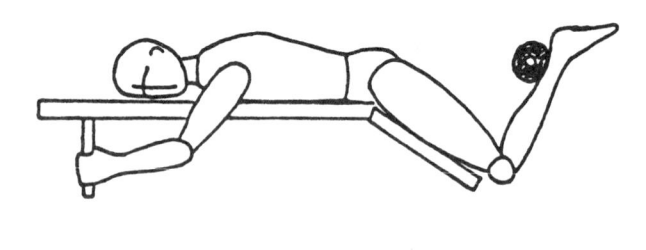

Exercise 29

Start/Finish **Movement**

Movement: Seated knee flexion
Target Muscles: Hamstrings
Instructions: Position yourself in the seat so that your knee joint is aligned with the axis about which the resistance arm rotates. You will begin with your knees extended and perform the movement by bending at your knees. Think of trying to touch your heels to your buttocks. Concentrate on using both legs equally.

Repetitions: _____
Goal: _____
Precautions/Comments: _____
_____
_____

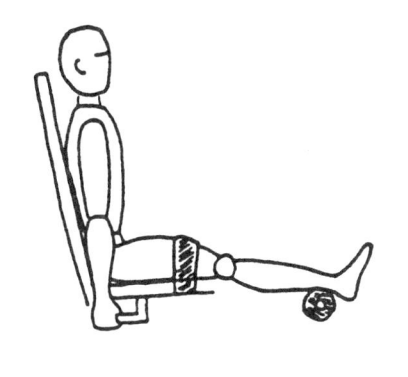

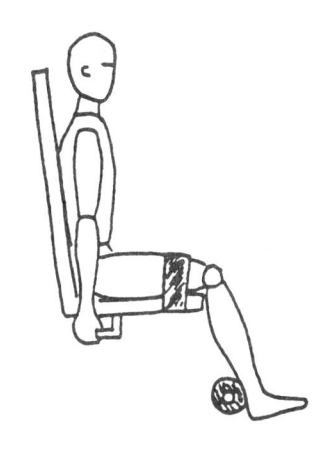

Exercise 30

Start/Finish   **Movement**

Movement: Standing knee flexion
Target Muscles: Hamstrings
Instructions: Stand with your thigh supported against the thigh pad. This is your Start/Finish position. Maintain your upper body and both thighs vertically throughout the movement. Adjust the thigh pad so that your kneecap does not contact the pad. Flex your knee, bringing your heel as close to your buttock as possible.

Repetitions: _____
Goal: _____
Precautions/Comments: _____
_____
_____
_____

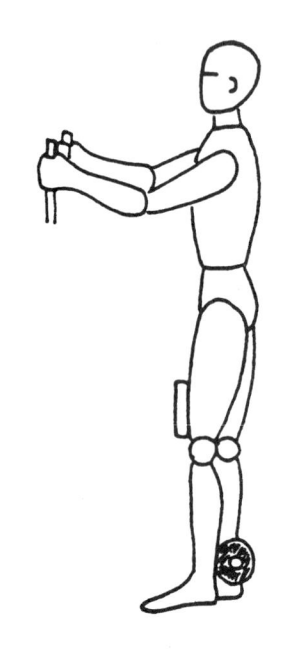

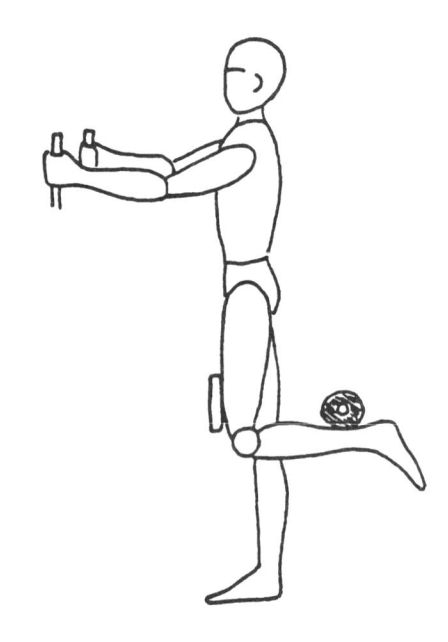

Exercise 31

Start/Finish **Movement**

Movement: Standing knee flexion with cuff weight
Target Muscles: Hamstrings
Instructions: Position yourself at the outside corner of two walls. Stand on a stable block (2 to 4 inches high). Use the wall to support yourself from falling backward and to support the thigh of the exercising lower extremity. Maintain your upper body and both thighs vertically throughout the movement. Keep the thigh of your exercising leg against the wall as you flex your knee fully.

Repetitions: _____
Goal: _____
Precautions/Comments: _____
_____
_____

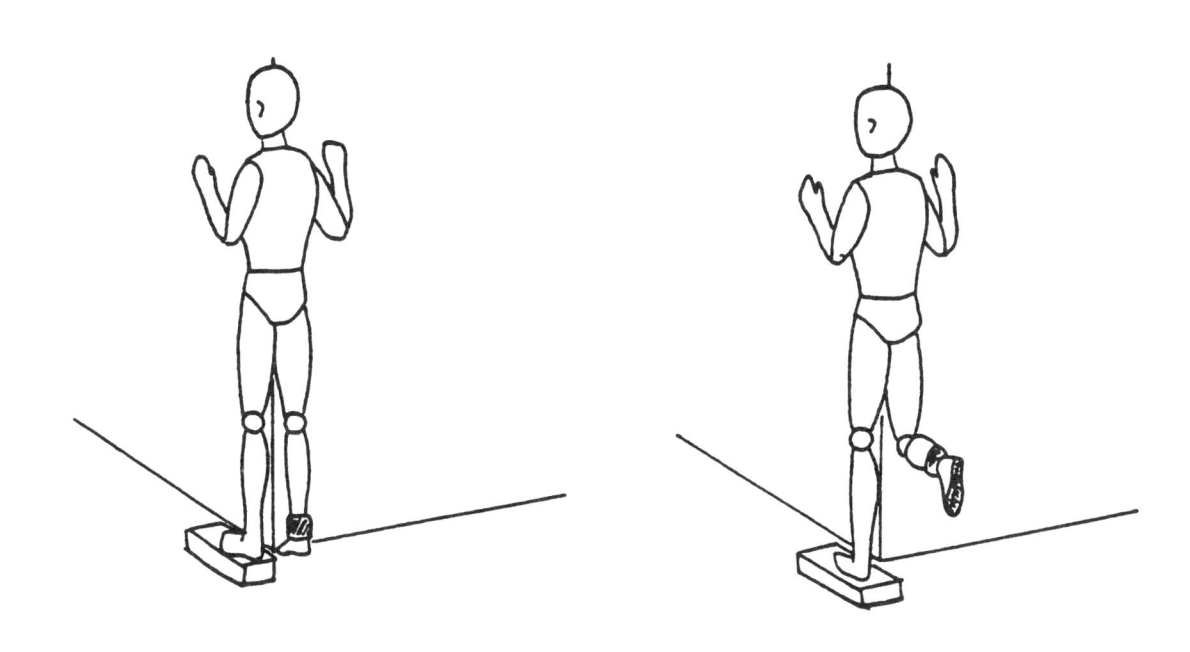

Exercise 32

Start/Finish **Movement**

Movement: Knee extension
Target Muscles: Quadriceps
Instructions: Position yourself on the seat with your knee joint aligned with the axis about which the resistance arm rotates. The Start/Finish position is with your knees at a right angle (90 degrees) or flexed just slightly past 90 degrees. Perform the movement by extending at the knees to 60 to 45 degrees of knee flexion. Think of this as moving from the Start/Finish position to between 1/3 and 1/2 the way to full extension. Exceeding this range unnecessarily increases patellofemoral pressure. The remaining part of the range is exercised with other movements such as the leg press.

Repetitions: _____
Goal: _____
Precautions/Comments: _____

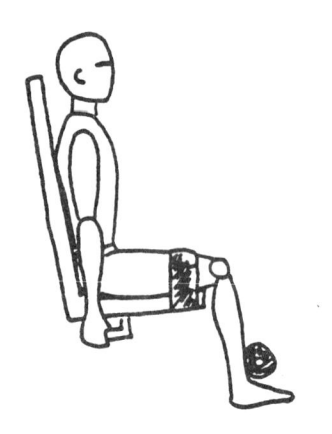

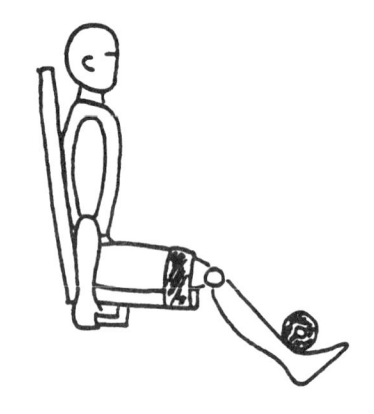

Exercise 33

Start/Finish   **Movement**

Movement: Heel raise with bodyweight/dumbbell
Target Muscles: Gastrocnemius
Instructions: Perform this movement while standing on a step to allow full range of motion. In the Start/Finish position, allow your heel to move below the level of the ball of your foot while concentrating on maintaining the arch in your foot. This will allow a full range movement without compromise to the arch. Raise up onto the ball of your foot as you fully extend the ankle. Like all other resistive movements, raise and lower slowly. Maintain the foot so that the toes are directed straight ahead rather than angled inward or outward.

Repetitions: _____
Goal: _____
Precautions/Comments: _____
_____
_____

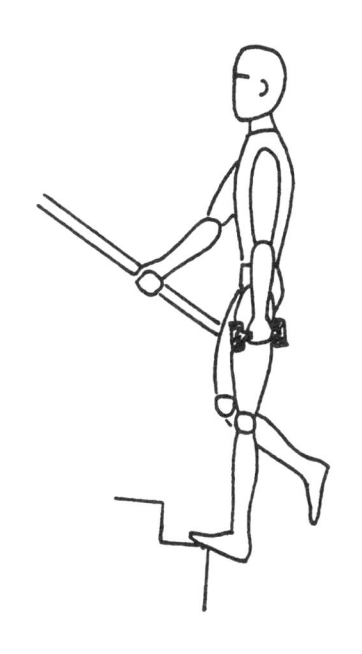

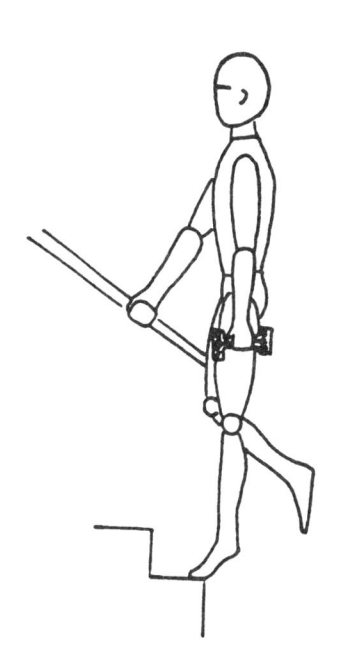

Exercise 34

Start/Finish **Movement**

Movement: Heel raise on leg press machine
Target Muscles: Gastrocnemius
Instructions: Concentrate on maintaining the arch in your feet as you allow the footplate to move toward you enough to allow a comfortable stretch behind the knees. Press the footplate by fully extending your ankles. Do not hyperextend the knees. Use each leg equally.

Repetitions: _____
Goal: _____
Precautions/Comments: _____
_____
_____
_____

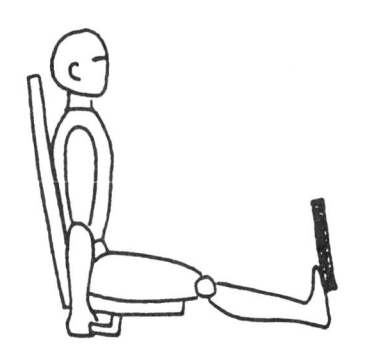

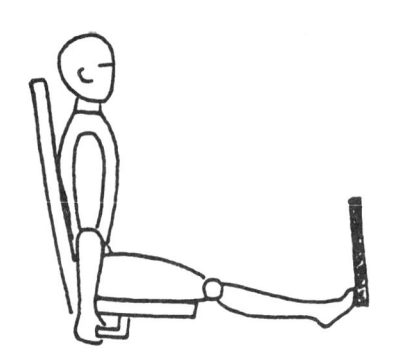

Exercise 35

Start/Finish   **Movement**

Movement: Seated heel raise
Target Muscles: Soleus
Instructions: Position yourself so that the balls of your feet are in contact with the footplate, and the thigh pad is at least six inches proximal to the kneecap. Concentrate on maintaining the arch in your feet as you allow the resistance to flex your ankles to the point of comfortable stretch. Lift the resistance by fully extending up onto the balls of your feet. Use each leg equally.

Repetitions: _____
Goal: _____
Precautions/Comments: _____
_____
_____

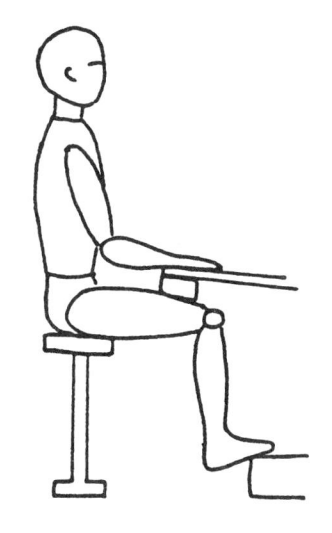

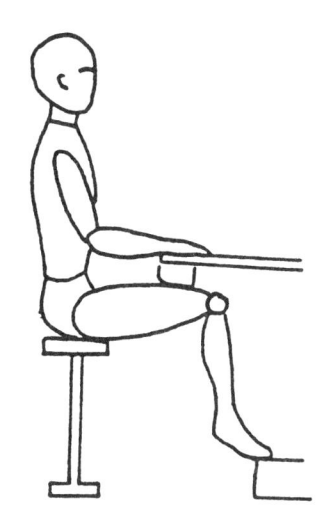

Exercise 36

Start/Finish   **Movement**

Movement: Ankle dorsiflexion with elastic band or tubing
Target Muscles: Tibialis anterior
Instructions: Attach the elastic band so that some tension remains even in the Start/Finish position. The band crosses over your foot just proximal to your toes. Flex your ankle as fully as possible, moving your toes toward your leg. Maintain your leg stationary. Allow the foot to extend *slowly* back to the Start/Finish position.

Repetitions: _____
Goal: _____
Precautions/Comments: _____
_____
_____

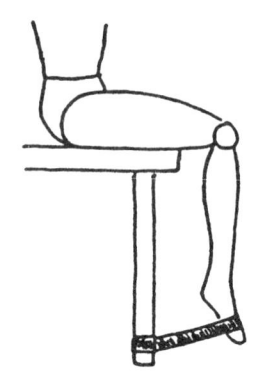

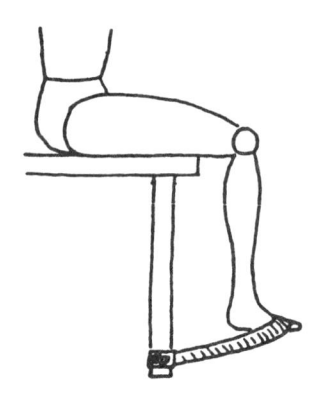

Copyright © 1997, Aspen Publishers, Inc.
Exercises for Health Promotion

Exercise 37

Start/Finish **Movement**

Movement: Ankle eversion with elastic band or tubing
Target Muscles: Peroneals
Instructions: Perform this movement from the seated position. A regular chair works fine. Tie the elastic at a length and position the chair such that there is tension even at the Start/Finish position. The elastic should contact your feet just proximal to your toes. Throughout the movement, hold your thighs and legs stationary. As you perform the movement, think of moving the big toes of each of your feet away from each other as far as possible. Move only the foot to isolate the evertors.

Repetitions: _____
Goal: _____
Precautions/Comments: _____
_____
_____
_____

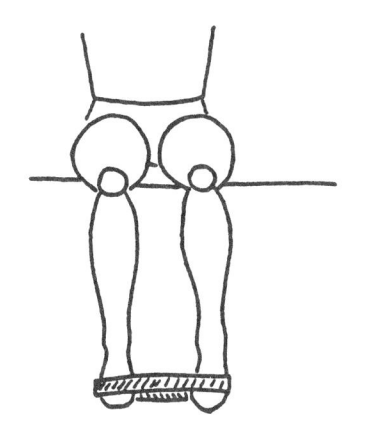

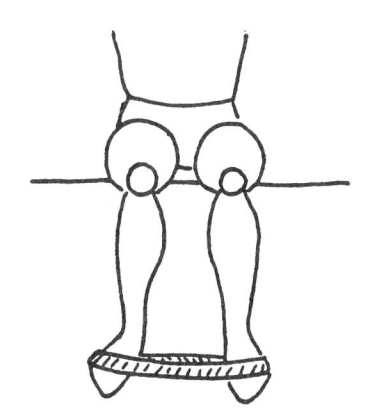

Exercise 38

Start/Finish   **Movement**

Movement: Ankle inversion with elastic tubing or resistance
Target Muscles: Tibialis posterior and anterior
Instructions: Perform this movement with one ankle at a time. Tie one end of your elastic tubing or band to a secure anchor, such as the leg of a bed or couch. Position your body in a sitting position so that as you move your left forefoot to the right, you will be moving against the resistance. Hold your thigh and leg stationary. Your foot is the only body part that moves.

Repetitions: _____
Goal: _____
Precautions/Comments: _____
_____
_____
_____

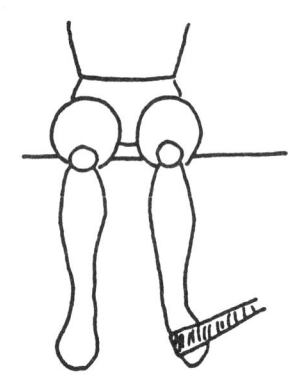

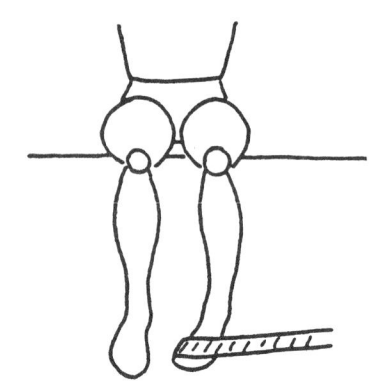

Exercise 39

Start/Finish **Movement**

Movement: Shoulder extension on lat row machine
Target Muscles: Latissimus dorsi, teres major
Instructions: Adjust the chest pad so that your chest is far enough away from the hand grips that in order to grasp both hand grips you must take one initially and pull it backward slightly to allow you to reach the other hand grip. This will allow full range movement, as the selected weight plates are lifted from the weight stack even in the starting positon. To perform the movement, think of pulling your elbows as far backward as possible. Maintain your upper body in erect posture. Do not shrug your shoulders upward. Keep them relaxed and downward as you move your elbows backward. Slowly lower the weight to a position of full stretch. When finished, carefully release one hand grip. This will allow you to turn your body slightly and lower the selected weight plates to the stack in a controlled, safe manner.

Repetitions: _____
Goal: _____
Precautions/Comments: _____
_____
_____
_____

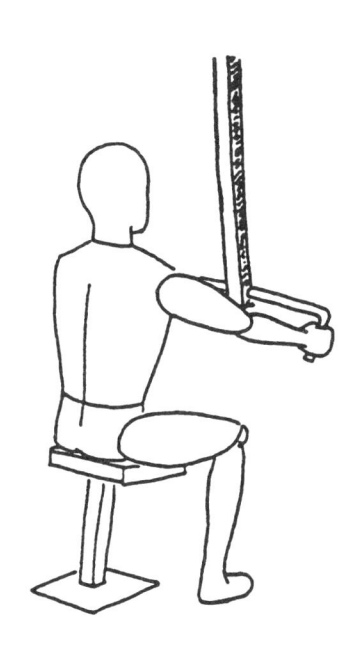

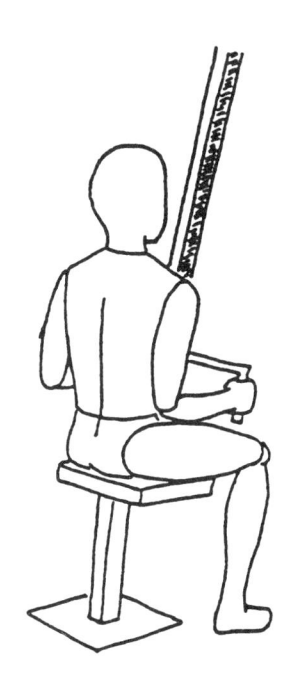

Exercise 40

Start/Finish   **Movement**

Movement: Pull up
Target Muscles: Latissimus dorsi, teres major, biceps
Instructions: Grasp the bar at shoulder width with an underhand (supinated) grip. Pull yourself upward until your chin is above the level of the bar, but not hooked over the bar. To achieve full contraction, think of pulling your elbows behind you. Lower fully to exercise your shoulder and elbow muscles through their full range of motion.

Repetitions: _____
Goal: _____
Precautions/Comments: _____
_____
_____

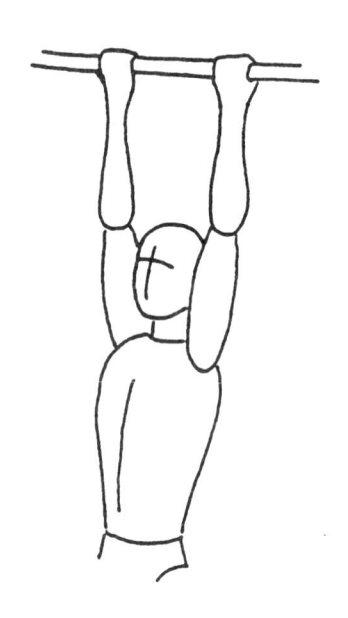

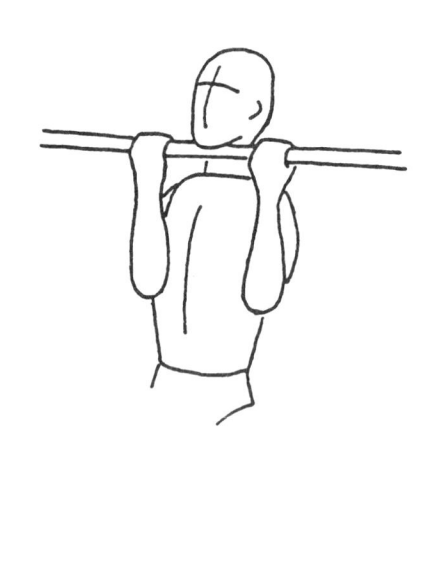

Exercise 41

Start/Finish **Movement**

Movement: Shoulder flexion
Target Muscles: Anterior deltoid
Instructions: Place your feet shoulder width apart with one foot staggered slightly forward to increase your stability. Maintain upright posture throughout the movement. Raise the weight forward until your arm is horizontal. You may alternate arms or raise both arms simultaneously. Movement takes place only at the shoulder joint. Do not swing the weight by invoking momentum from hip or back movement. Hand position is thumbs upward, knuckles outward.

Repetitions: _____
Goal: _____
Precautions/Comments: _____
_____
_____
_____

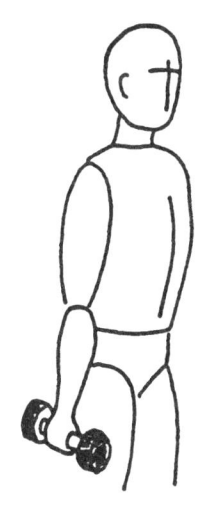

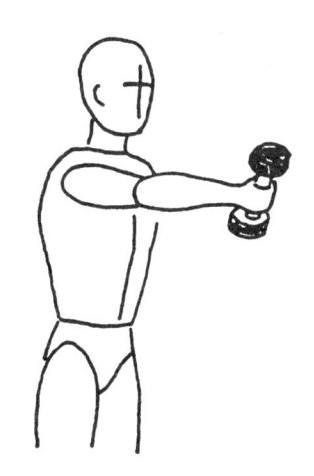

Exercise 42

Start/Finish **Movement**

Movement: Shoulder abduction
Target Muscles: Deltoid, rotator cuff muscles
Instructions: Place your feet shoulder width apart. Maintain upright posture throughout the movement. Raise the weights until your arms are horizontal. Concentrate on moving your arms out only to the sides. Do not let your arms drift forward as you fatigue. Move only at the shoulder. Do not swing the weight by using your legs or back.

Repetitions: _____
Goal: _____
Precautions/Comments: _____
_____
_____

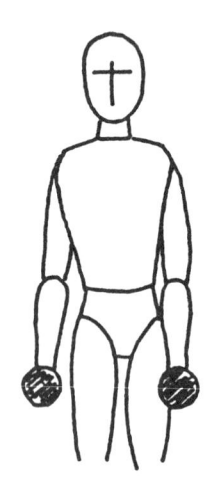

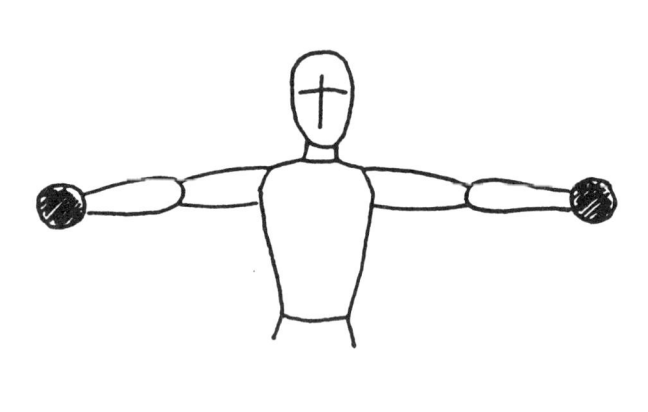

Exercise 43

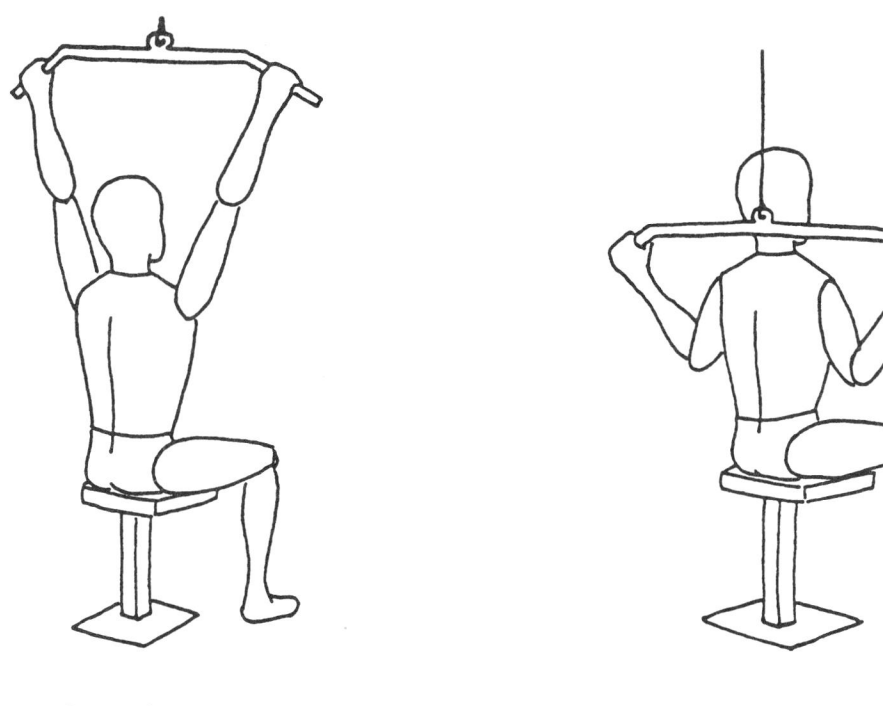

Start/Finish **Movement**

Movement: Shoulder adduction on lat pulldown machine
Target Muscles: Latissimus dorsi, pectoralis major
Instructions: Select the desired resistance. Grasp the bar at a comfortable width. Adjust the height of the seat so that as you carefully sit down on the seat and place your distal thighs under the thigh pad, you pull the selected plates slightly (1 to 2 inches) from the rest of the weight stack. This will allow you to achieve a full stretch and exercise through the full range of motion. From this starting position, pull the bar downward while maintaining erect posture with your upper body. Do not allow your torso to lean backward. Concentrate on pulling your elbows all the way to your ribs. You may pull the bar either in front of or behind your head, whichever is most comfortable.

Repetitions: ___
Goal: ___
Precautions/Comments: ___

Exercise 44

Start/Finish **Movement**

Movement: Pull up with wide, pronated grip
Target Muscles: Latissimus dorsi, pectoralis major
Instructions: Grasp the bar with an overhand (pronated) grip. Each hand will grip the bar approximately six inches wider than shoulder width. Pull yourself upward until your chin is above the level of the bar, but not hooked over the bar. To achieve full contraction, think of pulling your elbows toward your ribs. Lower fully to exercise your shoulder and elbow muscles through their full range of motion.

Repetitions: _____
Goal: _____
Precautions/Comments: _____
_____
_____
_____

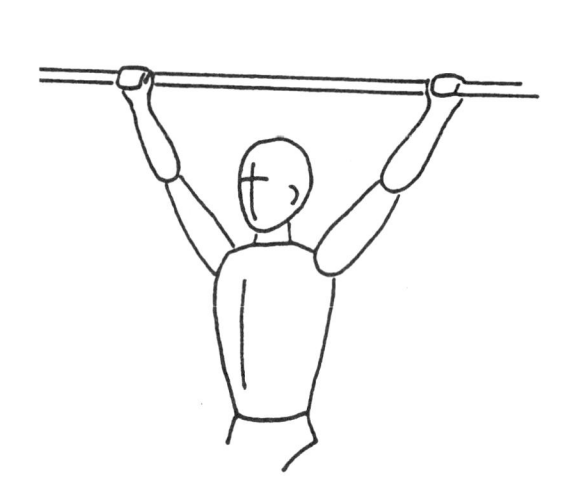

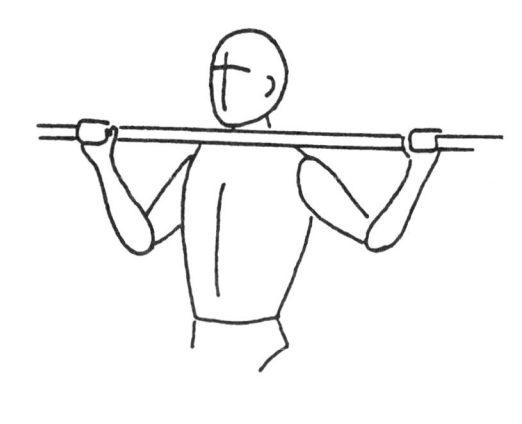

Copyright © 1997, Aspen Publishers, Inc.
Exercises for Health Promotion

Exercise 45

Start/Finish **Movement**

Movement: Supraspinatus raise
Target Muscles: Supraspinatus
Instructions: Rotate your shoulders so that your bicep is anterior. This position is called lateral shoulder rotation. You will raise your arms not to the side or to the front, but at an angle halfway between side and front (45 degrees anterior to the frontal plane). Elevate your arms to slightly (approximately 20 degrees) above horizontal. All movement occurs at the shoulder joint. Do not use your legs or back to swing the weight. Hand position is thumbs up.

Repetitions: _____
Goal: _____
Precautions/Comments: _____
_____
_____
_____

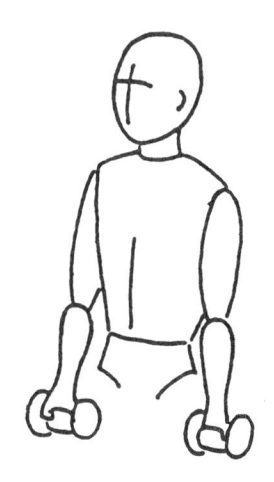

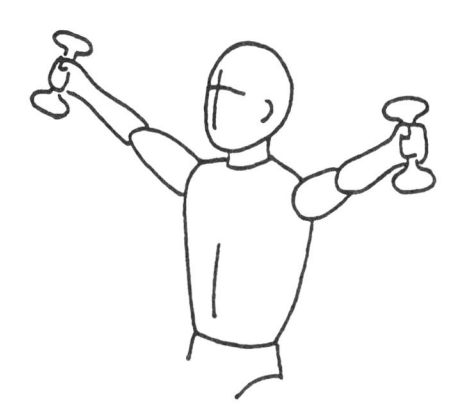

Exercise 46

Start/Finish **Movement**

Movement: Shoulder transverse adduction on chest fly machine
Target Muscles: Pectoralis major
Instructions: Adjust the seat so that your arms contact the pads with your arms horizontal and your forearms vertical. Move the pads together until they touch. Use both arms equally. As you complete the movement, concentrate on trying to touch your elbows together rather than internally rotating the shoulders or flexing at your wrists.

Repetitions: _____
Goal: _____
Precautions/Comments: _____
_____
_____

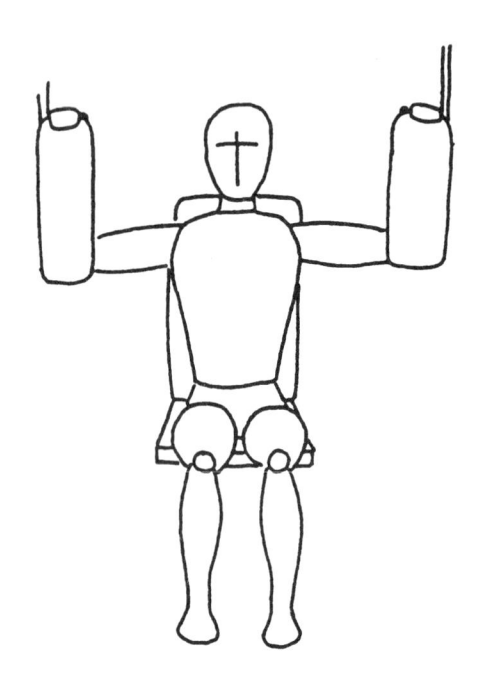

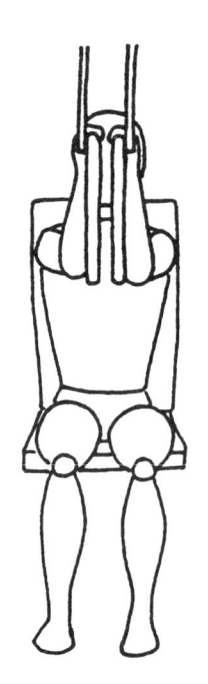

Exercise 47

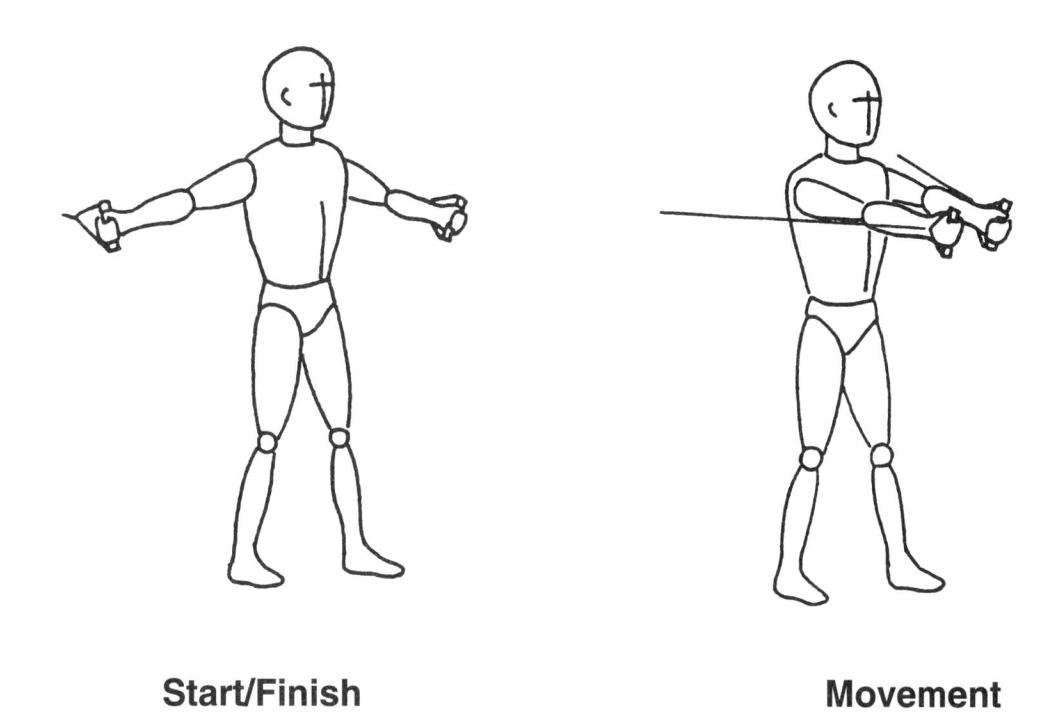

Start/Finish   **Movement**

Movement: Shoulder transverse adduction with pulleys/cables
Target Muscles: Pectoralis major
Instructions: Perform this movement in a standing position with your feet slightly wider than shoulder width. Stagger one foot slightly in front of the other to increase your stability. After selecting your resistance, begin with your arms to your sides and positioned horizontally. To exercise through the full range of motion, position yourself so the selected weight is slightly elevated (1 to 2 inches) from the rest of the weight stack in the Start/Finish position. While keeping your arms horizontal and your elbows straight, touch your hands together in front of your body. Stand up straight throughout the movement. Movement should take place only at the shoulder.

Repetitions: _____
Goal: _____
Precautions/Comments: _____
_____
_____

Exercise 48

Start/Finish **Movement**

Movement: Dumbbell bench press
Target Muscles: Pectoralis major, anterior deltoid, tricep
Instructions: To perform this movement, you must have a spotter carefully hand you the dumbbells, one at a time, as you lay on your back on a weight bench. From the Start/Finish position of comfortable stretch, raise the dumbbells vertically. Do not rotate the dumbbells as you raise them. Your spotter must maintain her or his hands loosely around your wrists throughout each repetition so assistance may be provided quickly if needed. Communication between you and your spotter is crucial throughout the exercise to ensure safety. When you have finished exercising, hold the dumbbells close to your body. The spotter then transfers the dumbbells carefully to the floor, one at a time. Immediately return the dumbbells to their place in the rack.

Repetitions: _____
Goal: _____
Precautions/Comments: _____
_____
_____

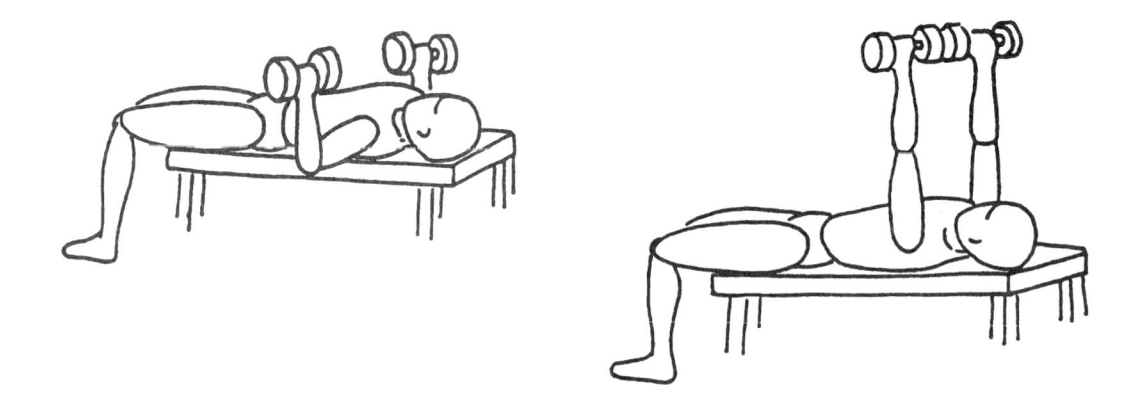

Exercise 49

Start/Finish **Movement**

Movement: Dumbbell incline press
Target Muscles: Pectoralis major, anterior deltoid, tricep
Instructions: To perform this movement, you must have a spotter carefully hand you the dumbbells, one at a time, as you lay on an adjustable bench set at approximately 45 degrees of inclination. From the Start/Finish position of comfortable stretch, raise the dumbbells vertically. Do not rotate the dumbbells as you raise them. Your spotter must maintain her or his hands loosely around your wrists throughout each repetition so assistance may be given quickly if needed. Communication between you and your spotter is crucial throughout the exercise to ensure safety. When you have finished exercising, hold the dumbbells close to your body. The spotter then transfers the dumbbells carefully to the floor, one at a time. Immediately return the dumbbells to their place in the rack.

Repetitions: _____
Goal: _____
Precautions/Comments: _____
_____
_____
_____

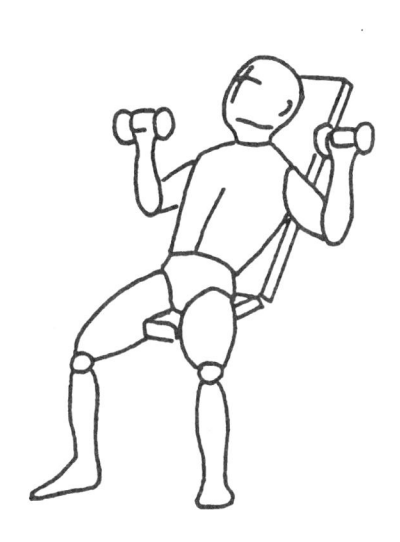

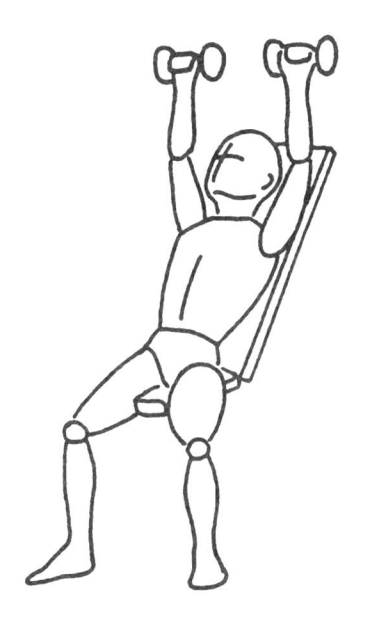

Exercise 50

Start/Finish   **Movement**

Movement: Bench press
Target Muscles: Pectoralis major, anterior deltoid, triceps
Instructions: Due to the number of spotters and learning time required to perform the barbell bench press movement safely, an alternative shoulder transverse adduction movement may be more practical. If you desire to perform this movement, secure extensive instructions in correct, safe performance and spotting prior to initiating the movement. Until correct technique is learned, the movement is practiced with the bar only. Subsequently, weight plates may be added.

Repetitions: _____
Goal: _____
Precautions/Comments: _____
_____
_____

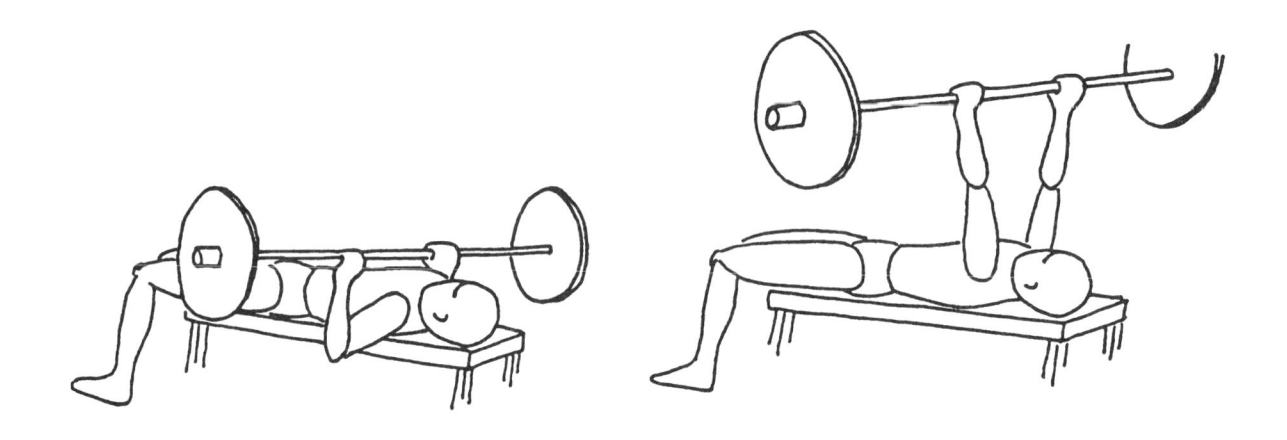

Exercise 51

Start/Finish **Movement**

Movement: Push up
Target Muscles: Pectoralis major, anterior deltoid, triceps
Instructions: Place your hands slightly wider than shoulder width. While maintaining straight alignment of legs, thighs, and trunk, lower your chest toward the floor. Press against the floor to return to the Start/Finish position. Avoid arching your back.

Repetitions: _____
Goal: _____
Precautions/Comments: _____
_____
_____

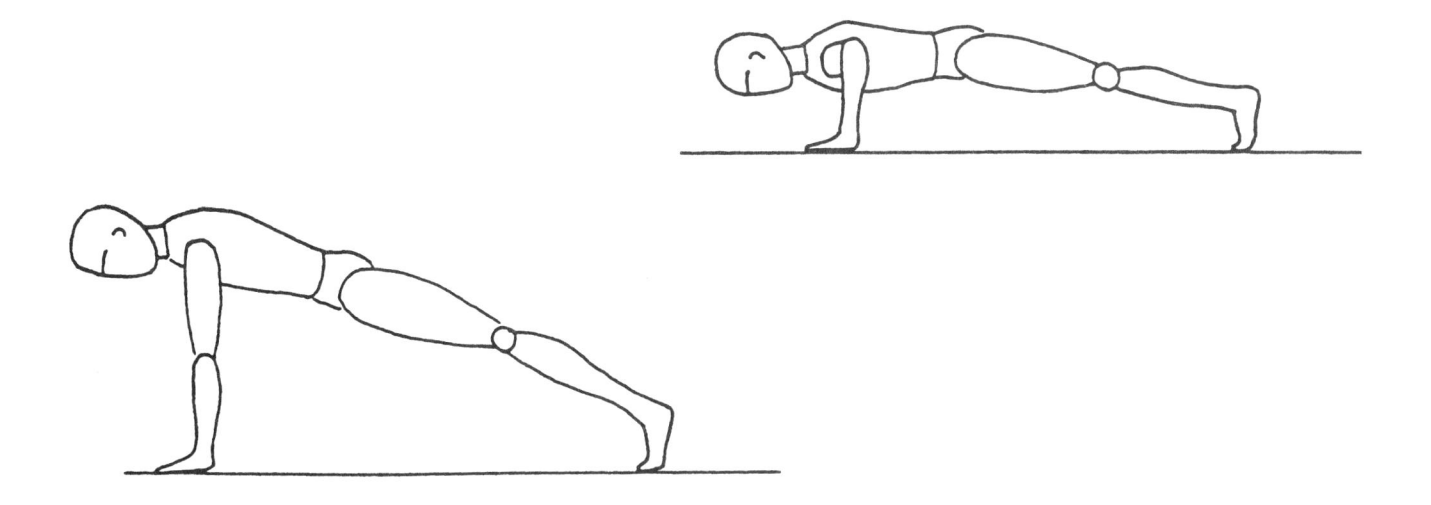

Exercise 52

Start/Finish **Movement**

Movement: Shoulder transverse abduction
Target Muscles: Posterior deltoid
Instructions: During this movement you will use the back support pad of an adjustable bench set at approximately 45 degrees. Before beginning, always check to make sure the back support pad is locked securely in position. With the dumbbells in your hands, bend your knees as you carefully lower your chest to the top of the back support pad. This is the Start/Finish position. To perform the movement, raise the dumbbells vertically. Maintain elbows extended, so movement occurs only at the shoulder. Although your arms may want to drift toward your hips, particularly as you fatigue, maintain arm movement at 90 degrees from your torso. At alternate sessions, perform this movement with knuckles upward (shoulder neutral) and with knuckles facing backward (lateral shoulder rotation).

Repetitions: _____
Goal: _____
Precautions/Comments: _____
_____
_____

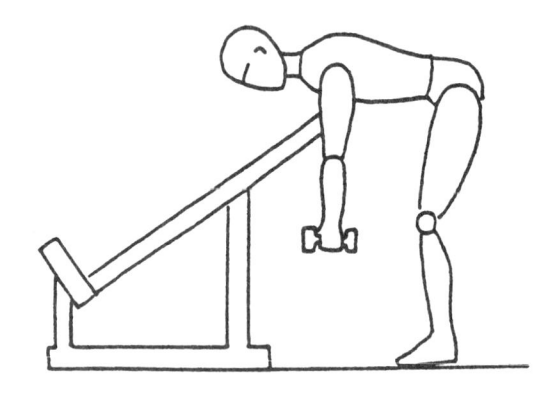

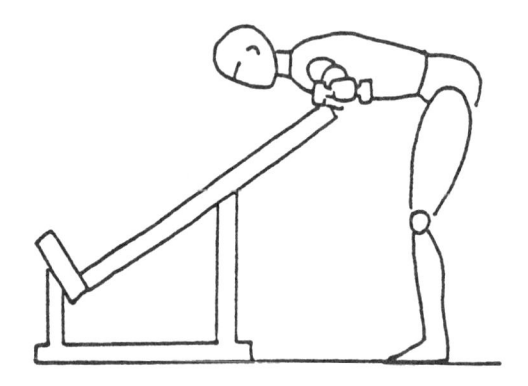

Exercise 53

Start/Finish **Movement**

Movement: Shoulder elevation
Target Muscles: Trapezius, levator scapulae
Instructions: Begin this movement by standing with dumbbells in your hands. Slightly flex your knees—just enough so they do not feel locked in extension. This is your Start/Finish position. From this point on, the only movement takes place at your shoulders. Do not use leg or back movement to elevate the weight. Elevate your shoulders straight upward as if performing a shrug. Think of trying to touch your ears with your shoulders. Maintain vertical stance. Slowly lower and repeat.

Repetitions: _____
Goal: _____
Precautions/Comments: _____
_____
_____

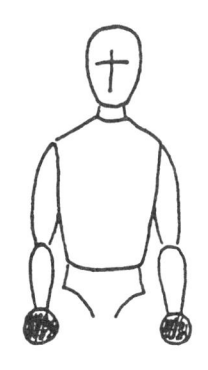

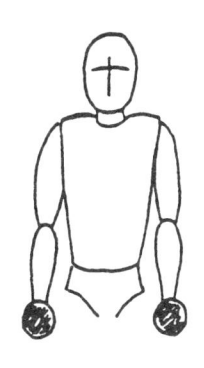

Exercise 54

Start/Finish   **Movement**

Movement: Shoulder depression using overhead bar
Target Muscles: Pectoralis minor, latissimus dorsi
Instructions: Begin this movement from a hanging position on the bar. Hand placement is approximately shoulder width. This is a short arc movement (even in performing the movement correctly you will not feel like you are moving very much). The movement is performed by moving your shoulders directly downward. You will feel your body elevate about an inch as you perform the movement correctly. To help visualize this movement, think of it as the opposite of shrugging your shoulders upward.

Repetitions: _____
Goal: _____
Precautions/Comments: _____
_____
_____

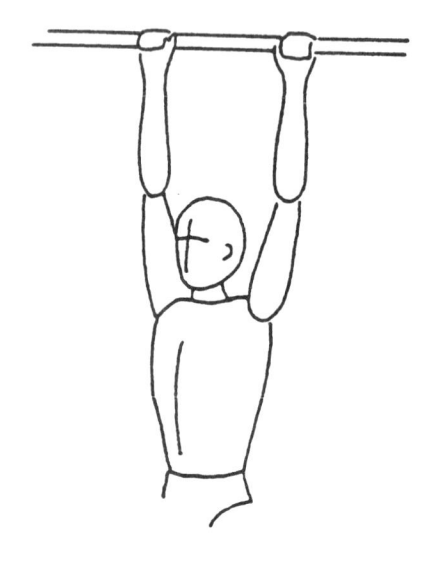

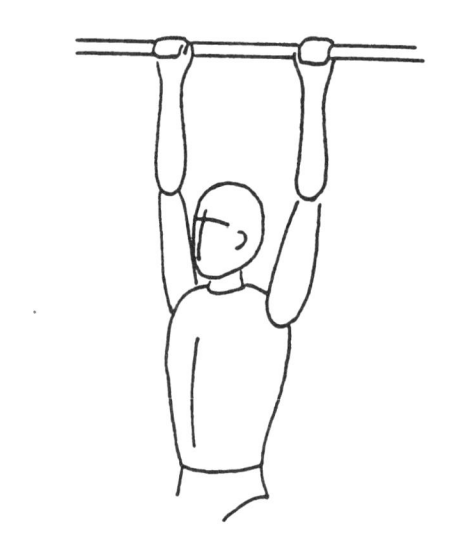

Exercise 55

Start/Finish **Movement**

Movement: Shoulder depression using dip bars
Target Muscles: Pectoralis minor, latissimus dorsi
Instructions: Begin this movement on the bars of the dip station with elbows straight. This is a short arc movement (even in performing the movement correctly you will not feel like you are moving very much). The movement is performed by moving your shoulders directly downward. You will feel your body elevate about an inch as you perform the movement correctly. To help you visualize this movement, think of it as the opposite of shrugging your shoulders upward. Remember to maintain elbows extended throughout the performance of this exercise.

Repetitions: _____
Goal: _____
Precautions/Comments: _____
_____
_____

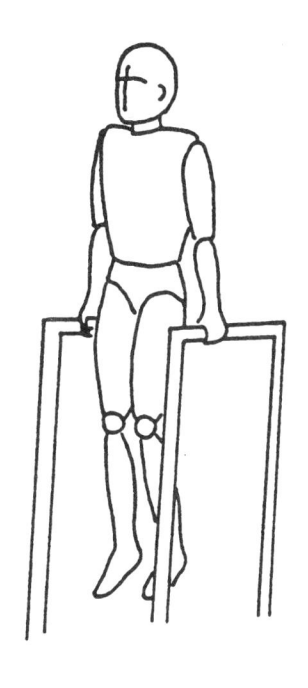

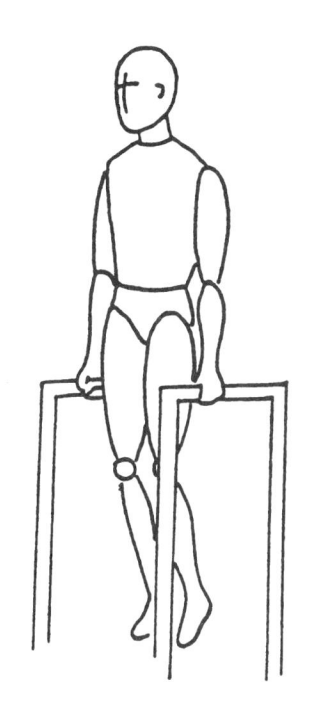

Exercise 56

Start/Finish **Movement**

Movement: Shoulder depression using weight bench
Target Muscles: Pectoralis minor, latissimus dorsi
Instructions: Begin this movement on the weight bench with elbows straight. This is a short arc movement (even in performing the movement correctly you will not feel like you are moving very much). The movement is performed by moving your shoulders directly downward. You will feel your body elevate about an inch as you perform the movement correctly. Your elbows should remain straight throughout this movement. Lower slowly to the Start/Finish position. To help you visualize this movement, think of it as the opposite of shrugging your shoulders upward.

Repetitions: _____
Goal: _____
Precautions/Comments: _____
_____
_____

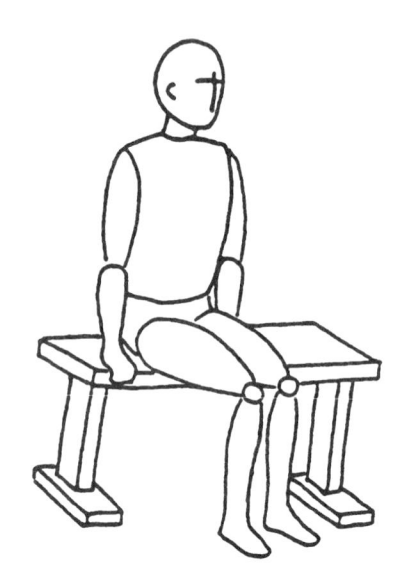

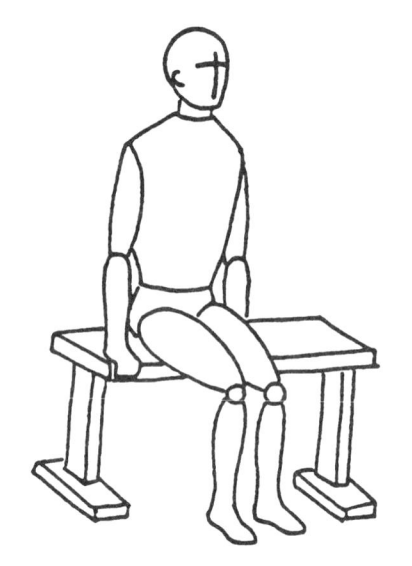

Exercise 57

Start/Finish **Movement**

Movement: Scapular protraction
Target Muscles: Serratus anterior
Instructions: To perform this movement, you must have a spotter carefully hand you the dumbbells, one at a time, as you lay on your back on a weight bench. Raise the dumbbells vertically with elbows extended. This is the Start/Finish position. This is a short arc movement (even in performing the movement correctly you will not feel like you are moving very much). Move the dumbbells vertically by protracting your shoulders. Your elbows remain extended throughout the set. To help visualize this movement, think of stretching toward an object that is just slightly out of reach. Do not arch with your back or neck. The dumbbells should rise about an inch if you are performing the movement correctly. Slowly lower the dumbbells back to the Start/Finish position. Your spotter must maintain her or his hands loosely around your wrists throughout each repetition so assistance may be given quickly if needed. Communication between you and your spotter is crucial throughout the exercise to ensure safety. When you have finished exercising, hold the dumbbells close to your body. The spotter then transfers the dumbbells carefully to the floor, one at a time. Immediately return the dumbbells to their place in the rack.

Repetitions: _____
Goal: _____
Precautions/Comments: _____
_____
_____

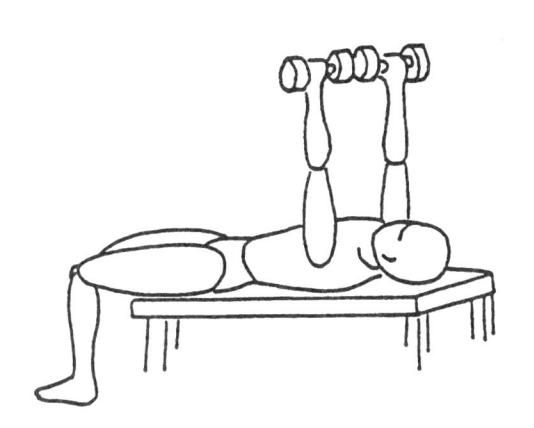

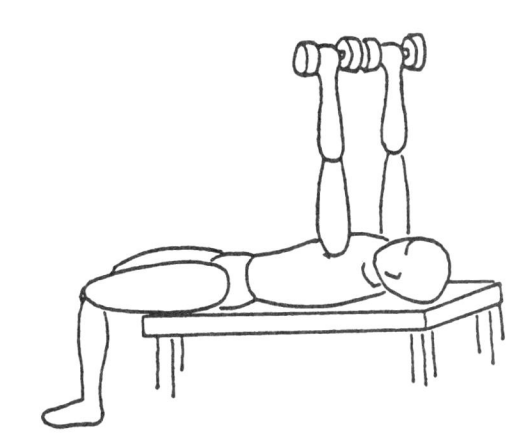

Exercise 58

Start/Finish **Movement**

Movement: Scapular retraction using lat rowing machine
Target Muscles: Middle trapezius, rhomboids
Instructions: Adjust the chest pad so that your chest is far enough away from the hand grips that in order to grasp both hand grips you must take one initially and pull it backward slightly to allow you to reach the other hand grip. This will allow full range movement as the selected weight plates are elevated from the weight stack even in the Start/Finish position. This is a short arc movement (even in performing the movement correctly you will not feel like you are moving very much). To perform the movement, retract your shoulders fully while maintaining elbow extension. Think of touching your shoulder blades together behind your back. Maintain your upper body in erect posture. When finished exercising, carefully release one hand grip. This will allow you to turn your body slightly and lower the selected weight plates to the stack in a controlled, safe manner.

Repetitions: _____
Goal: _____
Precautions/Comments: _____
_____
_____
_____

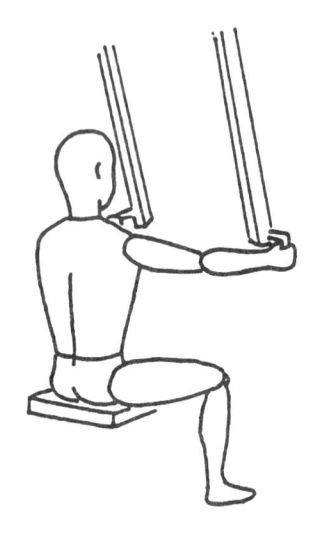

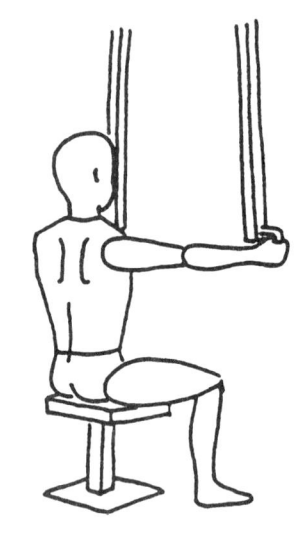

Exercise 59

Start/Finish **Movement**

Movement: Combined scapular retraction and shoulder elevation
Target Muscles: Middle trapezius, rhomboids
Instructions: Before you begin, secure an adjustable bench at an angle of approximately 45 degrees. Position yourself on the seat pad with your chest supported by the back support pad. Place your feet on the floor slightly wider than shoulder width. At this point ask your partner to hand you the dumbbells, one at a time. This is the Start/Finish position. This is a short arc movement (even in performing the movement correctly you will not feel like you are moving very much). To perform the movement, move your shoulders vertically while maintaining elbow extension. To visualize this movement, think of moving your shoulders toward the ceiling. When the exercise is completed, your spotter should transfer the dumbbells carefully to the floor, one at a time. Immediately return the dumbbells to their place in the rack.

Repetitions: _____
Goal: _____
Precautions/Comments: _____

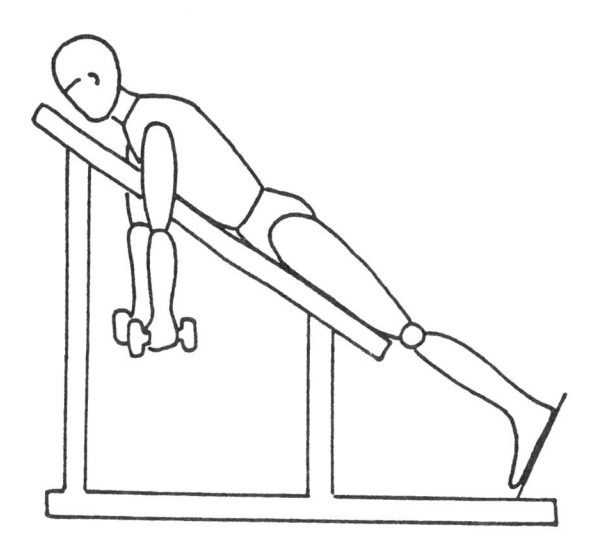

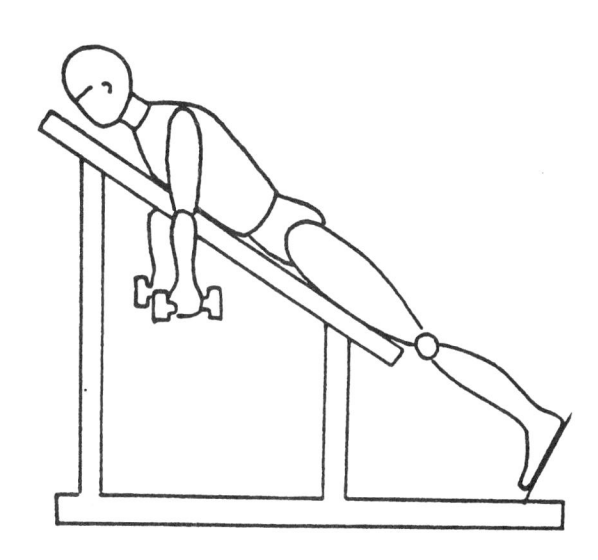

Exercise 60

Start/Finish **Movement**

Movement: Shoulder medial rotation with dumbbell
Target Muscles: Subscapularis, pectoralis major, latissimus dorsi, teres major
Instructions: To exercise the medial rotators of your left shoulder, assume a left side-lying position on a weight bench. Position your left elbow at a 90 degree angle. Hold your left elbow 4 to 6 inches from the side of your rib cage. You will maintain this elbow position throughout the movement. Gently lower the dumbbell until you feel a comfortable stretch in your left shoulder, but do not overstretch. This is your Start/Finish position. Rotating at the shoulder, bring the dumbbell upward until your forearm contacts your torso. Slowly return to the Start/Finish position. Reverse body position to address medial rotators of right shoulder.

Repetitions: _____
Goal: _____
Precautions/Comments: _____

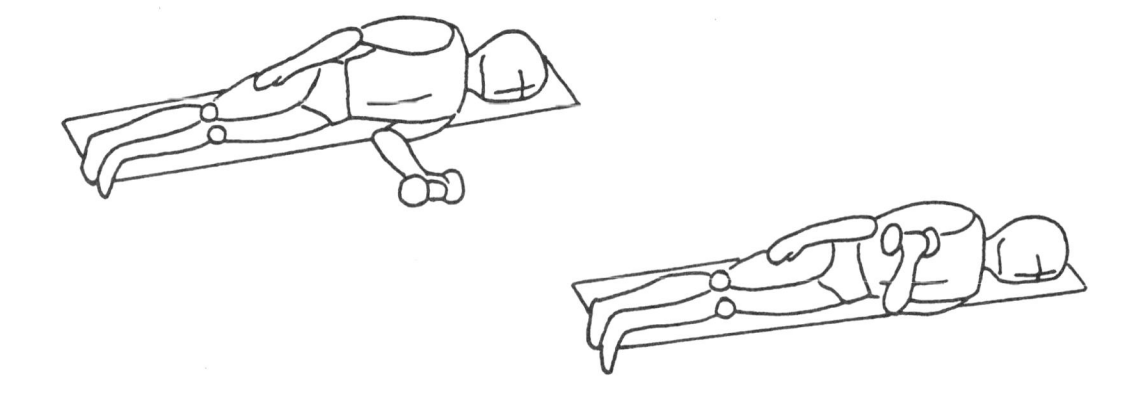

_____
_____
_____

Exercise 61

Start/Finish **Movement**

Movement: Shoulder medial rotation with elastic or cable resistance
Target Muscles: Subscapularis, pectoralis major, latissimus dorsi, teres major
Instructions: Stand upright with your right elbow flexed to 90 degrees and held approximately 4 to 6 inches from the side of your rib cage. Allow the resistance to pull your hand outward to the point of comfortable stretch. This is the Start/Finish position. Maintain your elbow in 90 degrees of flexion throughout the movement. Pull the resistance, bringing your forearm across to contact the front of your torso. Concentrate on rotating at your shoulder only. Slowly return to the Start/Finish position. Reverse body position to exercise your left shoulder.

Repetitions: _____
Goal: _____
Precautions/Comments: _____

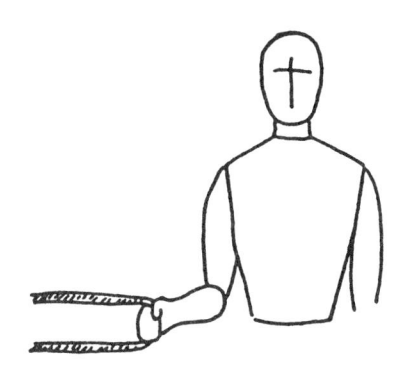

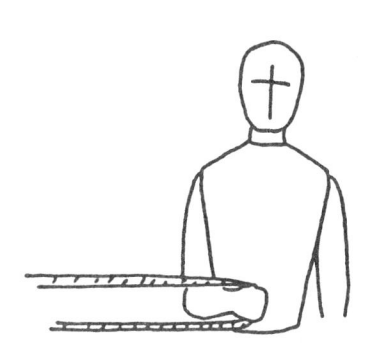

Exercise 62

Start/Finish   **Movement**

Movement: Shoulder lateral rotation with dumbbell
Target Muscles: Infraspinatus, teres minor
Instructions: To exercise the lateral rotators of your right shoulder, assume a left side-lying position on a weight bench. Position your right elbow 4 to 6 inches from the right side of your rib cage, in 90 degrees of flexion. Stagger your feet slightly to stabilize your body on the bench. Lower the weight to allow your right forearm to contact the front of your torso. This is the Start/Finish position. To elevate the dumbbell, rotate only at your right shoulder. Elevate the weight as high as you can while maintaining the elbow in the position described above. Reverse body position to address lateral rotators of left shoulder.

Repetitions: _____
Goal: _____
Precautions/Comments: _____
_____
_____
_____

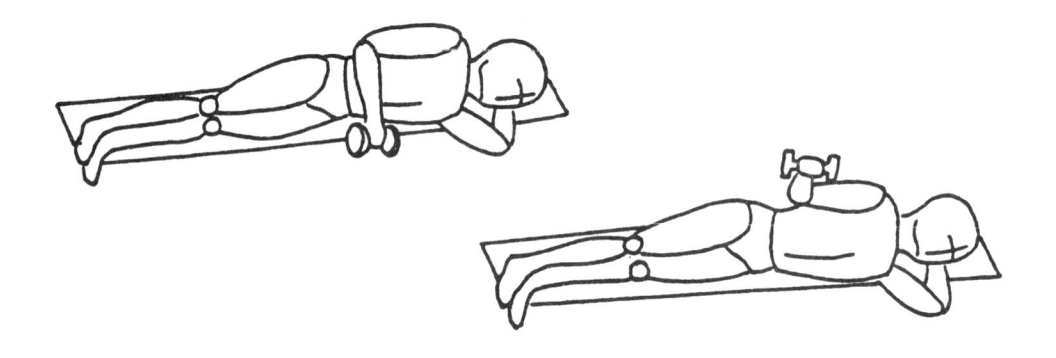

Exercise 63

Start/Finish **Movement**

Movement: Shoulder lateral rotation with elastic or cable
Target Muscles: Infraspinatus, teres minor
Instructions: To exercise the lateral rotators of your right shoulder, stand upright with your right elbow flexed to 90 degrees and positioned approximately 4 to 6 inches from the right side of your rib cage. Maintain this elbow position throughout the movement. Allow the resistance to pull your hand across the front of your body until your forearm contacts your torso. This is the Start/Finish position. Rotate only your right shoulder to pull your hand to the right against the resistance. Slowly return to the Start/Finish position. Reverse body position to exercise your left shoulder.

Repetitions: _____
Goal: _____
Precautions/Comments: _____

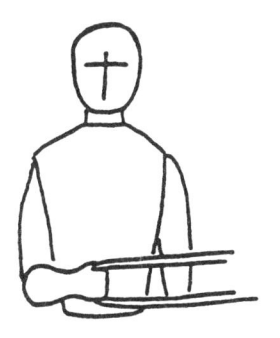

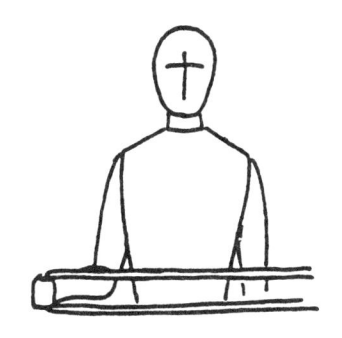

Exercise 64

Start/Finish   **Movement**

Movement: Elbow flexion with dumbbells
Target Muscles: Biceps, brachialis
Instructions: Place your feet at shoulder width with one foot slightly in front of the other to increase your base of stability. With dumbbells in hands, let your elbows slowly extend until you feel a comfortable stretch in your arms. This is the Start/Finish position. Maintain your elbows in contact with your torso. Flex your elbows fully bringing the dumbbells to your shoulders. Concentrate on keeping your arms vertical and stationary. Only your forearms should move. Maintain erect posture throughout the movement. Avoid swinging the weight with momentum generated by leg or back movement.

Repetitions: _____
Goal: _____
Precautions/Comments: _____
_____
_____
_____

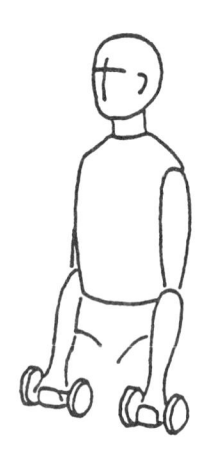

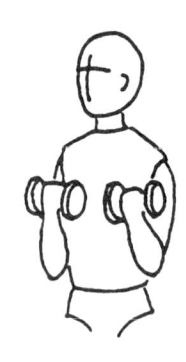

Exercise 65

Start/Finish **Movement**

Movement: Elbow flexion on machine
Target Muscles: Biceps, brachialis
Instructions: Adjust the seat height so that the arm pad provides support to the back of your entire upper arms. Your elbows should extend just off the pad. After selecting your resistance, grasp the handles. Your seat height should be such that when you have grasped the handles your elbows are extended, but not uncomfortably so. Do not hyperextend the elbows. This is the Start/Finish position. To perform the movement, bring your hands to your shoulders bending only at the elbows. Keep your upper arms supported on the pad. Maintain erect posture throughout the movement. As you fatigue, you may be tempted to increase movement speed, but you should maintain slow, controlled movements.

Repetitions: _____
Goal: _____
Precautions/Comments: _____

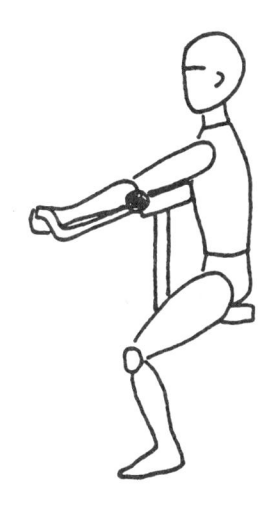

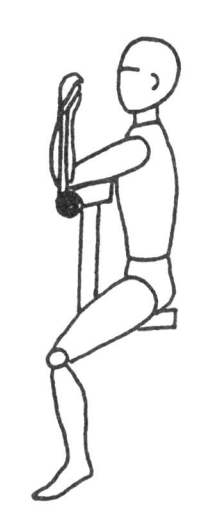

Exercise 66

Start/Finish **Movement**

Movement: Pronated elbow flexion
Target Muscles: Biceps, brachialis, brachioradialis
Instructions: Place your feet at shoulder width, with one foot slightly in front of the other to increase your base of stability. Your hand placement on the bar is at approximately shoulder width with an overhand grip (pronation). Let your elbows slowly extend until you feel a comfortable stretch in your arms. This is the Start/Finish position. Maintain your elbows in contact with your torso throughout the movement. Flex your elbows fully, bringing the bar to your shoulders. Concentrate on keeping your arms vertical and stationary. Only your forearms should move. Maintain erect posture throughout the movement. Avoid swinging the weight with leg or back movement. As you fatigue you may be tempted to increase movement speed, but maintain slow, controlled movements.

Repetitions: _____
Goal: _____
Precautions/Comments: _____
_____
_____

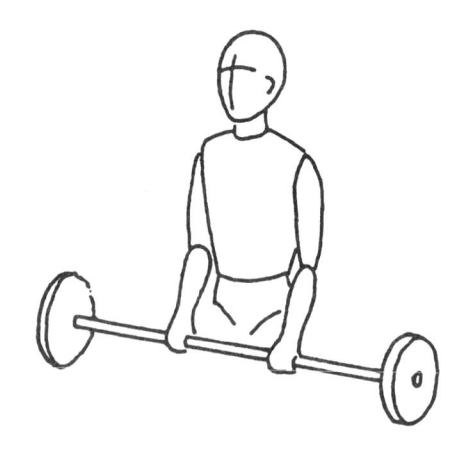

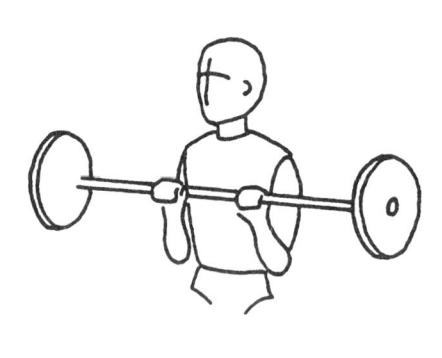

Exercise 67

Start/Finish   **Movement**

Movement: Elbow extension on machine
Target Muscles: Triceps
Instructions: Adjust the seat height so that the arm pad provides support to the backs of your upper arms. Your elbows should extend just off the pad. After selecting your resistance, grasp the handles. Your seat height should be such that when you have grasped the handles your elbows are flexed, placing a comfortable stretch on your triceps. This is the Start/Finish position. To perform the movement, fully extend your elbows. Keep your upper arms supported on the pad. Maintain erect posture throughout the movement.

Repetitions: _____
Goal: _____
Precautions/Comments: _____
_____
_____

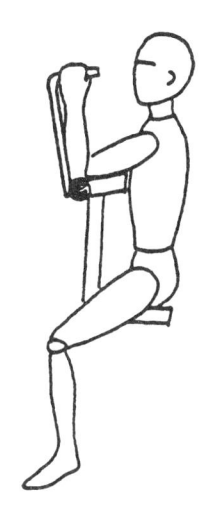

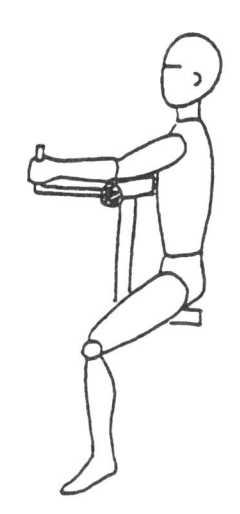

Exercise 68

Start/Finish **Movement**

Movement: Elbow extension with dumbbell
Target Muscles: Triceps
Instructions: With a suitable dumbbell in your left hand, begin by sitting on an exercise bench. Slowly and carefully ease yourself back so you are lying on the bench. Use your right hand to support your left arm vertically. This is the Start/Finish position. Raise the dumbbell toward the ceiling by extending your elbow. Only your forearm, not your upper arm, moves during this exercise.

Repetitions: _____
Goal: _____
Precautions/Comments: _____
_____
_____

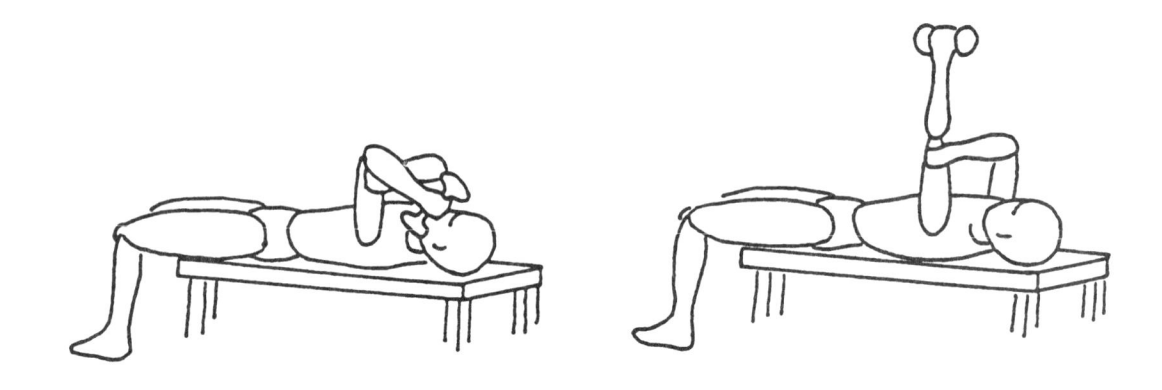

Exercise 69

Start/Finish   **Movement**

Movement: Forearm supination and pronation with dumbbell
Target Muscles: Pronator quadratus, pronator teres biceps, supinator
Instructions: For supination, grasp a dumbbell firmly at one end rather than at the dumbbell handle. Perform this movement from a seated position with your elbow supported on your distal thigh, your wrist extending just in front of your knee. Rotate at the elbow so your palm is downward. This is the Start/Finish position. To perform the movement, slowly rotate your forearm from palm down to palm up. Grasp the end of the dumbbell firmly so you will be able to control its descent. Slowly return to the palm down position. Now reverse the movement to perform pronation.

Repetitions: _____
Goal: _____
Precautions/Comments: _____
_____
_____
_____

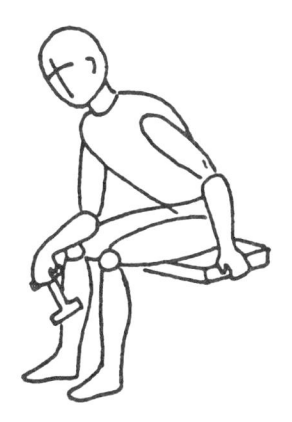

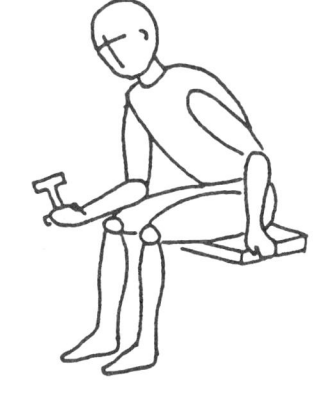

Exercise 70

Start/Finish　　　　　　　　　　　　**Movement**

Movement: Wrist flexion with bar or dumbbells
Target Muscles: Flexor carpi radialis and ulnaris
Instructions: Perform this movement from a seated position with your forearms resting on your thighs. Your grasp is underhand (supination) and hand spacing is approximately shoulder width. Lower the bar by allowing your wrists to extend until you feel a comfortable stretch. This is the Start/Finish position. The movement is performed by flexing your wrists fully. Concentrate on full range of motion. This movement can be performed with dumbbells as well as a bar.

Repetitions: _____
Goal: _____
Precautions/Comments: _____
_____
_____

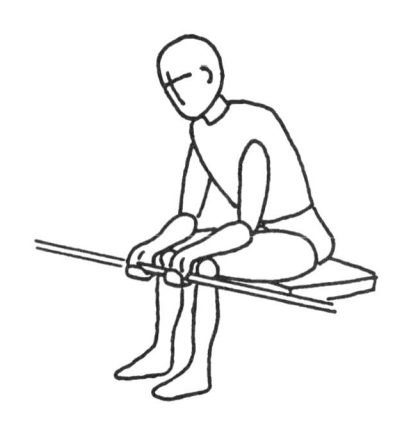

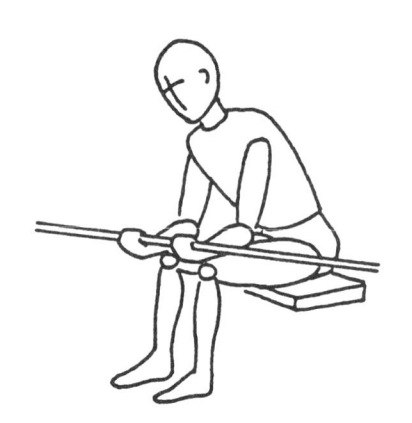

Copyright © 1997, Aspen Publishers, Inc.
Exercises for Health Promotion

Exercise 71

Start/Finish **Movement**

Movement: Wrist extension with bar or dumbbells
Target Muscles: Extensor carpi radialis and ulnaris
Instructions: Perform this movement from a seated position with your forearms resting on your thighs. Your grasp is overhand (pronation) and hand spacing is approximately shoulder width. Lower the bar by allowing your wrists to flex until you feel a comfortable stretch. This is the Start/Finish position. The movement is performed by extending your wrists fully. Concentrate on the full range of motion. This movement can be performed with dumbbells as well as a bar.

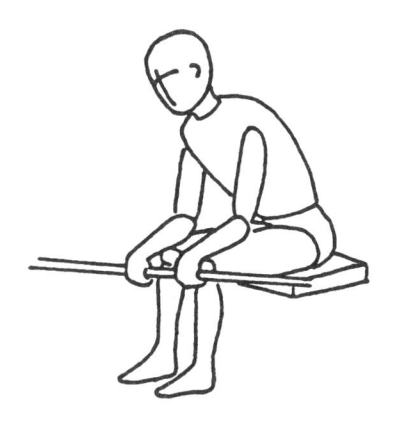

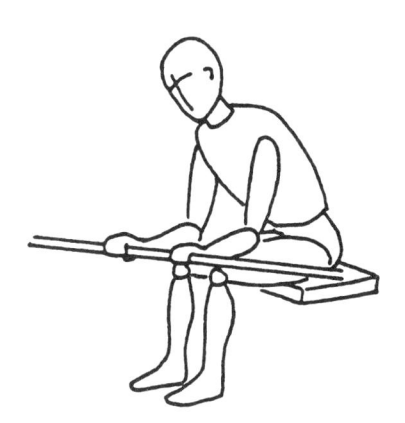

Repetitions: _____
Goal: _____
Precautions/Comments: _____
_____
_____

Exercise 72

Start/Finish   **Movement**

Movement: Radial deviation with dumbbell
Target Muscles: Flexor carpi radialis, extensor carpi radialis
Instructions: Firmly grasp a dumbbell at one end. Stand upright with your arm and forearm vertical, and your knuckles facing to the side. Allow the front end of the dumbbell to lower until you feel a comfortable stretch. This is the Start/Finish position. To perfom the movement, raise only the front end of the dumbbell by moving only at your wrist. Do not allow the front end of the dumbbell to move right or left, only upward.

Repetitions: _____
Goal: _____
Precautions/Comments: _____
_____
_____
_____

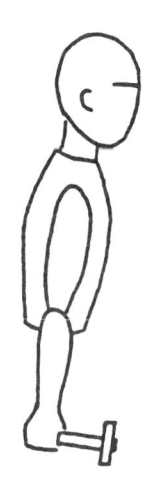

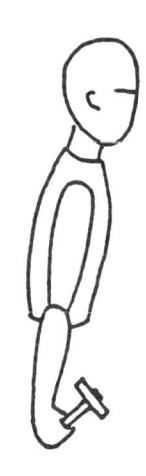

Exercise 73

Start/Finish **Movement**

Movement: Ulnar deviation with dumbbell
Target Muscles: Flexor carpi ulnaris, extensor carpi ulnaris
Instructions: Firmly grasp a dumbbell at one end such that the free end of the dumbbell is behind you. Stand upright with your arm and forearm vertical, and your knuckles facing to the side. This is the Start/Finish position. To perfom the movement, raise only the free end of the dumbbell with movement occurring only at your wrist. Do not allow the free end of the dumbbell to move right or left, only upward.

Repetitions: _____
Goal: _____
Precautions/Comments: _____
_____
_____

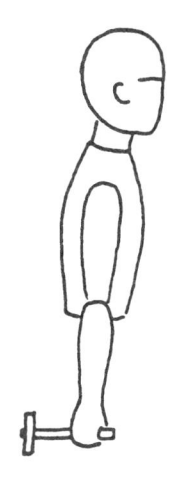

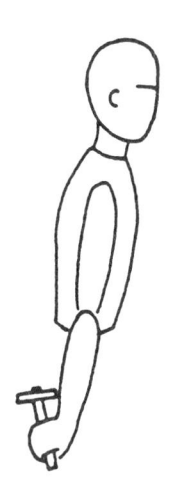

Exercise 74

Start/Finish   **Movement**

Movement: Cervical flexion with strap
Target Muscles: Sternocleidomastoid
Instructions: There are several types of strap apparatus for exercising the neck. In general, attach the resistance to the strap and then secure the head harness as per specific type. Carefully lie back on a weight bench, supporting the weight with one of your hands until you reach the supine position. Slowly take up the slack in the strap by lowering the weight with your hand. This allows you to make sure the resistance is appropriate. This is the Start/Finish position. To perform the movement, slowly flex your neck, bringing your chin to your chest. Emphasize full contraction and slow lowering to the point of comfortable stretch. Do not overstretch.

Repetitions: _____
Goal: _____
Precautions/Comments: _____
_____
_____

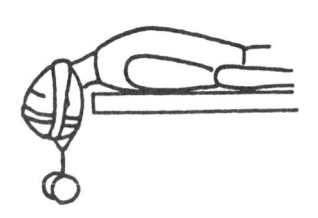

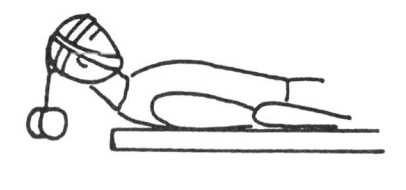

Exercise 75

Start/Finish   **Movement**

Movement: Cervical extension with strap
Target Muscles: Upper trapezius, splenius cervicis and capitis
Instructions: There are several types of strap apparatus for exercising the neck. In general, you will attach the resistance to the strap and then secure the head harness as per specific type. Carefully lie on your stomach on a weight bench, supporting the weight with one of your hands until you reach the prone position. Slowly take up the slack in the strap by lowering the weight with your hand. This will allow you to make sure the resistance is appropriate. This is the Start/Finish position. To perform the movement, slowly extend your neck as fully as possible. Think of trying to look to the ceiling. Do not rotate your head, only extend. Slowly return to the point of comfortable stretch.

Repetitions: _____
Goal: _____
Precautions/Comments: _____
_____
_____

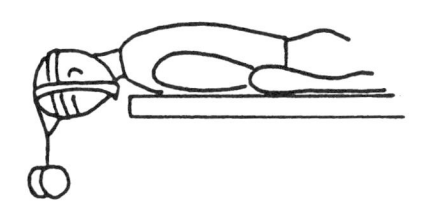

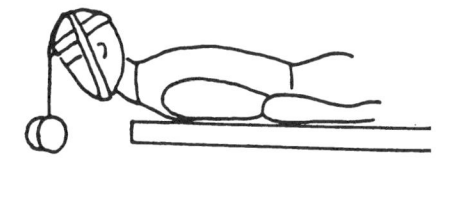

Exercise 76

Start/Finish **Movement**

Movement: Cervical lateral flexion with strap
Target Muscles: Sternocleidomastoid, scalenes
Instructions: There are several types of strap apparatus for exercising the neck. In general, you will attach the resistance to the strap and then secure the head harness as per specific type. Carefully lower yourself to a right side-lying position on the weight bench. As you move into position, support the weight with one of your hands. When you are in a comfortable position on the bench, take up the slack in the strap by slowly lowering the weight with your hand. This will allow you to make sure the resistance is appropriate. Allow your neck to bend sideways to the right to the point of comfortable stretch but do not overstretch. This is the Start/Finish position to perform the movement of lateral flexion to the left. To perform the movement, slowly bend your neck to the side, moving your left ear toward your left shoulder. Avoid rotating your head or bending it forward or backward. This movement involves side-bending only. Emphasize full contraction. To perform lateral flexion to the right, you will be in the left side-lying position and will laterally flex your neck to the right, moving your right ear toward your right shoulder.

Repetitions: _____
Goal: _____
Precautions/Comments: _____
_____
_____

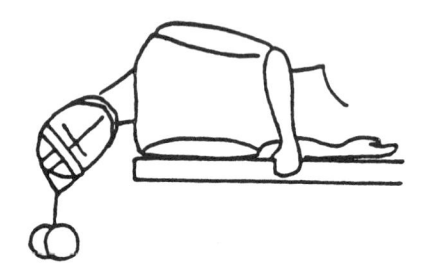

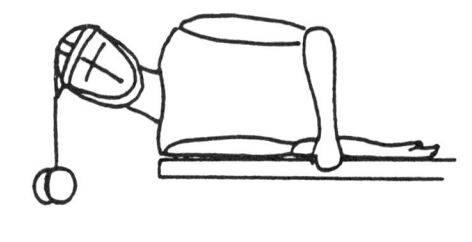

GUIDELINES FOR MANUAL RESISTIVE EXERCISE

1. Communication between exerciser and partner is crucial for safety and to maximize productivity.
2. The eccentric muscle action should be taken only to the point of a mild, comfortable stretch.
3. The partner must gauge resistance to allow smooth range of movement, particularly at the onset of the eccentric muscle action, and to allow the exerciser to complete each repetition within the approximate time frame of six seconds (three seconds concentric action and three seconds eccentric action or two seconds concentric action and four seconds eccentric action).
4. The partner must vary the direction of the resistance applied such that the resistance is applied perpendicular to the exerciser's moving body segment.
5. During the initial three or four repetitions of the set, the partner provides submaximal, but gradually increasing, resistance.
6. The principles outlined in Chapter 1 are followed.

Exercise 77

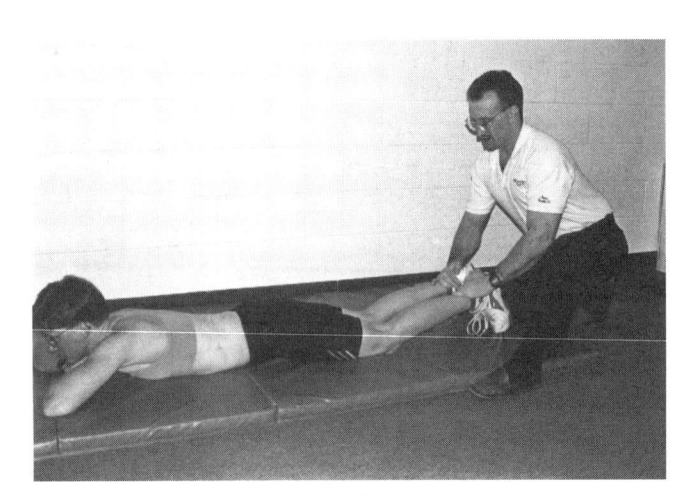

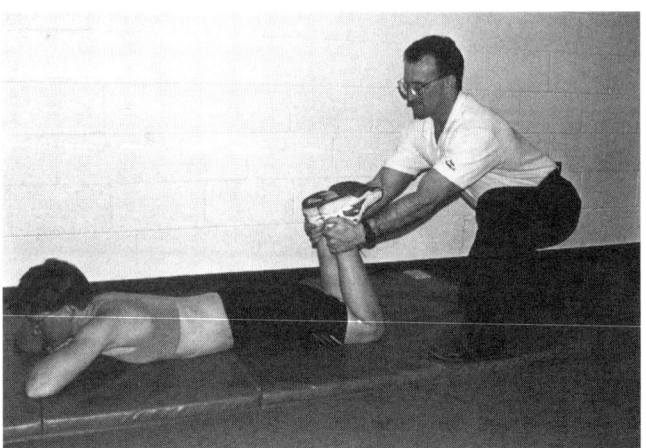

Start/Finish

Movement

Movement: Manual knee flexion
Target Muscles: Hamstrings
Instructions: Lie face down on a double thickness mat or weight bench. Your thighs are supported, but your knees extend off the end of the supporting surface. Your knees are fully extended. This is the Start/Finish position. To perform the movement, flex your knees as fully as possible against the resistance provided by your partner. Think of trying to touch your heels to your buttocks. Emphasize full range of motion. Your partner will now pull your legs back to the Start/Finish position as you resist in a controlled manner.

Repetitions: _____
Goal: _____
Precautions/Comments: _____

_____
_____

Copyright © 1997, Aspen Publishers, Inc.
Exercises for Health Promotion

Exercise 78

Start/Finish **Movement**

Movement: Manual knee extension
Target Muscles: Quadriceps
Instructions: This movement is performed from the side of a supportive table or weight bench. Your Start/Finish position is seated with upright torso, your thighs supported by the table or bench, and your knees at 90 degrees of flexion (legs vertical). Extend your right knee 30 to 45 degrees as your partner provides resistance. This is a short arc movement. You are now at a position of 60 to 45 degrees of knee flexion (full extension equals 0 degrees). Resist smoothly as your partner pushes your ankle back to the Start/Finish position. When finished, repeat with left leg.

Repetitions: _____
Goal: _____
Precautions/Comments: _____

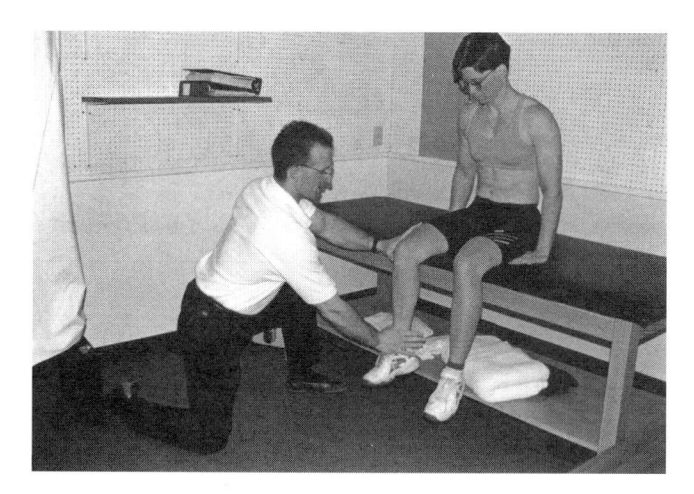

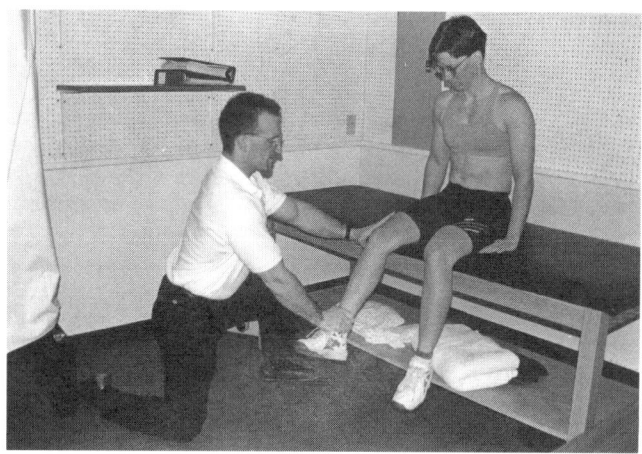

Exercise 79

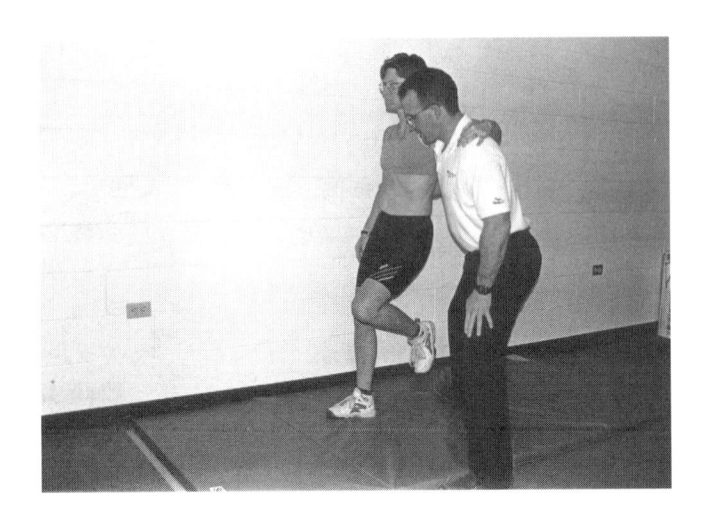

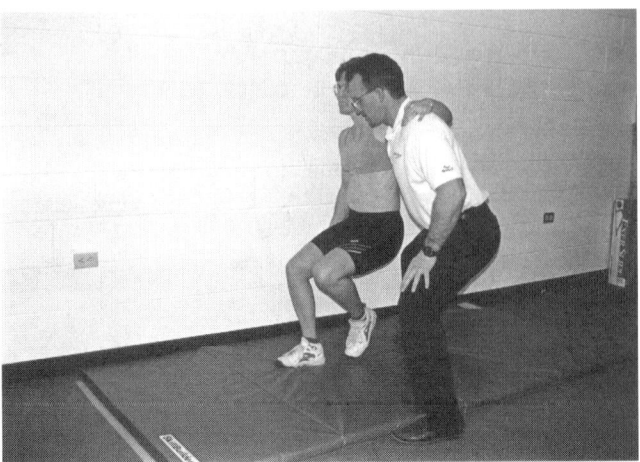

Start/Finish

Movement

Movement: Single leg squat
Target Muscles: Gluteals, quadriceps, hamstrings
Instructions: Stand on your right leg with your left thigh vertical and left knee flexed to 90 degrees. Place your left arm around your partner's shoulders for balance only. This is the Start/Finish position. To perform the movement, slowly lower your body by allowing your right knee and right hip to flex. *Important:* As you lower your body, maintain your right knee directly above your right ankle. Do not allow your right knee to move in front of your right ankle. To visualize this movement, think of sitting down and back as if you were sitting down on a chair. Use your partner only for balance. Do not pull on your partner's shoulders to help lower or raise yourself. Maintain relatively vertical trunk position throughout the movement. In the event the exerciser's final elevation needs assistance, the partner also must use correct body mechanics (flexing at the knees with pelvis and low back in stable position). To exercise the left lower extremity, both the exerciser and the partner reverse position.

Repetitions: _____
Goal: _____
Precautions/Comments: _____

Exercise 80

Start/Finish **Movement**

Movement: Manual hip abduction
Target Muscles: Gluteals, tensor fasciae latae
Instructions: To exercise your left hip abductors, begin in a right side-lying position on a mat or carpet. Flex your right hip and knee slightly to prevent your body from rolling forward or backward during the movement. Resistance is provided immediately proximal to the knee to avoid varus stress. This is the Start/Finish position. To perform the movement, raise your left thigh and leg. Lift as high as you can. Do not flex or laterally rotate your hip to substitute with your hip flexors/rotators. Smoothly resist as your partner returns your leg to the Start/Finish position. Reverse your body position to exercise your right hip abductors.

Repetitions: _____
Goal: _____
Precautions/Comments: _____
_____
_____

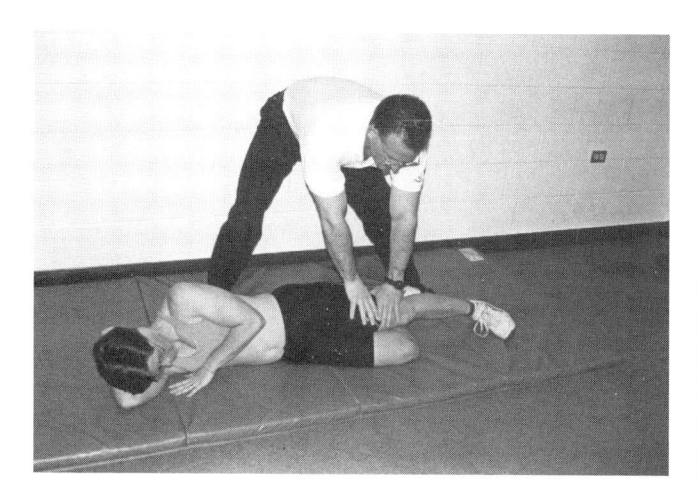

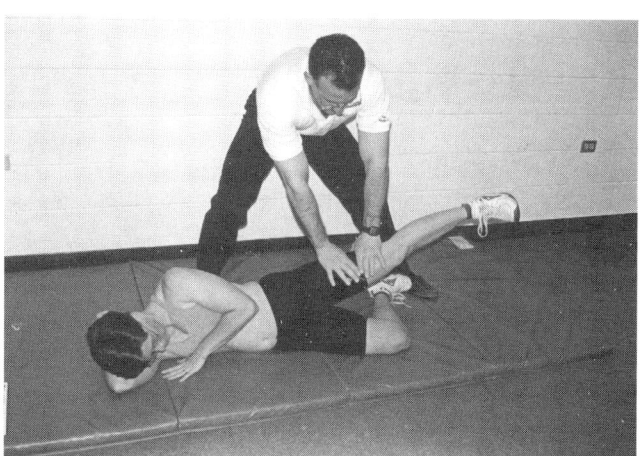

Exercise 81

Start/Finish **Movement**

Movement: Manual hip adduction
Target Muscles: Adductor magnus, longus, brevis
Instructions: To isolate your right hip adductors, begin in a right side-lying position on a mat or carpet. Your partner will support your left thigh and leg in an abducted position to allow unimpeded motion by the exercising extremity. This is the Start/Finish position. To perform the movement, raise your right thigh and leg vertically until contact is made with your left thigh. Emphasize straight alignment of your body, including both legs, throughout the movement. Often, the weight of the limb being raised will provide sufficient resistance. If additional resistance is desired, it is applied by your partner to the distal right thigh to avoid valgus stress at the knee. Slowly lower the right leg to the Start/Finish position. You will notice that the adductors of the thigh held stationary are isometrically active.

Repetitions: _____
Goal: _____
Precautions/Comments: _____
_____
_____

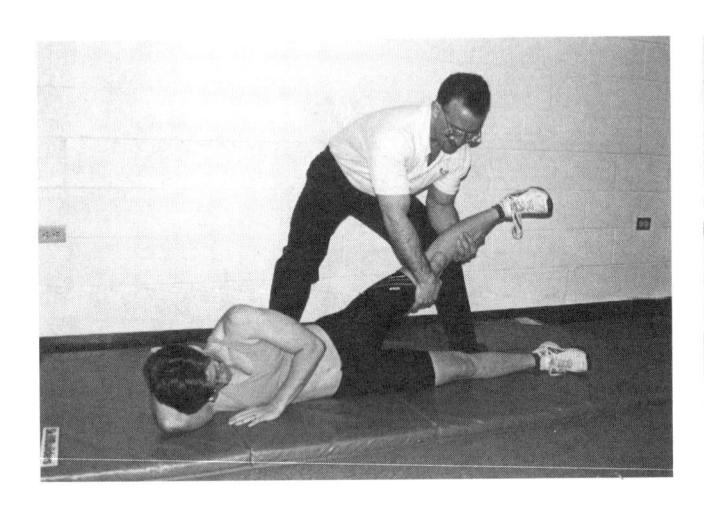

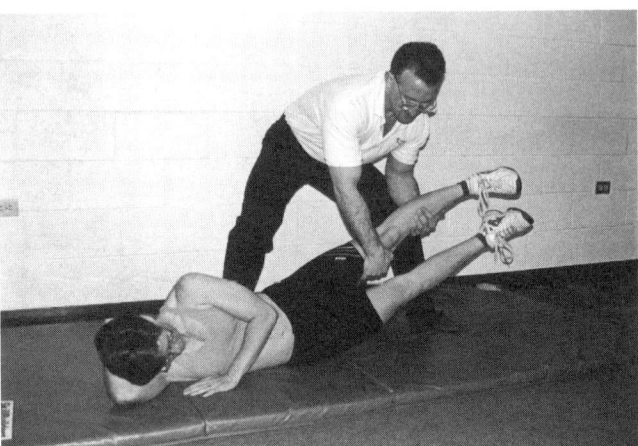

Exercise 82

Start/Finish **Movement**

Movement: Back extension
Target Muscles: Erector spinae
Instructions: Lie on your stomach on a padded surface. Place a pad or rolled up towel under your waist to allow you to begin the movement in some degree of lumbar flexion. Your partner will stabilize your thighs in contact with the support surface. This is the Start/Finish position. To perform the movement, move upward from the pad until your upper and lower body have formed a straight line (180 degrees). Do not hyperextend.

Repetitions: _____
Goal: _____
Precautions/Comments: _____
_____
_____

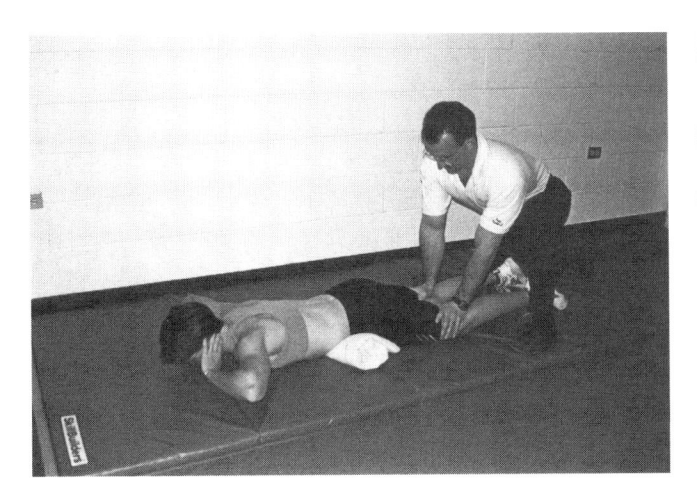

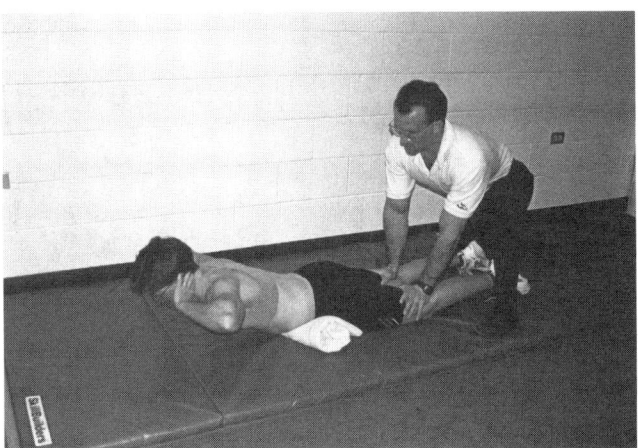

Exercise 83

Start/Finish   **Movement**

Movement: Abdominal curl
Target Muscles: Abdominals, obliques
Instructions: Begin on your back on a padded surface. Place your feet flat on the surface, slightly wider than shoulder width. Flex your knees to 90 degrees. Place your arms across your chest with each hand on the opposite shoulder, or, for increased resistance, place your hands behind your head. This is the Start/Finish position. To perform the movement, contract your stomach muscles to raise your shoulder blades up from the mat. Your partner may apply additional resistance to the front of your shoulders. Lower your shoulders in a controlled manner as you resist your partner with your abdominal muscles. Exhale as you rise, inhale as you lower.

Repetitions: _____
Goal: _____
Precautions/Comments: _____
_____
_____

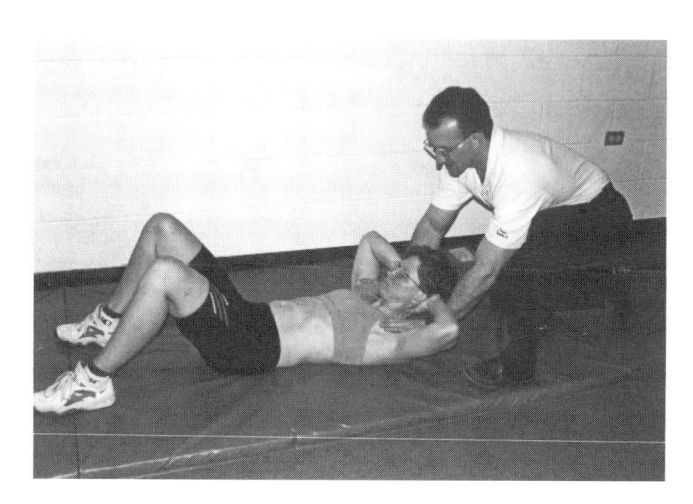

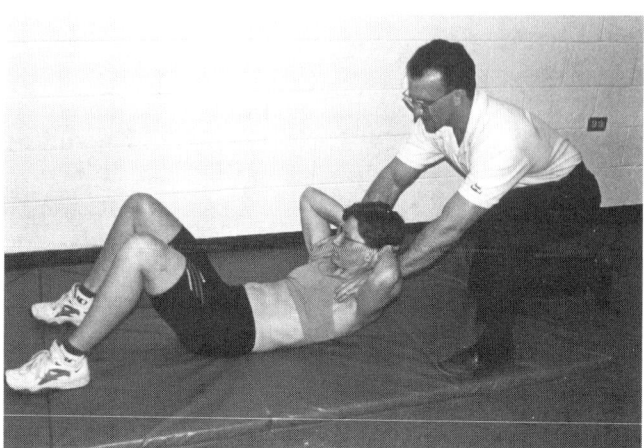

Exercise 84

Start/Finish **Movement**

Movement: Manual shoulder extension
Target Muscles: Latissimus dorsi, teres major, rhomboids
Instructions: Position an adjustable weight bench so that the back support pad is just slightly angled from vertical. Sit on the seat with your chest to the pad. Flex your right shoulder to horizontal. Your partner will provide resistance using a towel, as it provides for easy grasp by both individuals. When you have grasped the towel, you are in the Start/Finish position. Perform the movement by extending your shoulder. Concentrate on pulling your elbow as far behind you as possible. Provide controlled resistance as your partner pulls your arm back to the Start/Finish position. Communication is essential through both concentric and eccentric portions of the movement.

Repetitions: _____
Goal: _____
Precautions/Comments: _____
_____
_____
_____

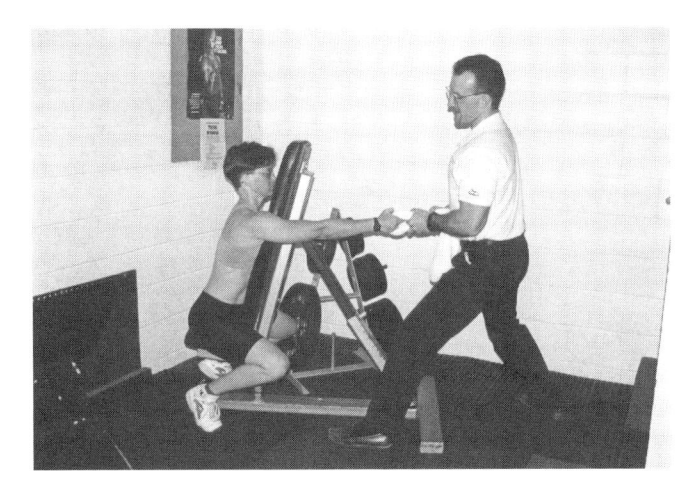

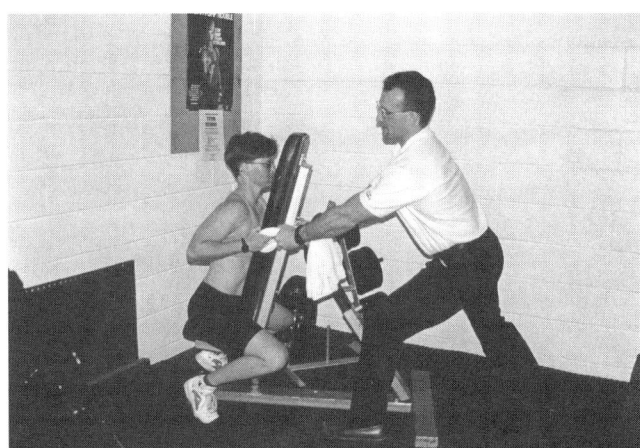

Exercise 85

Start/Finish **Movement**

Movement: Manual shoulder transverse adduction
Target Muscles: Pectoralis major
Instructions: Lie on your back on a weight bench. Place your hands to the side of your head, cupped over your ears. Allow your elbows to lower until you feel a comfortable stretch through your chest and shoulders. At this point your partner will place the palms of his or her hands over the medial aspect of your elbows. This is the Start/Finish position. To perform the movement, touch your elbows together above your head while maintaining your hands cupped over your ears. Your partner applies resistance to your movement. When you reach full contraction, perform graded resistance as your partner returns your elbows back to a position of comfortable stretch.

Repetitions: _____
Goal: _____
Precautions/Comments: _____
_____
_____
_____

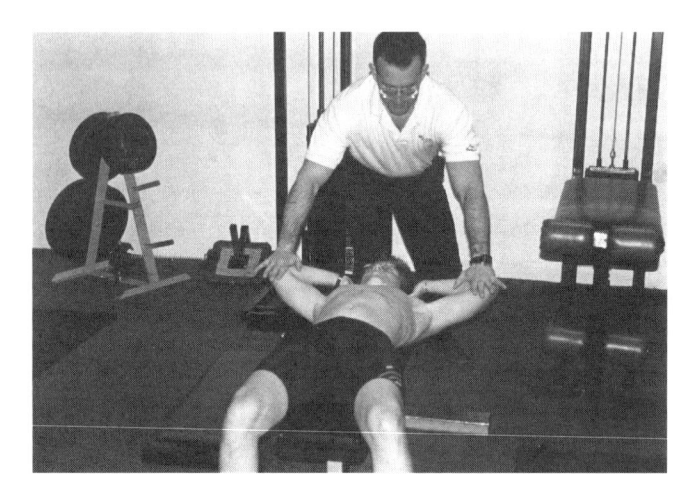

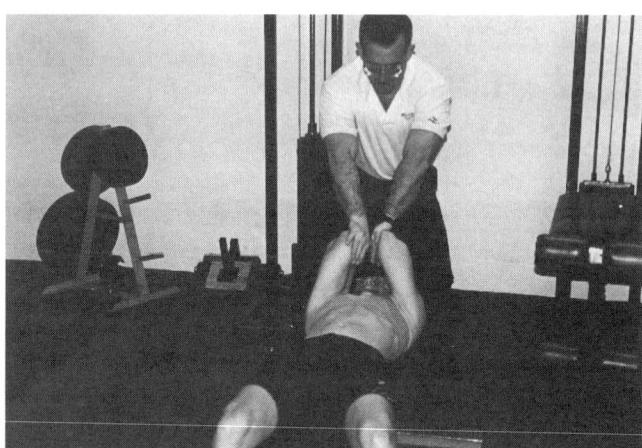

Exercise 86

Start/Finish **Movement**

Movement: Manual shoulder transverse abduction
Target Muscles: Posterior deltoid
Instructions: Support your chest on the seat top of an adjustable bench angled to about 45 degrees. Place your right hand either on your right knee or on the bench for support. Your left arm and forearm are resting in downward position. Your partner places one hand just proximal to your left elbow. This is the Start/Finish position. To perform the movement, raise your arm and forearm upward. Do not allow your arm to drift back toward your partner, only upward. To visualize, think of moving the back of your left hand toward the ceiling. Raise your arm and forearm as high as you can without compensating by raising your left shoulder. Your back remains horizontal. Lower to the Start/Finish position in a controlled manner as you resist your partner's downward force.

Repetitions: _____
Goal: _____
Precautions/Comments: _____

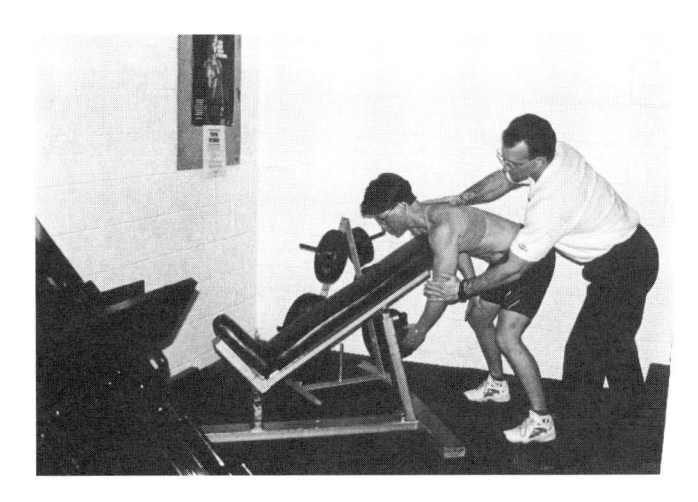

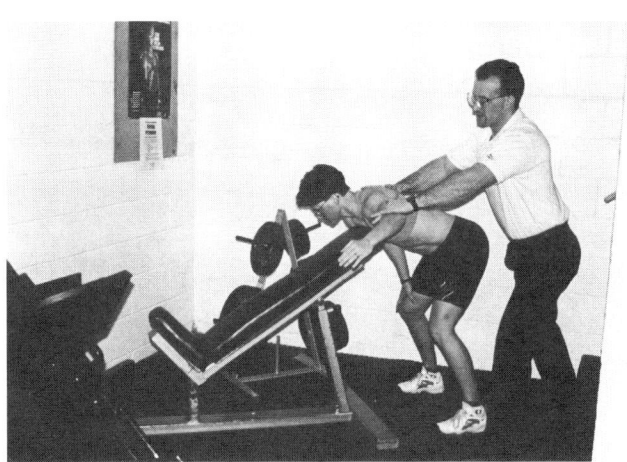

Exercise 87

Start/Finish   **Movement**

Movement: Manual cervical flexion
Target Muscles: Sternocleidomastoid
Instructions: Lie on your back on a weight bench. Position yourself so that the tops of your shoulders are at the edge of the bench. Allow your neck and head to extend over the edge of the bench. Slowly allow your neck to extend until you feel a comfortable stretch. Now flex your head upward one inch. This is the Start/Finish position. To perform the movement, flex your neck, bringing your chin to your chest. Your partner's hand placed on your forehead will serve as added resistance. Smoothly resist as you allow your partner to slowly lower your head to the Start/Finish position. Communicate often, and maintain the one inch cushion in extension in order to safeguard against hyperextension.

Repetitions: _____
Goal: _____
Precautions/Comments: _____
_____
_____

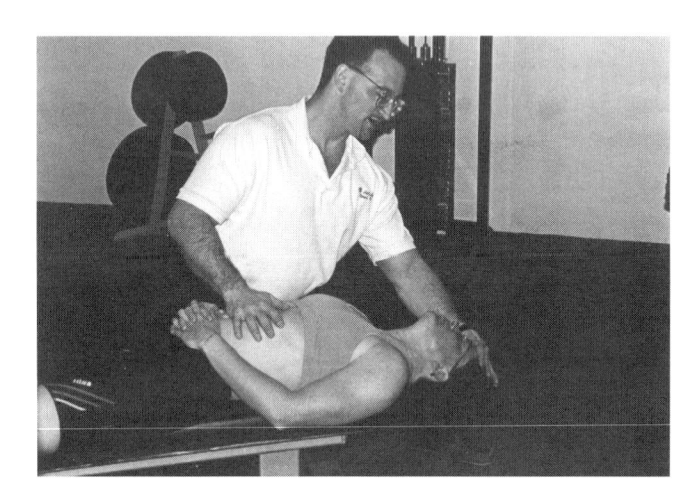

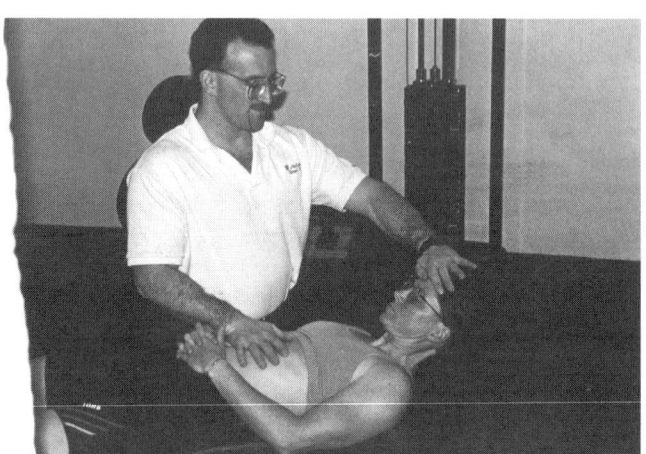

Exercise 88

Start/Finish   **Movement**

Movement: Manual cervical extension
Target Muscles: Upper trapezius, splenius cervicus and capitus
Instructions: Lie on your stomach on a weight bench. Position yourself so that the tops of your shoulders are at the edge of the bench. Allow your neck and head to extend over the edge of the bench. Slowly allow your neck to flex until you feel a comfortable stretch. Your partner now places one hand on the back of your head to provide resistance and the other hand on your back to help stabilize. This is the Start/Finish position. To perform the movement, extend your neck fully. Think of trying to look up to the ceiling. Do not allow your head to rotate during the movement, only extend. When full contraction has been reached, smoothly resist as you allow your partner to return your neck to a flexed position. Communicate often with your partner to avoid hyperflexion and to provide feedback about appropriate resistance.

Repetitions: _____
Goal: _____
Precautions/Comments: _____
_____
_____

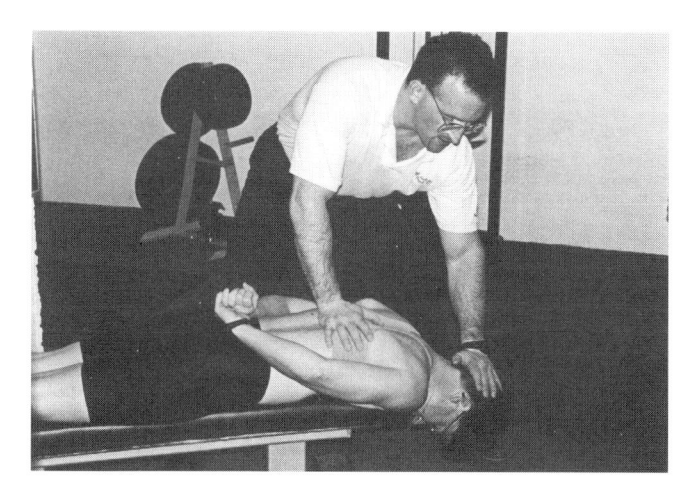

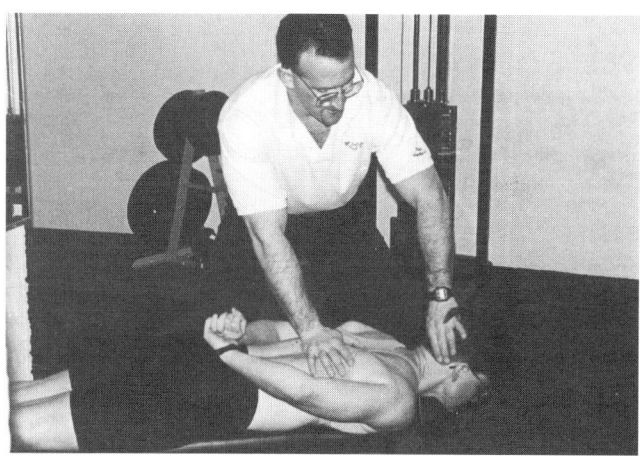

Exercise 89

Start/Finish **Movement**

Movement: Manual cervical lateral flexion
Target Muscles: Sternocleidomastoid, scalenes
Instructions: Position yourself sitting upright on a weight bench. Flex your neck to the left. Your partner now places one hand to the left of your left shoulder and the other hand on the right side of your head just above ear level. This is the Start/Finish position. To perform the movement, bend your neck sideways to the right against your partner's resistance. Maintain your torso upright and do not substitute with neck flexion or rotation. When you reach full contraction, resist as your partner returns your head to the Start/Finish position. Communicate often to avoid overstretching as you return to the left. Reverse the procedure to exercise the muscles that laterally flex the neck to the left.

Repetitions: _____
Goal: _____
Precautions/Comments: _____

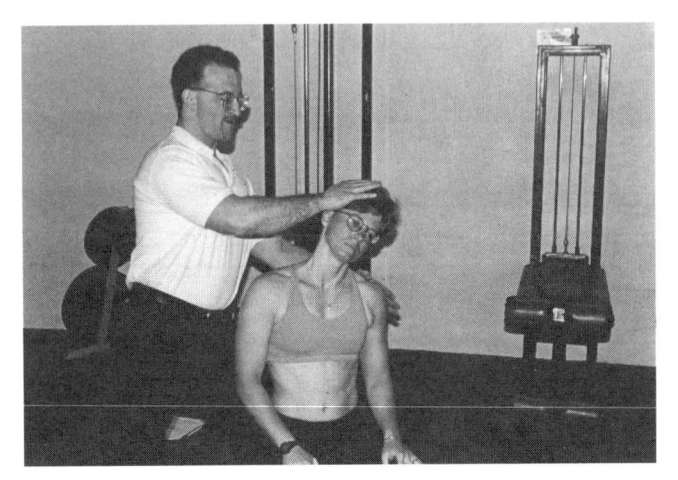

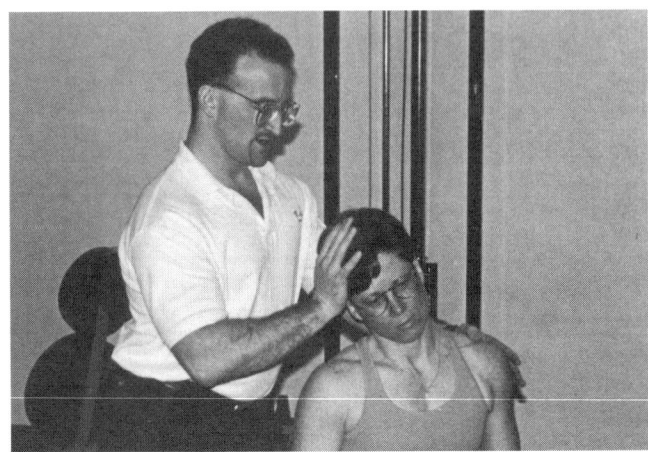

Exercise 90

Start/Finish   **Movement**

Movement: Manual tricep extension
Target Muscles: Triceps
Instructions: Position yourself comfortably on your back on a weight bench. You will be exercising each arm individually. Flex your right shoulder so your elbow is directed vertically. Flex your right elbow bringing your palm to ear level. Your partner places his or her right hand on the distal aspect of your right arm to stabilize the arm vertically, and places his or her left hand on the distal aspect of your right forearm to provide resistance. This is the Start/Finish position. To perform the movement, extend your elbow fully, working against your partner's resistance. The key to the movement is to hold your arm stationary and move only the forearm at the elbow. Do not rotate your shoulder. Resist in a smooth, controlled manner as your partner returns your forearm to the Start/Finish position. Reverse sides to exercise the left tricep.

Repetitions: _____
Goal: _____
Precautions/Comments: _____
_____
_____

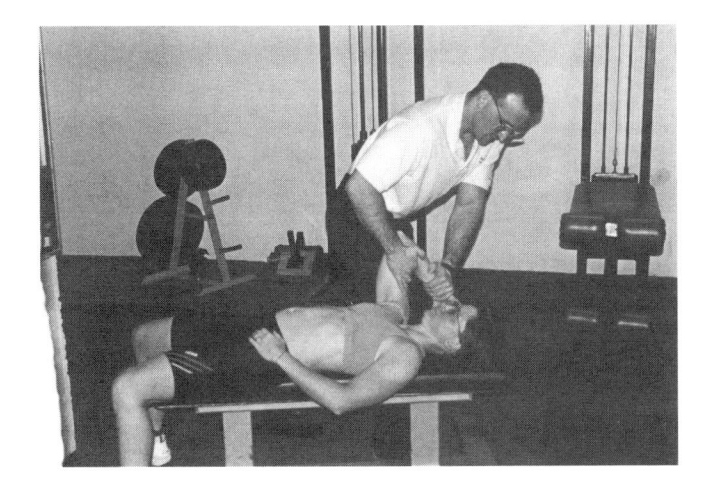

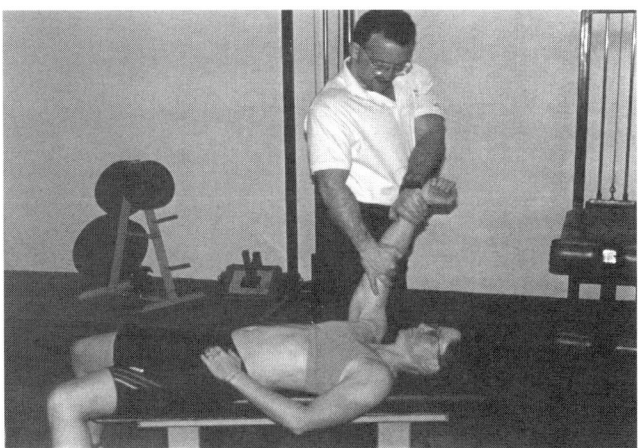

Exercise 91

Start/Finish **Movement**

Movement: Manual elbow flexion
Target Muscles: Biceps, brachialis
Instructions: Position an adjustable bench to a seat angle of 45 degrees. Make sure it is locked in place. Assume a staggered stance and bend both knees to lower your body. Support your arm on the seat pad with your shoulder rotated so that your bicep is directed upward. Grasp the middle of a rolled up towel with your partner grasping both ends of the towel. Extend your elbow to the point of comfortable stretch. This is the Start/Finish position. To perform the movement, flex your elbow bringing your right hand to your right shoulder. Maintain your bicep directed upward. Do not rotate your shoulder medially as you fatigue. Emphasize full contraction. Slowly resist your partner as he or she pulls your forearm back to the Start/Finish position. Communicate with your partner to prevent overstretch in extension.

Repetitions: _____
Goal: _____
Precautions/Comments: _____
_____
_____

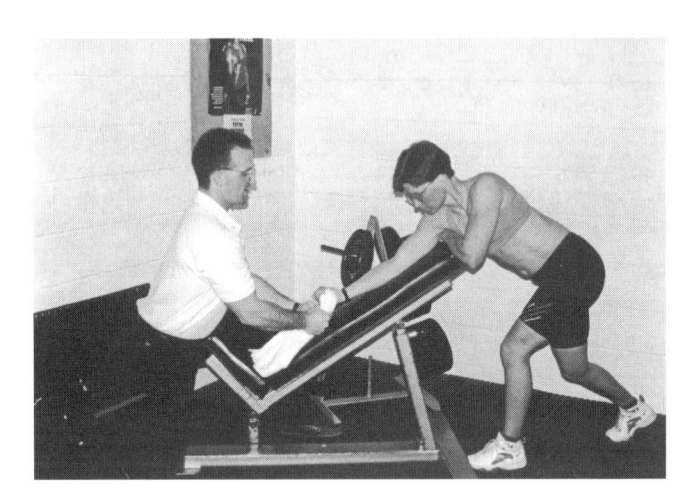

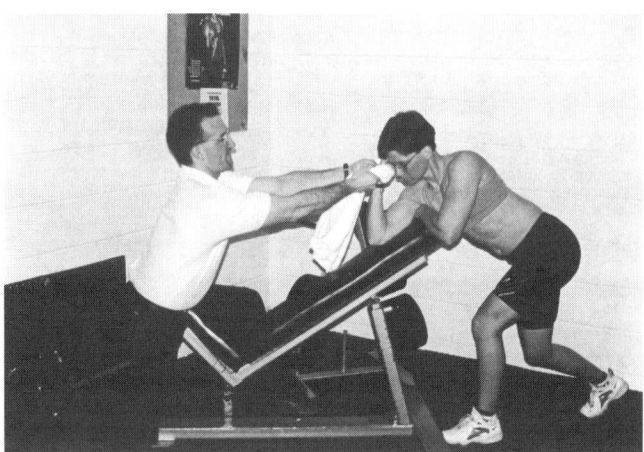

CHAPTER 16

Flexibility Exercise Movements

Caren J. Werlinger

FLEXIBILITY PROGRAM

An appropriate level of flexibility is required for the safe performance of any exercise activity, whether it be strength training or aerobics. If there is an asymmetry in flexibility, then there also exists an imbalance that predisposes a joint or soft tissues to injury. Even without the existence of a specific imbalance, muscles that have been properly warmed up and stretched are less likely to sustain injury during an exercise session. A static, slowly applied stretch usually will be more beneficial than a ballistic type of stretch. In addition, ballistic or bouncing stretches have a greater potential for tissue microtrauma. The following is a time-efficient flexibility program that covers most of the major muscle groups likely to be called upon in most exercise programs. This program, however, should be supplemented by additional stretching, if needed, for particularly tight muscles.

ACTIVITY-SPECIFIC STRETCHES

The stretch program that follows is designed to cover most of the major muscle groups of the body. Most sports activities require a general approach to stretching, with perhaps some additional emphasis on certain muscle groups specific to that activity. The following are some sports-specific stretches.

1. *Cycling*—Most of the muscle groups used during cycling are covered in the stretches that follow: back extensors, quads, hamstrings, gastrocnemius/soleus. One of the areas most often complained about by cyclists is the cervical spine. With the weight of the upper body supported by the arms, the cervical spine is usually in extension for long periods of time, often with the shoulders shrugging up about the ears. Before and during the ride, stretch the neck, especially into flexion and into a chin tuck to target the upper cervical spine. Periodically depress and protract the scapulae to pull the shoulders back down into position.

2. *Ball sports*—This category includes baseball, football, tennis, racquetball, volleyball, or any other sport in which the upper extremities must be used, especially in overhead positions requiring combined abduction and external rotation. This is the shoulder's most vulnerable position for rotator cuff strains. The shoulder should be stretched carefully into external rotation, perhaps more than that provided by the corner or wall stretches explained on the following pages. In addition, internal rotation can be performed by reaching each arm behind the back, trying to get the fingers to the opposite scapula. Normally the dominant shoulder will be tighter than the nondominant side.

   These sports often require a rapid deceleration from the triceps as a throw or serve is completed, so attention should also be paid to stretching the triceps by reaching overhead with the elbow flexed and pulling the stretch side into end range shoulder flexion.

3. *Golf*—Because of the strong rotational component of a golf swing, the spine is at particular risk of a strain. To stretch the spine, perform the flexion and extension stretches outlined on the following pages. In addition, lie supine with the knees bent. Keeping the shoulders flat on the floor, roll the knees to one side, allowing them to fall gently toward the floor. Repeat on the other side. It must be stressed that stretching alone will not protect the spine from the strong forces caused by a full golf swing; the abdominal and back extensor muscles must also be strengthened with exercises such as those outlined in Chapter 15.

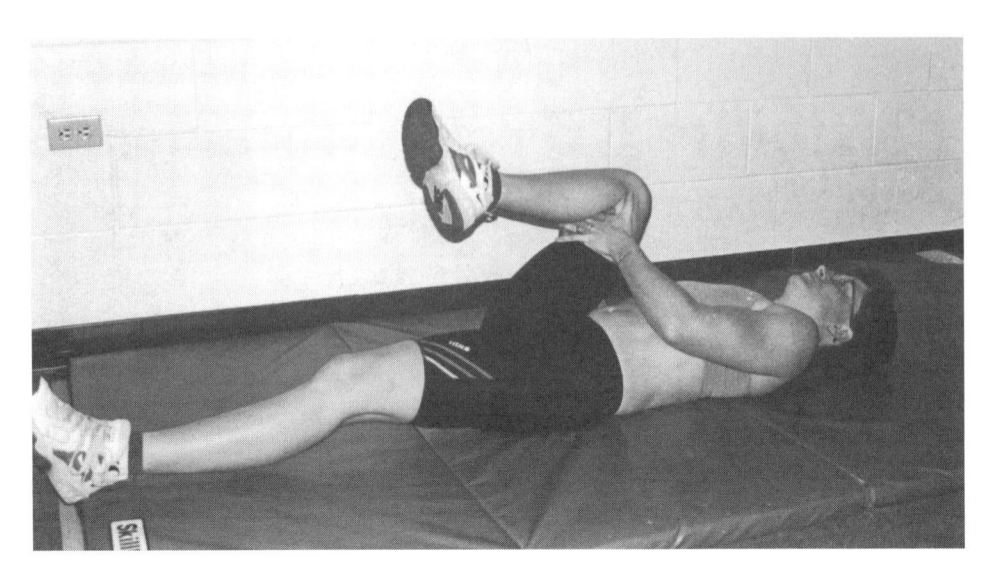

Exercise 16–1 Single Knee to Chest. This is a good stretch for the gluteus maximus. By lying supine with the knees bent, the spine is held in a flattened position. Gently pull one thigh at a time toward the chest and hold for 30 seconds. Switch.

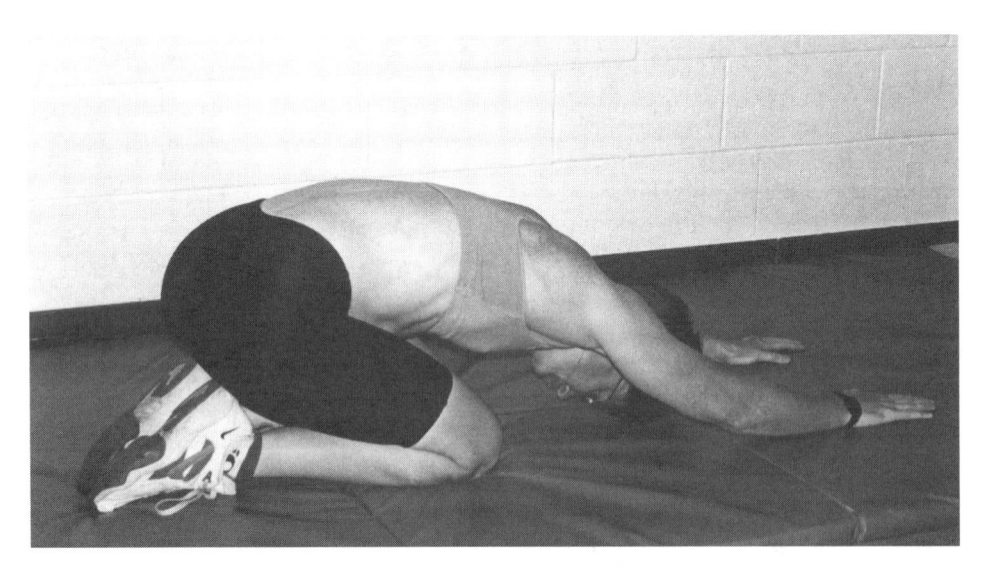

Exercise 16–2 Sit on Heels. Rather than doing a supine double knees to chest, this exercise allows a gentle flexion stretch of the entire length of the spine with no excessive external force applied at any isolated motion segment. In quadruped position, leave the hands in place and slowly lower the buttocks toward the heels, allowing the head to sink forward so the cervical spine is also in flexion. Hold for 30 seconds and release.

Copyright © 1997, Aspen Publishers, Inc.
Exercises for Health Promotion

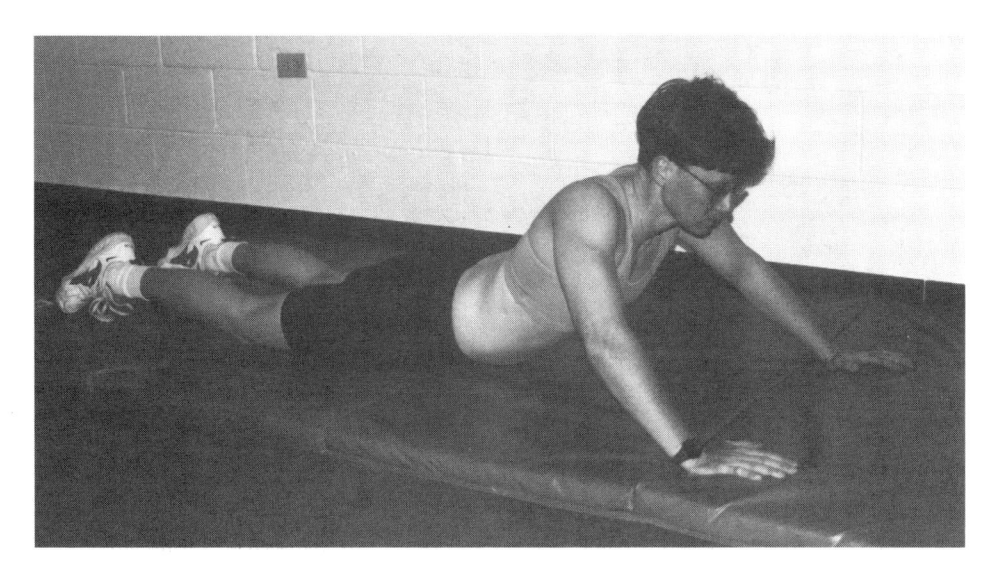

Exercise 16–3 Prone Press Up. The spine should be stretched carefully into extension. In prone position, place the hands about six inches in front of the shoulders, shoulder width apart. Gently extend the elbows, raising the trunk. It is very important that the pelvis stay in contact with the floor. If the pelvis cannot stay in contact with the floor with full elbow extension, the hands may be placed further in front. As the trunk becomes more flexible, greater stretch can be obtained by moving the hands closer to the shoulders.

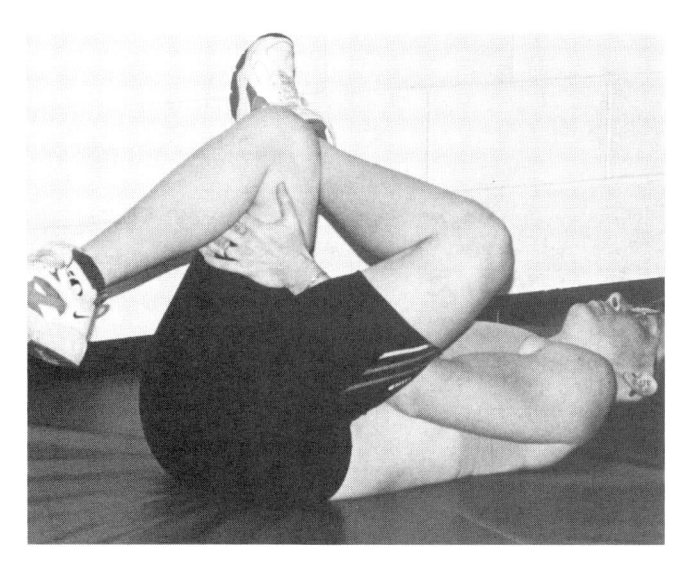

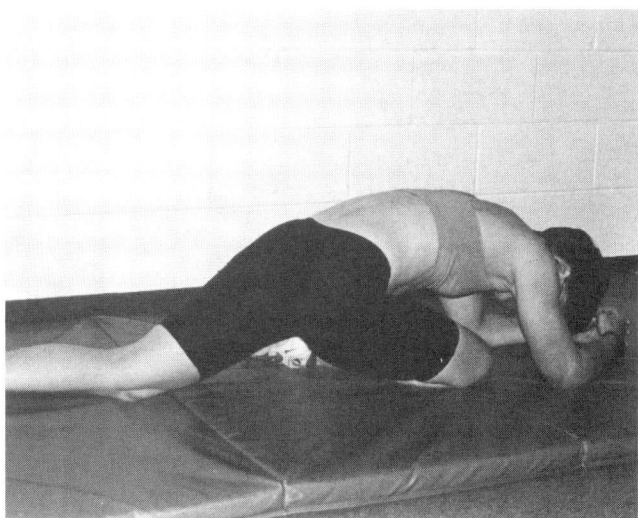

Exercise 16–4 Piriformis Stretch. This stretch obviously stretches the other external rotators in addition to the piriformis, and can be performed two ways. The more common way is in supine position with the stretch leg crossed over the opposite thigh. The opposite thigh can then be pulled manually toward the chest until a stretch is felt in the stretch-side buttock. The other method utilizes the passive force of gravity on body weight. Start in quadruped position. Place the stretch-side knee forward and externally rotate the hip so that the ankle is in front of the opposite knee. Extend the nonstretch extremity behind and go down on elbows so that body weight is supplying the stretch force. Hold 30 seconds and switch.

Copyright © 1997, Aspen Publishers, Inc.
Exercises for Health Promotion

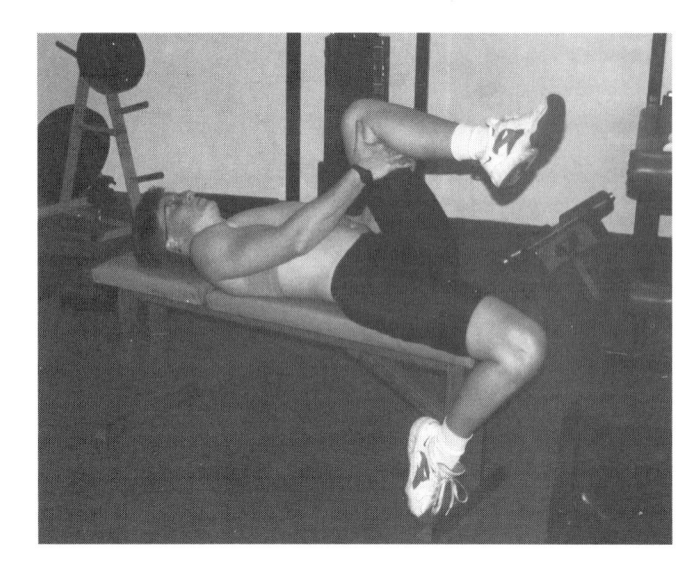

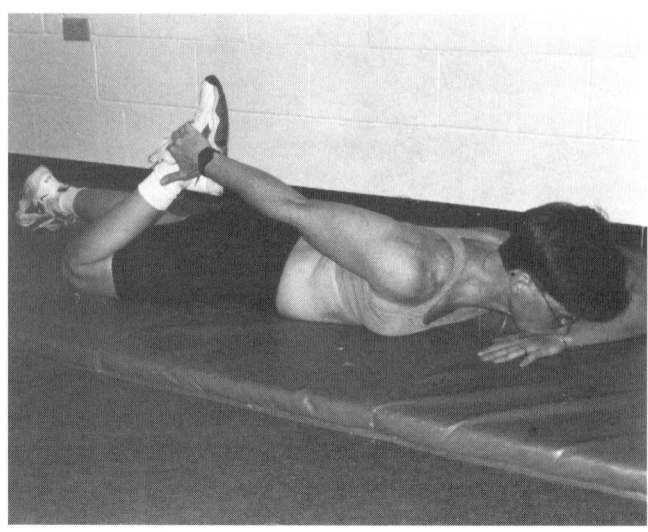

Exercise 16–5 Hip Flexor Stretch. Stretches for the hip flexors need to differentiate one-joint (iliopsoas) from two-joint (rectus femoris) muscles. It is very common for individuals with excessively tight hip flexors to substitute with excessive lumbar lordosis to create the appearance of hip extension. For this reason the safest position for stretching these muscles is the so-called (but somewhat inaccurately named) Thomas test position. Lying supine on a workout bench, the nonstretch thigh is pulled toward the chest only until the lumbar spine is flattened and no further to avoid excessive posterior pelvic tilt. Then the stretch-side extremity can be lowered with the knee extended to stretch the iliopsoas, if needed, but more commonly the rectus femoris will need to be stretched by flexing the knee. If another person is not available to push the knee gently into flexion, the individual can place the toe of the shoe behind the crossbar of the bench support and the stretch can be done without assistance. Hold 30 seconds and switch. If a bench is not available, the subject can lie prone, being sure to keep the pelvis in contact with the floor to safeguard against increasing the lordosis, and gently pull on the ankle to bring the knee into flexion.

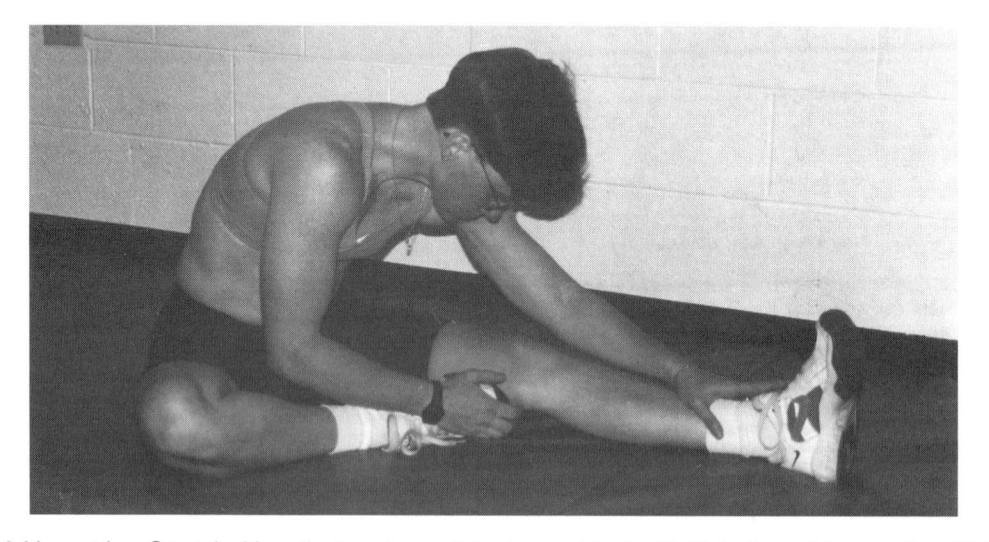

Exercise 16–6 Hamstring Stretch. Usually, in a long-sit test, a subject with tight hamstrings will exhibit excessive posterior pelvic tilt, perhaps accompanied by excessive thoracic kyphosis to reach the goal of touching the toes. Subjects should be instructed not to strive for a specific goal, but rather to maintain an anteriorly rotated pelvis and fairly flat back to isolate the hamstrings, stretching to the point of discomfort in the hamstrings and disregarding how close they get to touching their toes. Better pelvic control can be achieved by doing a unilateral, rather than bilateral, stretch. With the non-stretch extremity abducted and externally rotated with the knee flexed, the stretch side is extended, and the knee kept straight. To isolate medial or external hamstrings, the hip can be internally or externally rotated, respectively.

Copyright © 1997, Aspen Publishers, Inc.
Exercises for Health Promotion

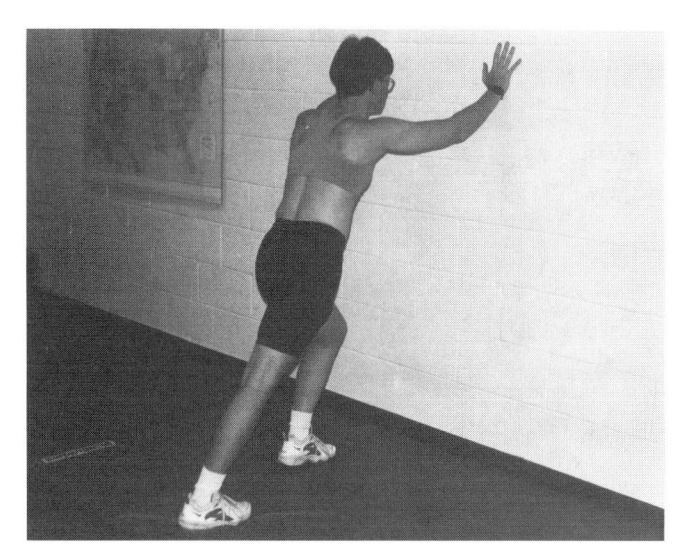

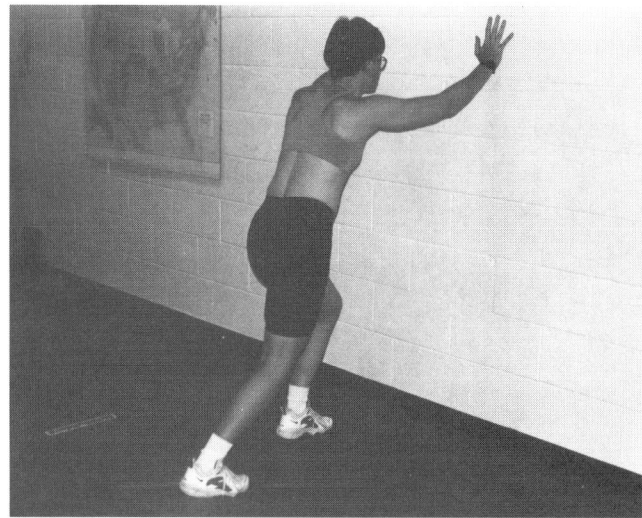

Exercise 16–7 Gastrocnemius/Soleus Stretch. Because tightness in these muscles can interfere with ankle function, it can also cause problems further up the kinetic chain, so these stretches should not be neglected. The gastrocnemius, being a two-joint muscle, needs to be stretched over both the knee and the ankle. The easiest position for this is standing, leaning against a wall, with the stretch extremity extended behind and the heel pressed toward the floor, keeping the knee extended. For the soleus, keep the same position as for the gastrocnemius, but flex the knee slightly to isolate a stretch at the ankle. Hold for 30 seconds each and switch.

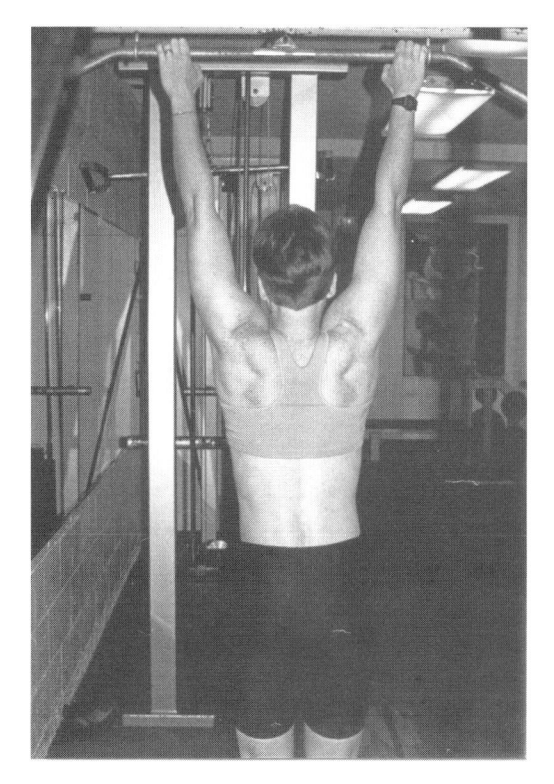

Exercise 16–8 Hanging Stretch. This is a general stretch that affects the latissimus, teres major, and subscapularis along with the rib cage as a whole. By hanging from a pull-up bar, body weight is used to pull the shoulders into end-range flexion. Care should be taken if there are other shoulder problems present; this stretch does not offer sufficient isolation if one or more of the target muscles is especially tight or if there is any capsular tightness present.

Copyright © 1997, Aspen Publishers, Inc.
Exercises for Health Promotion

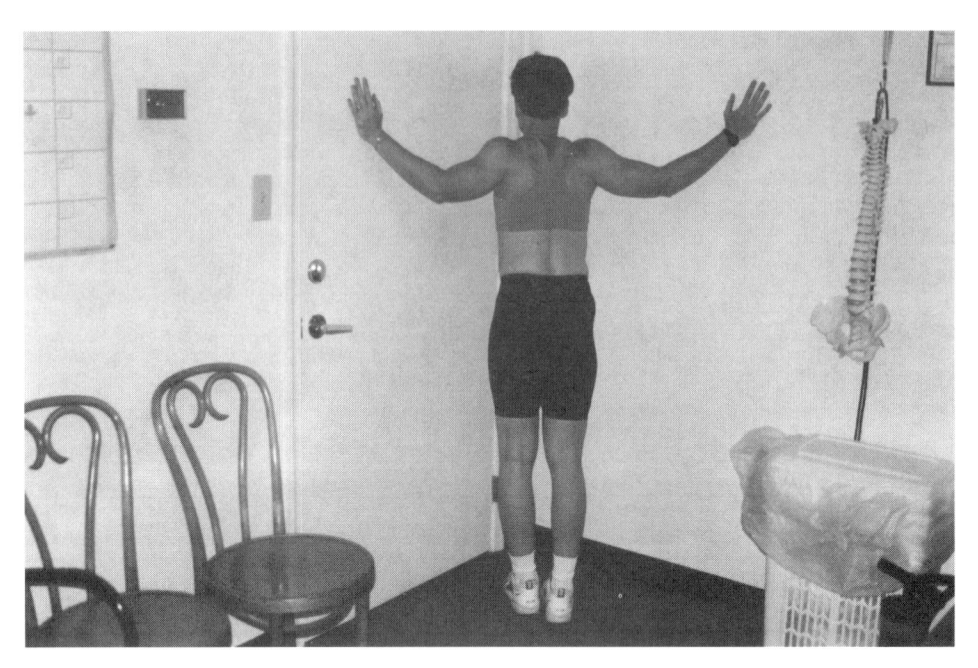

Exercise 16–9 Corner Stretch. Because of the prevalence of forward head posture and its accompanying scapular protraction, many people have developed tightness in the pectoral and internal rotator muscles of the shoulder. This stretch is most easily performed by standing in a corner and placing the upper extremities against the two walls at shoulder height, then leaning into the corner until a stretch is felt. If this stretch is applied with a gradual force, the chest will move toward the corner as the pectoral muscles lengthen.

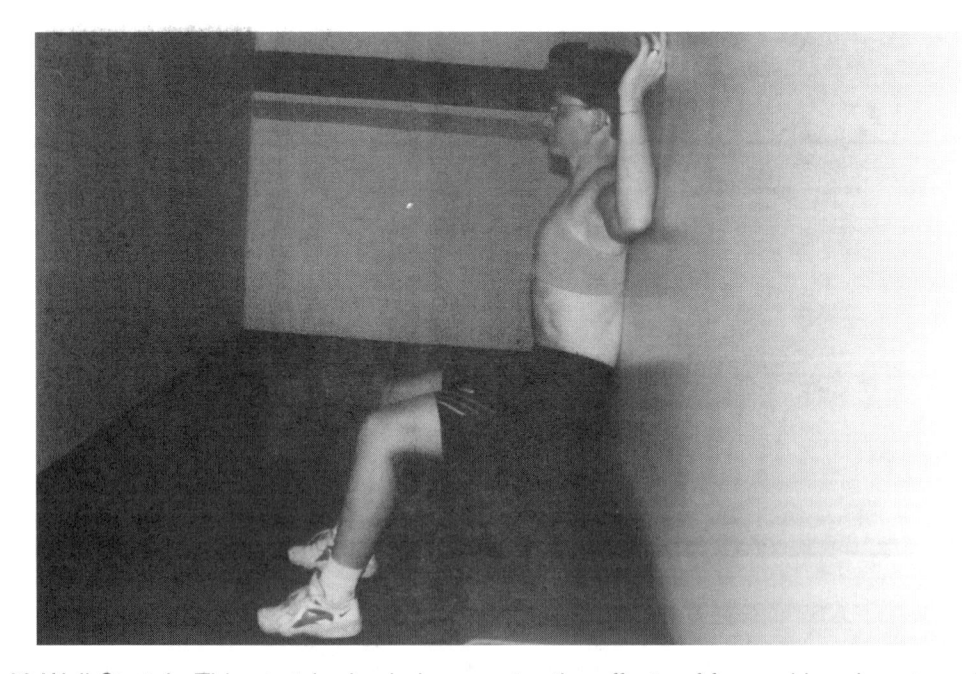

Exercise 16–10 Wall Stretch. This stretch also helps counter the effects of forward head posture. Sitting on a backless chair or bench with the spine pressed against a wall, press the lumbar curve flat against the wall. Maintaining a flat spine, abduct the shoulders to 90 degrees, and externally rotate so that both the wrists and the elbows are in contact with the wall. Rub the upper extremities up and down against the wall while keeping the elbows and wrists in contact and the spine flat. If the latissimus, teres major, or subscapularis is tight, the spine will tend to pull away from the wall.

Copyright © 1997, Aspen Publishers, Inc.
Exercises for Health Promotion

APPENDIX A

The Recommended Quantity and Quality of Exercise for Developing and Maintaining Cardiorespiratory and Muscular Fitness in Healthy Adults

This Position Stand replaces the 1978 ACSM position paper, "The Recommended Quantity and Quality of Exercise for Developing and Maintaining Fitness in Healthy Adults."

Increasing numbers of persons are becoming involved in endurance training and other forms of physical activity, and, thus, the need for guidelines for exercise prescription is apparent. Based on the existing evidence concerning exercise prescription for healthy adults and the need for guidelines, the American College of Sports Medicine (ACSM) makes the following recommendations for the quantity and quality of training for developing and maintaining cardiorespiratory fitness, body composition, and muscular strength and endurance in the healthy adult:

1. Frequency of training: 3–5 d · wk^{-1}.
2. Intensity of training: 60–90% of maximum heart rate (HR_{max}), or 50–85% of maximum oxygen uptake ($\dot{V}O_{2max}$) or HR_{max} reserve.*
3. Duration of training: 20–60 min of continuous aerobic activity. Duration is dependent on the intensity of the activity; thus, lower intensity activity should be conducted over a longer period of time. Because of the importance of "total fitness" and the fact that it is more readily attained in longer duration programs, and because of the potential hazards and compliance problems associated with high intensity activity, lower to moderate intensity activity of longer duration is recommended for the nonathletic adult.
4. Mode of activity: any activity that uses large muscle groups, can be maintained continuously, and is rhythmical and aerobic in nature, e.g., walking-hiking, running-jogging, cycling-bicycling, cross-country skiing, dancing, rope skipping, rowing, stair climbing, swimming, skating, and various endurance game activities.
5. Resistance training: Strength training of a moderate intensity, sufficient to develop and maintain fat-free weight (FFW), should be an integral part of an adult fitness program. One set of 8–12 repetitions of eight to ten exercises that condition the major muscle groups at least 2 d · wk^{-1} is the recommended minimum.

RATIONALE AND RESEARCH BACKGROUND

Introduction

The questions "How much exercise is enough," and "What type of exercise is best for developing and maintaining fitness?" are frequently asked. It is recognized that the term "physical fitness" is composed of a variety of characteristics included in the broad categories of cardiovascular-respiratory fitness, body composition, muscular strength and endurance, and flexibility. In this context fitness is defined as the ability to perform moderate to vigorous levels of physical activity without undue fatigue and the capability of maintaining such ability throughout life.[167] It is also recognized that the adaptive response to training is complex and includes peripheral, central, structural, and functional factors.[5,172] Although many such variables and their adaptive response to training have been documented, the lack of sufficient in-depth and comparative data relative to frequency,

---

Source: Reprinted with permission from The Recommended Quantity and Quality of Exercise for Developing and Maintaining Cardiorespiratory and Muscular Fitness in Healthy Adults, *Medicine and Science in Sports and Exercise,* Vol. 22, pp. 265–274, © 1990, American College of Sports Medicine.

*Maximum heart rate reserve is calculated from the difference between resting and maximum heart rate. To estimate training intensity, a percentage of this value is added to the resting heart rate and is expressed as a percentage of HR_{max} reserve.[85]

intensity, and duration of training makes them inadequate to use as comparative models. Thus, in respect to the above questions, fitness is limited mainly to changes in $\dot{V}O_{2max}$, muscular strength and endurance, and body composition, which includes total body mass, fat weight (FW), and FFW. Further, the rationale and research background used for this position stand will be divided into programs for cardiorespiratory fitness and weight control and programs for muscular strength and endurance.

Fitness versus Health Benefits of Exercise

Since the original position statement was published in 1978, an important distinction has been made between physical activity as it relates to health versus fitness. It has been pointed out that the quantity and quality of exercise needed to attain health-related benefits may differ from what is recommended for fitness benefits. It is now clear that lower levels of physical activity than recommended by this position statement may reduce the risk for certain chronic degenerative diseases and yet may not be of sufficient quantity or quality to improve $\dot{V}O_{2max}$.[71,72,98,167] ACSM recognizes the potential health benefits of regular exercise performed more frequently and for a longer duration, but at lower intensities than prescribed in this position statement.[13A,71,100,120,160] ACSM will address the issue concerning the proper amount of physical activity necessary to derive health benefits in another statement.

Need for Standardization of Procedures and Reporting Results

Despite an abundance of information available concerning the training of the human organism, the lack of standardization of testing protocols and procedures, of methodology in relation to training procedures and experimental design, and of a preciseness in the documentation and reporting of the quantity and quality of training prescribed make interpretation difficult.[123,133,139,164,167] Interpretation and comparison of results are also dependent on the initial level of fitness,[42,43,58,114,148,151,156] length of time of the training experiment,[17,45,125,128,139,145,150] and specificity of the testing and training.[5,43,130,139,145A,172] For example, data from training studies using subjects with varied levels of $\dot{V}O_{2max}$, total body mass, and FW have found changes to occur in relation to their initial values[14,33,109,112,113,148,151]; i.e., the lower the initial $\dot{V}O_{2max}$ the larger the percentage of improvement found, and the higher the FW the greater the reduction. Also, data evaluating trainability with age, comparison of the different magnitudes and quantities of effort, and comparison of the trainability of men and women may have been influenced by the initial fitness levels.

In view of the fact that improvement in the fitness variables discussed in this position statement continues over many months of training,[27,86,139,145,150] it is reasonable to believe that short-term studies conducted over a few weeks have certain limitations. Middle-aged sedentary and older participants may take several weeks to adapt to the initial rigors of training, and thus need a longer adaptation period to get the full benefit from a program. For example, Seals et al.[150] exercise trained 60–69-yr-olds for 12 months. Their subjects showed a 12% improvement in $\dot{V}O_{2max}$ after 6 months of moderate intensity walking training. A further 18% increase in $\dot{V}O_{2max}$ occurred during the next 6 months of training when jogging was introduced. How long a training experiment should be conducted is difficult to determine, but 15–20 wk may be a good minimum standard. Although it is difficult to control exercise training experiments for more than 1 yr, there is a need to study this effect. As stated earlier, lower doses of exercise may improve $\dot{V}O_{2max}$ and control or maintain body composition, but at a slower rate.

Although most of the information concerning training described in this position statement has been conducted on men, the available evidence indicates that women tend to adapt to endurance training in the same manner as men.[19,38,46,47,49,62,65,68,90,92,122,166]

Exercise Prescription for Cardiorespiratory Fitness and Weight Control

Exercise prescription is based upon the frequency, intensity, and duration of training, the mode of activity (aerobic in nature, e.g., listed under No. 4 above), and the initial level of fitness. In evaluating these factors, the following observations have been derived from studies conducted for up to 6–12 months with endurance training programs.

Improvement in $\dot{V}O_{2max}$ is directly related to frequency,[3,6,50,75-77,125,126,152,154,164] intensity,[3,6,26,29,58,61,75-77,80,85,93,118,152,164] and duration[3,29,60,61,70,75-77,101,109,118,152,162,164,168] of training. Depending upon the quantity and quality of training, improvement in $\dot{V}O_{2max}$ ranges from 5 to 30%.[8,29,30,48,59,61,65,67,69,75-77,82,84,96,99,101,102,111,115,119,123,127,139,141,143,149,150,152,153,158,164,168,173] These studies show that a minimum increase in $\dot{V}O_{2max}$ of 15% is generally attained in programs that meet the above stated guidelines. Although changes in $\dot{V}O_{2max}$ greater than 30% have been shown, they are usually associated with large total body mass and FW loss, in cardiac patients, or in persons with a very low initial level of fitness. Also, as a result of leg fatigue or a lack of motivation, persons with low initial fitness may have spuriously low initial $\dot{V}O_{2max}$ values. Klissouras[94A] and Bouchard[16A] have shown that human variation in the trainability of $\dot{V}O_{2max}$ is important and related to current phenotype level. That is, there is a genetically determined pretraining status of the trait and capacity to adapt to physical training. Thus, physiological results should be interpreted with respect to both genetic variation and the quality and quantity of training performed.

Intensity-Duration

Intensity and duration of training are interrelated, with total amount of work accomplished being an important factor in improvement in fitness.[12,20,27,48,90,92,123,127,128,136,149,151,164] Although more comprehensive inquiry is necessary, present evidence suggests that, when exercise is performed above the minimum intensity threshold, the total amount of work accomplished is an important factor in fitness development[19,27,126,127,149,151] and maintenance.[134] That is, improvement will be similar for activities performed at a lower intensity-longer duration compared to higher intensity-shorter duration if the total energy costs of the activities are equal. Higher intensity exercise is associated with greater cardiovascular risk,[156A] orthopedic injury,[124,139] and lower compliance to training than lower intensity exercise.[36,105,124,146] Therefore, programs emphasizing low to moderate intensity training with longer duration are recommended for most adults.

The minimal training intensity threshold for improvement in $\dot{V}O_{2max}$ is approximately 60% of the HR_{max} (50% of $\dot{V}O_{2max}$ or HR_{max} reserve).[80,85] The 50% of HR_{max} reserve represents a heart rate of approximately 130–135 beats · min^{-1} for young persons. As a result of the age-related change in maximum heart rate, the absolute heart rate to achieve this threshold is inversely related to age and can be as low as 105–115 beats · min^{-1} for older persons.[35,65,150] Patients who are taking beta-adrenergic blocking drugs may have significantly lower heart rate values.[171] Initial level of fitness is another important consideration in prescribing exercise.[26,90,104,148,151] The person with a low fitness level can achieve a significant training effect with a sustained training heart rate as low as 40–50% of HR_{max} reserve, while persons with higher fitness levels require a higher training stimulus.[35,58,152,164]

Classification of Exercise Intensity

The classification of exercise intensity and its standardization for exercise prescription based on a 20–60 min training session has been confusing, misinterpreted, and often taken out of context. The most quoted exercise classification system is based on the energy expenditure (kcal · min^{-1} · kg^{-1}) of industrial tasks.[40,89] The original data for this classification system were published by Christensen[24] in 1953 and were based on the energy expenditure of working in the steel mill for an 8-h day. The classification of industrial and leisure-time tasks by using absolute values of energy expenditure have been valuable for use in the occupational and nutritional setting. Although this classification system has broad application in medicine and, in particular, making recommendations for weight control and job placement, it has little or no meaning for preventive and rehabilitation exercise training programs. To extrapolate absolute values of energy expenditure for completing an industrial task based on an 8-h work day to 20–60 min regimens of exercise training does not make sense. For example, walking and jogging/running can be accomplished at a wide range of speeds; thus, the relative intensity becomes important under these conditions. Because the endurance training regimens recommended by ACSM for nonathletic adults are geared for 60 min or less of physical activity, the system of classification of exercise training intensity shown in Table 1 is recommended.[139] The use of a realistic time period for training and an individual's relative exercise intensity makes this system amenable to young, middle-aged, and elderly participants, as well as patients with a limited exercise capacity.[3,137,139]

Table 1 also describes the relationship between relative intensity based on percent HR_{max}, percentage of HR_{max} reserve or percentage of $\dot{V}O_{2max}$, and the rating of perceived exertion (RPE).[15,16,137] The use of heart rate as an estimate of intensity of training is the common standard.[3,139]

The use of RPE has become a valid tool in the monitoring of intensity in exercise training programs.[11,37,137,139] It is generally considered an adjunct to heart rate in monitoring relative exercise intensity, but once the relationship between heart rate and RPE is known, RPE can be used in place of heart rate.[23,139] This would not be the case in certain patient populations where a more precise knowledge of heart rate may be critical to the safety of the program.

Frequency

The amount of improvement in $\dot{V}O_{2max}$ tends to plateau when frequency of training is increased above 3 d · wk^{-1}.[50,123,139] The value of the added improvement found with train-

Table 1 Classification of intensity of exercise based on 20–60 min of endurance training.

	Relative Intensity (%)		
HR_{max}*	$\dot{V}O_{2max}$* or HR_{max} Reserve	Rating of Perceived Exertion	Classification of Intensity
<35%	<30%	<10	Very light
35–59%	30–49%	10–11	Light
60–79%	50–74%	12–13	Moderate (somewhat hard)
80–89%	75–84%	14–16	Heavy
≥90%	≥85%	>16	Very heavy

*HR_{max} = maximum heart rate; $\dot{V}O_{2max}$ = maximum oxygen uptake.

Source: Reprinted with permission from M.L. Pollock and J.H. Wilmore, *Exercise in Health and Disease: Evaluation and Prescription for Prevention and Rehabilitation,* 2nd Edition, © 1990, W.B. Saunders.

ing more than 5 d · wk^{-1} is small to not apparent in regard to improvement in $\dot{V}O_{2max}$.[75-77,106,123] Training of less than 2 d · wk^{-1} does not generally show a meaningful change in $\dot{V}O_{2max}$.[29,50,118,123,152,164]

Mode

If frequency, intensity, and duration of training are similar (total kcal expenditure), the training adaptations appear to be independent of the mode of aerobic activity.[101A,118,130] Therefore, a variety of endurance activities, e.g., those listed above, may be used to derive the same training effect.

Endurance activities that require running and jumping are considered high impact types of activity and generally cause significantly more debilitating injuries to beginning as well as long-term exercisers than do low impact and non-weight bearing type activities.[13,93,117,124,127,135,140,142] This is particularly evident in the elderly.[139] Beginning joggers have increased foot, leg, and knee injuries when training is performed more than 3 d · wk^{-1} and longer than 30 min duration per exercise session.[135] High intensity interval training (run-walk) compared to continuous jogging training was also associated with a higher incidence of injury.[124,136] Thus, caution should be taken when recommending the type of activity and exercise prescription for the beginning exerciser. Orthopedic injuries as related to overuse increase linearly in runners/joggers when performing these activities.[13,140] Thus, there is a need for more inquiry into the effect that different types of activities and the quantity and quality of training has on injuries over short-term and long-term participation.

An activity such as weight training should not be considered as a means of training for developing $\dot{V}O_{2max}$, but it has significant value for increasing muscular strength and endurance and FFW.[32,54,107,110,165] Studies evaluating circuit weight training (weight training conducted almost continuously with moderate weights, using 10–15 repetitions per exercise session with 15–30 s rest between bouts of activity) show an average improvement in $\dot{V}O_{2max}$ of 6%.[1,51-54,83,94,108,170] Thus, circuit weight training is not recommended as the only activity used in exercise programs for developing $\dot{V}O_{2max}$.

Age

Age in itself does not appear to be a deterrent to endurance training. Although some earlier studies showed a lower training effect with middle-aged or elderly participants,[9,34,79,157,168] more recent studies show the relative change in $\dot{V}O_{2max}$ to be similar to younger age groups.[7,8,65,132,150,161,163] Although more investigation is necessary concerning the rate of improvement in $\dot{V}O_{2max}$ with training at various ages, at present it appears that elderly participants need longer periods of time to adapt.[34,132,150] Earlier studies showing moderate to no improvement in $\dot{V}O_{2max}$ were conducted over a short time span,[9] or exercise was conducted at a moderate to low intensity,[34] thus making the interpretation of the results difficult.

Although $\dot{V}O_{2max}$ decreases with age and total body mass and FW increase with age, evidence suggests that this trend can be altered with endurance training.[22,27,86-88,139] A 9% reduction in $\dot{V}O_{2max}$ per decade for sedentary adults after age 25 has been shown,[31,73] but for active individuals the reduction may be less than 5% per decade.[21,31,39,73] Ten or more yr follow-up studies where participants continued training at a similar level showed maintenance of cardiorespiratory fitness.[4,87,88,138] A cross-sectional study of older competitive runners showed progressively lower values in $\dot{V}O_{2max}$ from the fourth to seventh decades of life, but also showed less training in the older groups.[129] More recent 10-yr follow-up data on these same athletes (50–82 yr of age) showed $\dot{V}O_{2max}$ to be unchanged when training quantity and quality remained unchanged.[138] Thus, lifestyle plays a significant role in the maintenance of fitness. More inquiry into the relationship of long-term training (quantity and quality), for both competitors and noncompetitors, and physiological function with increasing age is necessary before more definitive statements can be made.

Maintenance of Training Effect

In order to maintain the training effect, exercise must be continued on a regular basis.[18,25,28,47,97,111,144,147] A significant reduction in cardiorespiratory fitness occurs after 2 wk of detraining,[25,144] with participants returning to near pretraining levels of fitness after 10 wk[47] to 8 months of detraining.[97] A loss of 50% of their initial improvement in $\dot{V}O_{2max}$ has been shown after 4–12 wk of detraining.[47,91,144] Those individuals who have undergone years of continuous training maintain some benefits for longer periods of detraining than subjects from short-term training studies.[25] While stopping training shows dramatic reductions in $\dot{V}O_{2max}$, reduced training shows modest to no reductions for periods of 5–15 wk.[18,75-77,144] Hickson et al., in a series of experiments where frequency,[75] duration,[76] or intensity[77] of training were manipulated, found that, if intensity of training remained unchanged, $\dot{V}O_{2max}$ was maintained for up to 15 wk when frequency and duration of training were reduced by as much as $^2/_3$. When frequency and duration of training remained constant and intensity of training was reduced by $^1/_3$ or $^2/_3$, $\dot{V}O_{2max}$ was significantly reduced. Similar findings were found in regards to reduced strength training exercise. When strength training exercise was reduced from 3 or 2 d · wk^{-1} to at least 1 d · wk^{-1}, strength was maintained for 12 wk of reduced training.[62] Thus, it appears that missing an exercise session periodically or reducing training for up to 15 wk will not adversely effect $\dot{V}O_{2max}$ or muscular strength and endurance as long as training intensity is maintained.

Even though many new studies have given added insight into the proper amount of exercise, investigation is necessary to evaluate the rate of increase and decrease of fitness when varying training loads and reduction in training in relation to level of fitness, age, and length of time in training. Also, more information is needed to better identify the minimal level of exercise necessary to maintain fitness.

Weight Control and Body Composition

Although there is variability in human response to body composition change with exercise, total body mass and FW are generally reduced with endurance training programs,[133,139,171A] while FFW remains constant[123,133,139,169] or increases slightly.[116,174] For example, Wilmore[171A] reported the results of 32 studies that met the criteria for developing cardiorespiratory fitness that are outlined in this position stand and found an average loss in total body mass of 1.5 kg and percent fat of 2.2%. Weight loss programs using dietary manipulation that result in a more dramatic decrease in total body mass show reductions in both FW and FFW.[2,78,174] When these programs are conducted in conjunction with exercise training, FFW loss is more modest than in programs using diet alone.[78,121] Programs that are conducted at least 3 d · wk^{-1},[123,125,126,128,169] of at least 20 min duration,[109,123,169] and of sufficient intensity to expend approximately 300 kcal per exercise session (75 kg person)* are suggested as a threshold level for total body mass and FW loss.[27,64,77,123,133,139] An expenditure of 200 kcal per session has also been shown to be useful in weight reduction if the exercise frequency is at least 4 d · wk^{-1}.[155] If the primary purpose of the training program is for weight loss, then regimens of greater frequency and duration of training and low to moderate intensity are recommended.[2,139] Programs with less participation generally show little or no change in body composition.[44,57,93,123,133,159,162,169] Significant increases in $\dot{V}O_{2max}$ have been shown with 10–15 min of high intensity training[6,79,109,118,123,152,153]; thus, if total body mass and FW reduction are not considerations, then shorter duration, higher intensity programs may be recommended for healthy individuals at low risk for cardiovascular disease and orthopedic injury.

Exercise Prescription for Muscular Strength and Endurance

The addition of resistance/strength training to the position statement results from the need for a well-rounded program that exercises all the major muscle groups of the body. Thus, the inclusion of resistance training in adult fitness programs should be effective in the development and maintenance of FFW. The effect of exercise training is specific to the area of the body being trained.[5,43,145A,172] For example, training the legs will have little or no effect on the arms, shoulders, and trunk muscles. A 10-yr follow-up of master runners who continued their training regimen, but did no upper body exercise, showed maintenance of $\dot{V}O_{2max}$ and a 2-kg reduction in FFW.[138] Their leg circumference remained unchanged, but arm circumference was significantly lower. These data indicate a loss of muscle mass in the untrained areas. Three of the athletes who practiced weight training exercise for the upper body and trunk muscles maintained their FFW. A comprehensive review by Sale[145A] carefully documents available information on specificity of training.

Specificity of training was further addressed by Graves et al.[63] Using a bilateral knee extension exercise, they trained four groups: group A, first ½ of the range of motion; group B, second ½ of the range of motion; group AB, full range of motion; and a control group that did not train. The results clearly showed that the training result was specific to the range of motion trained, with group AB getting the best full range effect. Thus, resistance training should be performed through a full range of motion for maximum benefit.[63,95]

Muscular strength and endurance are developed by the overload principle, i.e., by increasing more than normal the resistance to movement or frequency and duration of activity.[32,41,43,74,145] Muscular strength is best developed by using heavy weights (that require maximum or nearly maximum tension development) with few repetitions, and muscular endurance is best developed by using lighter weights with a greater number of repetitions.[10,41,43,145] To some extent, both muscular strength and endurance are developed under each condition, but each system favors a more specific type of development.[43,145] Thus, to elicit improvement in both muscular strength and endurance, most experts recommend 8–12 repetitions per bout of exercise.

Any magnitude of overload will result in strength development, but higher intensity effort at or near maximal effort will give a significantly greater effect.[43,74,101B,103,145,172] The intensity of resistance training can be manipulated by varying the weight load, repetitions, rest interval between exercises, and number of sets completed.[43] Caution is advised for training that emphasizes lengthening (eccentric) contractions, compared to shortening (concentric) or isometric contractions, as the potential for skeletal muscle soreness and injury is accentuated.[3A,84A]

Muscular strength and endurance can be developed by means of static (isometric) or dynamic (isotonic or isokinetic) exercises. Although each type of training has its favorable and weak points, for healthy adults, dynamic resistance exercises are recommended. Resistance training for the average participant should be rhythmical, performed at a moderate to slow speed, move through a full range of motion, and not impede normal forced breathing. Heavy resis-

---

*Haskell and Haskell et al.[71,72] have suggested the use of 4 kcal · kg^{-1} of body weight of energy expenditure per day for a minimum standard for use in exercise programs.

tance exercise can cause a dramatic acute increase in both systolic and diastolic blood pressure.[100A,101C]

The expected improvement in strength from resistance training is difficult to assess because increases in strength are affected by the participants' initial level of strength and their potential for improvement.[43,66,74,114,172] For example, Mueller and Rohmert[114] found increases in strength ranging from 2 to 9% per week depending on initial strength levels. Although the literature reflects a wide range of improvement in strength with resistance training programs, the average improvement for sedentary young and middle-aged men and women for up to 6 months of training is 25–30%. Fleck and Kraemer,[43] in a review of 13 studies representing various forms of isotonic training, showed an average improvement in bench press strength of 23.3% when subjects were tested on the equipment with which they were trained and 16.5% when tested on special isotonic or isokinetic ergometers (six studies). Fleck and Kraemer[43] also reported an average increase in leg strength of 26.6% when subjects were tested with the equipment that they trained on (six studies) and 21.2% when tested with special isotonic or isokinetic ergometers (five studies). Results of improvement in strength resulting from isometric training have been of the same magnitude as found with isotonic training.[17,43,62,63]

In light of the information reported above, the following guidelines for resistance training are recommended for the average healthy adult. A minimum of 8–10 exercises involving the major muscle groups should be performed a minimum of two times per week. A minimum of one set of 8–12 repetitions to near fatigue should be completed. These minimal standards for resistance training are based on two factors. First, the time it takes to complete a comprehensive, well-rounded exercise program is important. Programs lasting more than 60 min per session are associated with higher dropout rates.[124] Second, although greater frequencies of training[17,43,56] and additional sets or combinations of sets and repetitions elicit larger strength gains,[10,32,43,74,145,172] the magnitude of difference is usually small. For example, Braith et al.[17] compared training 2 d · wk^{-1} with 3 d · wk^{-1} for 18 wk. The subjects performed one set of 7–10 repetitions to fatigue. The 2 d · wk^{-1} group showed a 21% increase in strength compared to 28% in the 3 d · wk^{-1} group. In other words, 75% of what could be attained in a 3 d · wk^{-1} program was attained in 2 d · wk^{-1}. Also, the 21% improvement in strength found by the 2 d · wk^{-1} regimen is 70–80% of the improvement reported by other programs using additional frequencies of training and combinations of sets and repetitions.[43] Graves et al.,[62,63] Gettman et al.,[55] Hurley et al.[83] and Braith et al.[17] found that programs using one set to fatigue showed a greater than 25% increase in strength. Although resistance training equipment may provide a better graduated and quantitative stimulus for overload than traditional calisthenic exercises, calisthenics and other resistance types of exercise can still be effective in improving and maintaining strength.

SUMMARY

The combination of frequency, intensity, and duration of chronic exercise has been found to be effective for producing a training effect. The interaction of these factors provide the overload stimulus. In general, the lower the stimulus the lower the training effect, and the greater the stimulus the greater the effect. As a result of specificity of training and the need for maintaining muscular strength and endurance, and flexibility of the major muscle groups, a well-rounded training program including resistance training and flexibility exercises is recommended. Although age in itself is not a limiting factor to exercise training, a more gradual approach in applying the prescription at older ages seems prudent. It has also been shown than endurance training of fewer than 2 d · wk^{-1}, at less than 50% of maximum oxygen uptake and for less than 10 min · d^{-1}, is inadequate for developing and maintaining fitness for healthy adults.

In the interpretation of this position statement, it must be recognized that the recommendations should be used in the context of participants' needs, goals, and initial abilities. In this regard, a sliding scale as to the amount of time allotted and intensity of effort should be carefully gauged for both the cardiorespiratory and muscular strength and endurance components of the program. An appropriate warm-up and cool-down, which would include flexibility exercises, is also recommended. The important factor is to design a program for the individual to provide the proper amount of physical activity to attain maximal benefit at the lowest risk. Emphasis should be placed on factors that result in permanent lifestyle change and encourage a lifetime of physical activity.

REFERENCES

1. Allen TE, Byrd RJ, Smith DP. Hemodynamic consequences of circuit weight training. *Res. Q.* 43:299–306, 1976.

2. American College of Sports Medicine. Proper and improper weight loss programs. *Med. Sci. Sports Exerc.* 15:ix–xiii, 1983.

3. American College of Sports Medicine. *Guidelines for Graded Exercise Testing and Exercise Prescription*, 3rd Ed. Philadelphia: Lea and Febiger, 1986.

3A. Armstrong RB. Mechanisms of exercise-induced delayed onset muscular soreness: a brief review. *Med. Sci. Sports Exerc.* 16:529–538, 1984.

4. Astrand PO. Exercise physiology of the mature athlete. In: *Sports Medicine for the Mature Athlete*, Sutton JR, Brock RM (Eds.). Indianapolis, IN: Benchmark Press, Inc., 1986, pp. 3–16.

5. Astrand PO, Rodahl K. *Textbook of Work Physiology*, 3rd Ed. New York: McGraw-Hill, 1986, pp. 412–485.

6. Atomi Y, Ito K, Iwasaski H, Miyashita M. Effects of intensity and frequency of training on aerobic work capacity of young females. *J. Sports Med.* 18:3–9, 1978.
7. Badenhop DT, Cleary PA, Schaal SF, Fox EL, Bartels RL. Physiological adjustments to higher- or lower-intensity exercise in elders. *Med. Sci. Sports Exerc.* 15:496–502, 1983.
8. Barry AJ, Daly JW, Pruett EDR, et al. The effects of physical conditioning on older individuals. I. Work capacity circulatory-respiratory function, and work electrocardiogram. *J. Gerontol.* 21:182–191, 1966.
9. Benestad AM. Trainability of old men. *Acta Med. Scand.* 178:321–327, 1965.
10. Berger RA. Effect of varied weight training programs on strength. *Res. Q.* 33:168–181, 1962.
11. Birk TJ, Birk CA. Use of ratings of perceived exertion for exercise prescription. *Sports Med.* 4:1–8, 1987.
12. Blair SN, Chandler JV, Ellisor DB, Langley J. Improving physical fitness by exercise training programs. *South. Med. J.* 73:1594–1596, 1980.
13. Blair SN, Kohl HW, Goodyear NN. Rates and risks for running and exercise injuries: studies in three populations. *Res. Q. Exerc. Sports* 58:221–228, 1987.
13A. Blair SN, Kohl HW, III, Paffenbarger RS, Clark DG, Cooper KH, Gibbons LH. Physical fitness and all-cause mortality. A prospective study of healthy men and women. *J.A.M.A.* 262:2395–2401, 1989.
14. Boileau RA, Buskirk ER, Horstman DH, Mendez J, Nicholas W. Body composition changes in obese and lean men during physical conditioning. *Med. Sci. Sports* 3:183–189, 1971.
15. Borg GAV. Psychophysical bases of perceived exertion. *Med. Sci. Sports Exerc.* 14:377–381, 1982.
16. Borg G, Ottoson D (Eds.). *The Perception of Exertion in Physical Work.* London, England: The MacMillan Press, Ltd., 1986, pp. 4–7.
16A. Bouchard C. Gene-environment interaction in human adaptability. In: *The Academy Papers.* Malina RB, Eckert HM (Eds.). Champaign, IL: Human Kinetics Publishers, 1988, pp. 56–66.
17. Braith RW, Graves JE, Pollock ML, Leggett SL, Carpenter DM, Colvin AB. Comparison of two versus three days per week of variable resistance training during 10 and 18 week programs. *Int. J. Sports Med.* 10:450–454, 1989.
18. Brynteson P, Sinning WE. The effects of training frequencies on the retention of cardiovascular fitness. *Med. Sci. Sports* 5:29–33, 1973.
19. Burke EJ. Physiological effects of similar training programs in males and females. *Res. Q.* 48:510–517, 1977.
20. Burke EJ, Franks BD. Changes in VO_{2max} resulting from bicycle training at different intensities holding total mechanical work constant. *Res. Q.* 46:31–37, 1975.
21. Buskirk ER, Hodgson JL. Age and aerobic power: the rate of change in men and women. *Fed. Proc.* 46:1824–1829, 1987.
22. Carter JEL, Phillips WH. Structural changes in exercising middle-aged males during a 2-year period. *J. Appl. Physiol.* 27:787–794, 1969.
23. Chow JR, Wilmore JH. The regulation of exercise intensity by ratings of perceived exertion. *J. Cardiac Rehabil.* 4:382–387, 1984.
24. Christensen EH. Physiological evaluation of work in the Nykroppa iron works. In: *Ergomonics Society Symposium on Fatigue*, Floyd WF, Welford AT (Eds.). London, England: Lewis, 1953, pp. 93–108.
25. Coyle EF, Martin WH, Sinacore DR, Joyner MJ, Hagberg JM, Holloszy JO. Time course of loss of adaptation after stopping prolonged intense endurance training. *J. Appl. Physiol.* 57:1857–1864, 1984.
26. Crews TR, Roberts JA. Effects of interaction of frequency and intensity of training. *Res. Q.* 47:48–55, 1976.
27. Cureton TK. *The Physiological Effects of Exercise Programs upon Adults.* Springfield, IL: Charles C Thomas Co., 1969, pp. 3–6, 33–77.
28. Cureton TK, Phillips EE. Physical fitness changes in middle-aged men attributable to equal eight-week periods of training, non-training and retraining. *J. Sports Med. Phys. Fitness* 4:1–7, 1964.
29. Davies CTM, Knibbs AV. The training stimulus, the effects of intensity, duration and frequency of effort on maximum aerobic power output. *Int. Z. Angew. Physiol.* 29:299–305, 1971.
30. Davis JA, Frank MH, Whipp BJ, Wasserman K. Anaerobic threshold alterations caused by endurance training in middle-aged men. *J. Appl. Physiol.* 46:1039–1049, 1979.
31. Dehn MM, Bruce RA. Longitudinal variations in maximal oxygen intake with age and activity. *J. Appl. Physiol.* 33:805–807, 1972.
32. Delorme TL. Restoration of muscle power by heavy resistance exercise. *J. Bone Joint Surg.* 27:645–667, 1945.
33. Dempsey JA. Anthropometrical observations on obese and nonobese young men undergoing a program of vigorous physical exercise. *Res. Q.* 35:275–287, 1964.
34. Devries HA. Physiological effects of an exercise training regimen upon men aged 52 to 88. *J. Gerontol.* 24:325–336, 1970.
35. Devries HA. Exercise intensity threshold for improvement of cardiovascular-respiratory function in older men. *Geriatrics* 26:94–101, 1971.
36. Dishman RK, Sallis J, Orenstein D. The determinants of physical activity and exercise. *Public Health Rep.* 100:158–180, 1985.
37. Dishman RK, Patton RW, Smith J, Weinberg R, Jackson A. Using perceived exertion to prescribe and monitor exercise training heart rate. *Int. J. Sports Med.* 8:208–213, 1987.
38. Drinkwater BL. Physiological responses of women to exercise. In: *Exercise and Sports Sciences Reviews.* Vol. 1, Wilmore JH (Ed.). New York: Academic Press, 1973, pp. 126–154.
39. Drinkwater BL, Horvath SM, Wells CL. Aerobic power of females, ages 10 to 68. *J. Gerontol.* 30:385–394, 1975.
40. Durnin JVGA, Passmore R. *Energy, Work and Leisure*, London, England: Heinemann Educational Books, Ltd., 1967, pp. 47–82.
41. Edstrom L, Grimby L. Effect of exercise on the motor unit. *Muscle Nerve* 9:104–126, 1986.
42. Ekblom B, Astrand PO, Saltin B, Stenberg J, Wallstrom B. Effect of training on circulatory response to exercise. *J. Appl. Physiol.* 24:518–528, 1968.
43. Fleck SJ, Kraemer WJ. *Designing Resistance Training Programs.* Champaign, IL: Human Kinetics Books, 1987, pp. 15–46, 161–162.
44. Flint MM, Drinkwater BL, Horvath SM. Effects of training on women's response to submaximal exercise. *Med. Sci. Sports* 6:89–94, 1974.
45. Fox EL, Bartels RL, Billings CE, O'Brien R, Bason R, Mathews DK. Frequency and duration of interval training programs and changes in aerobic power. *J. Appl. Physiol.* 38:481–484, 1975.
46. Franklin B, Buskirk E, Hodgson J, Gahagan H, Kollias J, Mendez J. Effects of physical conditioning on cardiorespiratory function, body composition and serum lipids in relatively normal weight and obese middle-age women. *Int. J. Obes.* 3:97–109, 1979.
47. Fringer MN, Stull AG. Changes in cardiorespiratory parameters during periods of training and detraining in young female adults. *Med. Sci. Sports* 6:20–25, 1974.
48. Gaesser GA, Rich RG. Effects of high- and low-intensity exercise training on aerobic capacity and blood lipids. *Med. Sci. Sports Exerc.* 16:269–274, 1984.
49. Getchell LH, Moore JC. Physical training: comparative responses of middle-aged adults. *Arch. Phys. Med. Rehabil.* 56:250–254, 1975.

50. Gettman LR, Pollock ML, Durstine JL, Ward A, Ayres J, Linnerud A.C. Physiological responses of men to 1, 3, and 5 day per week training programs. *Res. Q.* 47:638–646, 1976.
51. Gettman LR, Ayres JJ, Pollock ML, Jackson A. The effect of circuit weight training on strength, cardiorespiratory function, and body composition of adult men. *Med. Sci. Sports* 10:171–176, 1978.
52. Gettman LR, Ayres J, Pollock ML, Durstine JL, Grantham W. Physiological effects of circuit strength training and jogging. *Arch. Phys. Med. Rehabil.* 60:115–120, 1979.
53. Gettman LR, Culter LA, Strathman T. Physiologic changes after 20 weeks of isotonic vs. isokinetic circuit training. *J. Sports Med. Phys. Fitness* 20:265–274, 1980.
54. Gettman LR, Pollock ML. Circuit weight training: a critical review of its physiological benefits. *Phys. Sports Med.* 9:44–60, 1981.
55. Gettman LR, Ward P, Hagman RD. A comparison of combined running and weight training with circuit weight training. *Med. Sci. Sports Exerc.* 14:229–234, 1982.
56. Gillam GM. Effects of frequency of weight training on muscle strength enhancement. *J. Sports Med.* 21:432–436, 1981.
57. Girandola RN. Body composition changes in women: effects of high and low exercise intensity. *Arch. Phys. Med. Rehabil.* 57:297–300, 1976.
58. Gledhill N, Eynon RB. The intensity of training. In: *Training Scientific Basis and Application*, Taylor AW, Howell ML (Eds.). Springfield, IL: Charles C Thomas Co., 1972, pp. 97–102.
59. Golding L. Effects of physical training upon total serum cholesterol levels. *Res. Q.* 32:499–505, 1961.
60. Goode RC, Virgin A, Romet TT, et al. Effects of a short period of physical activity in adolescent boys and girls. *Can. J. Appl. Sports Sci.* 1:241–250, 1976.
61. Gossard D, Haskett WL, Taylor B, et al. Effects of low- and high-intensity home-based exercise training on functional capacity in healthy middle-age men. *Am. J. Cardiol.* 57:446–449, 1986.
62. Graves JE, Pollock ML, Leggett SH, Braith RW, Carpenter DM, Bishop LE. Effect of reduced training frequency on muscular strength. *Int. J. Sports Med.* 9:316–319, 1988.
63. Graves JE, Pollock ML, Jones AE, Colvin AB, Leggett SH. Specificity of limited range of motion variable resistance training. *Med. Sci. Sports Exerc.* 21:84–89, 1989.
64. Gwinup G. Effect of exercise alone on the weight of obese women. *Arch. Int. Med.* 135:676–680, 1975.
65. Hagberg JM, Graves JE, Limacher M, et al. Cardiovascular responses of 70–79 year old men and women to exercise training. *J. Appl. Physiol.* 66:2589–2594, 1989.
66. Hakkinen K. Factors influencing trainability of muscular strength during short term and prolonged training. *Natl. Strength Cond. Assoc. J.* 7:32–34, 1985.
67. Hanson JS, Tabakin BS, Levy AM, Nedde W. Long-term physical training and cardiovascular dynamics in middle-aged men. *Circulation* 38:783–799, 1968.
68. Hanson JS, Nedde WH. Long-term physical training effect in sedentary females. *J. Appl. Physiol.* 37:112–116, 1974.
69. Hartley LH, Grimby G, Kilbom A, et al. Physical training in sedentary middle-aged and older men. *Scand. J. Clin. Lab. Invest.* 24:335–344, 1969.
70. Hartung GH, Smolensky MH, Harrist RB, Runge R. Effects of varied durations of training on improvement in cardiorespiratory endurance. *J. Hum. Ergol.* 6:61–68, 1977.
71. Haskell WL. Physical activity and health: need to define the required stimulus. *Am. J. Cardiol.* 55:4D–9D, 1985.
72. Haskell WL, Montoye HJ, Orenstein D. Physical activity and exercise to achieve health-related physical fitness components. *Public Health Rep.* 100:202–212, 1985.
73. Heath GW, Hagberg JM, Ehsani AA, Holloszy JO. A physiological comparison of young and older endurance athletes. *J. Appl. Physiol.* 51:634–640, 1981.
74. Hettinger T. *Physiology of Strength*. Springfield, IL: Charles C Thomas Publisher, 1961, pp. 18–40.
75. Hickson RC, Rosenkoetter MA. Reduced training frequencies and maintenance of increased aerobic power. *Med. Sci. Sports Exerc.* 13:13–16, 1981.
76. Hickson RC, Kanakis C, Davis JR, Moore AM, Rich S. Reduced training duration effects on aerobic power, endurance, and cardiac growth. *J. Appl. Physiol.* 53:225–229, 1982.
77. Hickson RC, Foster C, Pollock ML, Galassi TM, Rich S. Reduced training intensities and loss of aerobic power, endurance, and cardiac growth. *J. Appl. Physiol.* 58:492–499, 1985.
78. Hill JO, Sparling PB, Shields TW, Heller PA. Effects of exercise and food restriction on body composition and metabolic rate in obese women. *Am. J. Clin. Nutr.* 46:622–630, 1987.
79. Hollmann W. *Changes in the Capacity for Maximal and Continuous Effort in Relation to Age. Int. Res. Sports Phys. Ed.*, Jokl E, Simon E (Eds.). Springfield, IL: Charles C Thomas Co., 1964, pp. 369–371.
80. Hollmann W, Venrath H. Die Beinflussung von grösse, maximaler O_2—Aufnahme und Ausdauergranze ein Ausdauertraining mittlerer und hoher Intensität. *Der Sp* 9:189–193, 1963.
81. No reference 81 due to renumbering in proof.
82. Huibregtse WH, Hartley HH, Jones LR, Doolittle WD, Criblez TL. Improvement of aerobic work capacity following non-strenuous exercise. *Arch. Environ. Health* 27:12–15, 1973.
83. Hurley BF, Seals DR, Ehsani AA, et al. Effects of high-intensity strength training on cardiovascular function. *Med. Sci. Sports Exerc.* 16:483–488, 1984.
84. Ismail AH, Corrigan D, McLeod DF. Effect of an eight-month exercise program on selected physiological, biochemical, and audiological variables in adult men. *Br. J. Sports Med.* 7:230–240, 1973.
84A. Jones DA, Newman DJ, Round JM, Tolfree SEL. Experimental human muscle damage: morphological changes in relation to other indices of damage. *J. Physiol. (Lond.)* 375:435–438, 1986.
85. Karvonen M, Kentala K, Mustala O. The effects of training heart rate: a longitudinal study. *Ann. Med. Exp. Biol. Fenn* 35:307–315, 1957.
86. Kasch FW, Phillips WH, Carter JEL, Boyer JL. Cardiovascular changes in middle-aged men during two years of training. *J. Appl. Physiol.* 314:53–57, 1972.
87. Kasch FW, Wallace JP. Physiological variables during 10 years of endurance exercise. *Med. Sci. Sports* 8:5–8, 1976.
88. Kasch FW, Wallace JP, Van Camp SP. Effects of 18 years of endurance exercise on physical work capacity of older men. *J. Cardiopulmonary Rehabil.* 5:308–312, 1985.
89. Katch FI, McArdle WD. *Nutrition, Weight Control and Exercise*, 3rd Ed. Philadelphia: Lea and Febiger, 1988, pp. 110–112.
90. Kearney JT, Stull AG, Ewing JL, Strein JW. Cardiorespiratory responses of sedentary college women as a function of training intensity. *J. Appl. Physiol.* 41:822–825, 1976.
91. Kendrick ZB, Pollock ML, Hickman TN, Miller HS. Effects of training and detraining on cardiovascular efficiency. *Am. Corr. Ther. J.* 25:79–83, 1971.
92. Kilbom A. Physical training in women. *Scand. J. Clin. Lab. Invest.* 119 (Suppl.):1–34, 1971.

93. Kilbom A, Hartley L, Saltin B, Bjure J, Grimby G, Åstrand I. Physical training in sedentary middle-aged and older men. *Scand. J. Clin. Lab. Invest.* 24:315–322, 1969.
94. Kimura Y, Itow H, Yamazakie S. The effects of circuit weight training on VO_{2max} and body composition of trained and untrained college men. *J. Physiol. Soc. Jpn.* 43:593–596, 1981.
94A. Klissouras V, Pirnay F, Petit J. Adaptation to maximal effort: genetics and age. *J. Appl. Physiol.* 35:288–293, 1973.
95. Knapik JJ, Maudsley RH, Rammos NV. Angular specificity and test mode specificity of isometric and isokinetic strength training. *J. Orthop. Sports Phys. Ther.* 5:58–65, 1983.
96. Knehr CA, Dill DB, Neufeld W. Training and its effect on man at rest and at work. *Am. J. Physiol.* 136:148–156, 1942.
97. Knuttgen HG, Nordesjo LO, Ollander B, Saltin B. Physical conditioning through interval training with young male adults. *Med. Sci. Sports* 5:220–226, 1973.
98. Laporte RE, Adams LL, Savage DD, Brenes G, Dearwater S, Cook T. The spectrum of physical activity, cardiovascular disease and health: an epidemiologic perspective. *Am. J. Epidemiol.* 120:507–517, 1984.
99. Leon AS, Conrad J, Hunninghake DB, Serfass R. Effects of a vigorous walking program on body composition, and carbohydrate and lipid metabolism of obese young men. *Am. J. Clin. Nutr.* 32:1776–1787, 1979.
100. Leon AS, Connett J, Jacobs DR, Rauramaa R. Leisure-time physical activity levels and risk of coronary heart disease and death: the multiple risk factor intervention trial. *J.A.M.A.* 258:2388–2395, 1987.
100A. Lewis SF, Taylor WF, Graham RM, Pettinger WA, Shutte JE, Blomqvist CG. Cardiovascular responses to exercise as function of absolute and relative work load. *J. Appl. Physiol.* 54:1314–1323, 1983.
101. Liang MT, Alexander JF, Taylor HL, Serfrass RC, Leon AS, Stull GA. Aerobic training threshold, intensity duration, and frequency of exercise. *Scand. J. Sports Sci.* 4:5–8, 1982.
101A. Lieber DC, Lieber RL, Adams WC. Effects of run-training and swim-training at similar absolute intensities on treadmill VO_{2max}. *Med. Sci. Sports Exerc.* 21:655–661, 1989.
101B. MacDougall JD, Ward GR, Sale DG, Sutton JR. Biochemical adaptation of human skeletal muscle to heavy resistance training and immobilization. *J. Appl. Physiol.* 43:700–703, 1977.
101C. MacDougall JD, Tuxen D, Sale DG, Moroz JR, Sutton JR. Arterial blood pressure response to heavy resistance training. *J. Appl. Physiol.* 58:785–790, 1985.
102. Mann GV, Garrett LH, Farhi A, et al. Exercise to prevent coronary heart disease. *Am. J. Med.* 46:12–27, 1969.
103. Marcinik EJ, Hodgdon JA, Mittleman U, O'Brien JJ. Aerobic/calisthenic and aerobic/circuit weight training programs for Navy men: a comparative study. *Med. Sci. Sports Exerc.* 17:482–487, 1985.
104. Marigold EA. The effect of training at predetermined heart rate levels for sedentary college women. *Med. Sci. Sports* 6:14–19, 1974.
105. Martin JE, Dubbert PM. Adherence to exercise. In: *Exercise and Sports Sciences Reviews,* Vol. 13, Terjung RL (Ed.). New York: MacMillan Publishing Co., 1985, pp. 137–167.
106. Martin WH, Montgomery J, Snell PG, et al. Cardiovascular adaptations to intense swim training in sedentary middle-aged men and women. *Circulation* 75:323–330, 1987.
107. Mayhew JL, Gross PM. Body composition changes in young women with high resistance weight training. *Res. Q.* 45:433–439, 1974.
108. Messier JP, Dill M. Alterations in strength and maximal oxygen uptake consequent to Nautilus circuit weight training. *Res. Q. Exerc. Sport* 56:345–351, 1985.
109. Milesis CA, Pollock ML, Bah MD, Ayres JJ, Ward A, Linnerud AC. Effects of different durations of training and cardiorespiratory function, body composition and serum lipids. *Res. Q.* 47:716–725, 1976.
110. Misner JE, Boileau RA, Massey BH, Mayhew JH. Alterations in body composition of adult men during selected physical training programs. *J. Am. Geriatr. Soc.* 22:33–38, 1974.
111. Miyashita M, Haga S, Mitzuta T. Training and detraining effects on aerobic power in middle-aged and older men. *J. Sports Med.* 18:131–137, 1978.
112. Moody DL, Kollias J, Buskirk ER. The effect of a moderate exercise program on body weight and skinfold thickness in overweight college women. *Med. Sci. Sports* 1:75–80, 1969.
113. Moody DL, Wilmore JH, Girandola RN, Royce JP. The effects of a jogging program on the body composition of normal and obese high school girls. *Med. Sci. Sports* 4:210–213, 1972.
114. Mueller EA, Rohmert W. Die geschwindigkeit der muskelkraft zunahme bein isometrischen training. *Int. Z. Angew. Physiol.* 19:403–419, 1963.
115. Naughton J, Nagle F. Peak oxygen intake during physical fitness program for middle-aged men. *J.A.M.A.* 191:899–901, 1965.
116. O'Hara W, Allen C, Shephard RJ. Loss of body weight and fat during exercise in a cold chamber. *Eur. J. Appl. Physiol.* 37:205–218, 1977.
117. Oja P, Teraslinna P, Partanen T, Karava R. Feasibility of an 18 months' physical training program for middle-aged men and its effect on physical fitness. *Am. J. Public Health* 64:459–465, 1975.
118. Olree HD, Corbin B, Penrod J, Smith C. Methods of achieving and maintaining physical fitness for prolonged space flight. Final Progress Rep. to NASA, Grant No. NGR-04-002-004, 1969.
119. Oscai LB, Williams T, Hertig B. Effects of exercise on blood volume. *J. Appl. Physiol.* 24:622–624, 1968.
120. Paffenbarger RS, Hyde RT, Wing AL, Hsieh C. Physical activity and all-cause mortality, and longevity of college alumni. *N. Engl. J. Med.* 314:605–613, 1986.
121. Pavlou KN, Steffee WP, Learman RH, Burrows BA. Effects of dieting and exercise on lean body mass, oxygen uptake, and strength. *Med. Sci. Sports Exerc.* 17: 466–471, 1985.
122. Pels AE, Pollock ML, Dohmeier TE, Lemberger KA, Oehrlein BF. Effects of leg press training on cycling, leg press, and running peak cardiorespiratory measures. *Med. Sci. Sports Exerc.* 19:66–70, 1987.
123. Pollock ML. The quantification of endurance training programs. In: *Exercise and Sport Sciences Reviews,* Wilmore JH. (Ed.). New York: Academic Press, 1973, pp. 155–188.
124. Pollock ML. Prescribing exercise for fitness and adherence. In: *Exercise Adherence: Its Impact on Public Health,* Dishman RK (Ed.). Champaign, IL: Human Kinetics Books, 1988, pp. 259–277.
125. Pollock ML, Cureton TK, Greninger L. Effects of frequency of training on working capacity, cardiovascular function, and body composition of adult men. *Med. Sci. Sports* 1:70–74, 1969.
126. Pollock ML, Tiffany J, Gettman L, Janeway R, Lofland H. Effects of frequency of training on serum lipids, cardiovascular function, and body composition. In: *Exercise and Fitness*, Franks BD (Ed.). Chicago: Athletic Institute, 1969, pp. 161–178.
127. Pollock ML, Miller H, Janeway R, Linnerud AC, Robertson B, Valentino R. Effects of walking on body composition and cardiovascular function of middle-aged men. *J. Appl. Physiol.* 30:126–130, 1971.
128. Pollock ML, Broida J, Kenrick Z, Miller HS, Janeway R, Linnerud AC. Effects of training two days per week at different intensities on middle-aged men. *Med. Sci. Sports* 4:192–197, 1972.

129. Pollock ML, Miller Jr. HS, Wilmore J. Physiological characteristics of champion American track athletes 40 to 70 years of age. *J. Gerontol.* 29:645–649, 1974.
130. Pollock ML, Dimmick J, Miller HS, Kendrick Z, Linnerud AC. Effects of mode of training on cardiovascular function and body composition of middle-aged men. *Med. Sci. Sports* 7:139–145, 1975.
131. No reference 131 due to renumbering in proof.
132. Pollock ML, Dawson GA, Miller Jr. HS, et al. Physiologic response of men 49 to 65 years of age to endurance training. *J. Am. Geriatr. Soc.* 24:97–104, 1976.
133. Pollock ML, Jackson A. Body composition: measurement and changes resulting from physical training. Proceedings National College Physical Education Association for Men and Women, January, 1977, pp. 125–137.
134. Pollock ML, Ayres J, Ward A. Cardiorespiratory fitness: response to differing intensities and durations of training. *Arch. Phys. Med. Rehabil.* 58:467–473, 1977.
135. Pollock ML, Gettman R, Milesis CA, Bah MD, Durstine JL, Johnson RB. Effects of frequency and duration of training on attrition and incidence of injury. *Med. Sci. Sports* 9:31–36, 1977.
136. Pollock ML, Gettman LR, Raven PB, Ayres J, Bah M, Ward A. Physiological comparison of the effects of aerobic and anaerobic training. In: *Physical Fitness Programs for Law Enforcement Officers: A Manual for Police Administrators*, Price CS, Pollock ML, Gettman LR, Kent DA (Eds.). Washington, D.C.: U.S. Government Printing Office, No. 027-000-00671-0, 1978, pp. 89–96.
137. Pollock ML, Jackson AS, Foster C. The use of the perception scale for exercise prescription. In: *The Perception of Exertion in Physical Work*, Borg G, Ottoson D (Eds.). London, England: The MacMillan Press, Ltd., 1986, pp. 161–176.
138. Pollock ML, Foster C, Knapp D, Rod JS, Schmidt DH. Effect of age and training on aerobic capacity and body composition of master athletes. *J. Appl. Physiol.* 62:725–713, 1987.
139. Pollock ML, Wilmore JH. *Exercise in Health and Disease: Evaluation and Prescription for Prevention and Rehabilitation*, 2nd Ed. Philadelphia: W. B. Saunders Co., 1990.
140. Powell KE, Kohl HW, Caspersen CJ, Blair SN. An epidemiological perspective of the causes of running injuries. *Phys. Sportsmed.* 14:100–114, 1986.
141. Ribisl PM. Effects of training upon the maximal oxygen uptake of middle-aged men. *Int. Z. Angew. Physiol.* 26:272–278, 1969.
142. Richie DH, Kelso SF, Bellucci PA. Aerobic dance injuries: a retrospective study of instructors and participants. *Phys. Sportsmed.* 13:130–140, 1985.
143. Robinson S, Harmon PM. Lactic acid mechanism and certain properties of blood in relation to training. *Am. J. Physiol.* 132:757–769, 1941.
144. Roskamm H. Optimum patterns of exercise for healthy adults. *Can. Med. Assoc. J.* 96:895–899, 1967.
145. Sale DG. Influence of exercise and training on motor unit activation. In: *Exercise and Sport Sciences Reviews*, Pandolf KB (Ed.). New York: MacMillan Publishing Co., 1987, pp. 95–152.
145A. Sale DG. Neural adaptation to resistance training. *Med. Sci. Sports Exerc.* 20:S135–S145, 1988.
146. Sallis JF, Haskell WL, Fortman SP, Vranizan KM, Taylor CB, Soloman DS. Predictors of adoption and maintenance of physical activity in a community sample. *Prev. Med.* 15:131–141, 1986.
147. Saltin B, Blomqvist G, Mitchell J, Johnson RL, Wildenthal K, Chapman CB. Response to exercise after bed rest and after training. *Circulation* 37, 38(Suppl. 7):1–78, 1968.
148. Saltin B, Hartley L, Kilbom A, Åstrand I. Physical training in sedentary middle-aged and older men. *Scand. J. Clin. Lab. Invest.* 24:323–334, 1969.
149. Santigo MC, Alexander JF, Stull GA, Serfrass RC, Hayday AM, Leon AS. Physiological responses of sedentary women to a 20-week conditioning program of walking or jogging. *Scand. J. Sports Sci.* 9:33–39, 1987.
150. Seals DR, Hagberg JM, Hurley BF, Ehsani AA, Holloszy JO. Endurance training in older men and women. I. Cardiovascular responses to exercise. *J. Appl. Physiol.* 57:1024–1029, 1984.
151. Sharkey BJ. Intensity and duration of training and the development of cardiorespiratory endurance. *Med. Sci. Sports* 2:197–202, 1970.
152. Shephard RJ. Intensity, duration, and frequency of exercise as determinants of the response to a training regime. *Int. Z. Angew. Physiol.* 26:272–278, 1969.
153. Shephard RJ. Future research on the quantifying of endurance training. *J. Hum. Ergol.* 3:163–181, 1975.
154. Sidney KH, Eynon RB, Cunningham DA. Effect of frequency of training of exercise upon physical working performance and selected variables representative of cardiorespiratory fitness. In: *Training Scientific Basis and Application*, Taylor AW (Ed.). Springfield, IL: Charles C Thomas Co., 1972, pp. 144–188.
155. Sidney KH, Shephard RJ, Harrison J. Endurance training and body composition of the elderly. *Am. J. Clin. Nutr.* 30:326–333, 1977.
156. Siegel W, Blomqvist G, Mitchell JH. Effects of a quantitated physical training program on middle-aged sedentary males. *Circulation* 41:19–29, 1970.
156A. Siscovick DS, Weiss NS, Fletcher RH, Lasky T. The incidence of primary cardiac arrest during vigorous exercise. *N. Engl. J. Med.* 311:874–877, 1984.
157. Skinner J. The cardiovascular system with aging and exercise. In: *Physical Activity and Aging*, Brunner D, Jokl E (Eds.). Baltimore: University Park Press, 1970, pp. 100–108.
158. Skinner J, Holloszy J, Cureton T. Effects of a program of endurance exercise on physical work capacity and anthropometric measurements of fifteen middle-aged men. *Am. J. Cardiol.* 14:747–752, 1964.
159. Smith DP, Stransky FW. The effect of training and detraining on the body composition and cardiovascular response of young women to exercise. *J. Sports Med.* 16:112–120, 1976.
160. Smith EL, Reddan W, Smith PE. Physical activity and calcium modalities for bone mineral increase in aged women. *Med. Sci. Sports Exerc.* 13:60–64, 1981.
161. Suominen H, Heikkinen E, Tarkatti T. Effect of eight weeks physical training on muscle and connective tissue of the m. vastus lateralis in 69-year-old men and women. *J. Gerontol.* 32:33–37, 1977.
162. Terjung RL, Baldwin KM, Cooksey J, Samson B, Sutter RA. Cardiovascular adaptation to twelve minutes of mild daily exercise in middle-aged sedentary men. *J. Am. Geriatr. Soc.* 21:164–168, 1973.
163. Thomas SG, Cunningham DA, Rechnitzer PA, Donner AP, Howard JH. Determinants of the training response in elderly men. *Med. Sci. Sports Exerc.* 17:667–672, 1985.
164. Wenger HA, Bell GJ. The interactions of intensity, frequency, and duration of exercise training in altering cardiorespiratory fitness. *Sports Med.* 3:346–356, 1986.
165. Wilmore JH. Alterations in strength, body composition, and anthropometric measurements consequent to a 10-week weight training program. *Med. Sci. Sports* 6:133–138, 1974.
166. Wilmore J. Inferiority of female athletes: myth or reality. *J. Sports Med.* 3:1–6, 1974.

167. Wilmore JH. Design issues and alternatives in assessing physical fitness among apparently healthy adults in a health examination survey of the general population. In: *Assessing Physical Fitness and Activity in General Population Studies*, Drury TF (Ed.). Washington, D.C.: U.S. Public Health Service, National Center for Health Statistics, 1988 (in press).

168. Wilmore JH, Royce J, Girandola RN, Katch FI, Katch VL. Physiological alternatives resulting from a 10-week jogging program. *Med. Sci. Sports* 2:7–14, 1970.

169. Wilmore JH, Royce J, Girandola RN, Katch FI, Katch VL. Body composition changes with a 10-week jogging program. *Med. Sci. Sports* 2:113–117, 1970.

170. Wilmore J, Parr RB, Vodak PA, et al. Strength, endurance, BMR, and body composition changes with circuit weight training. *Med. Sci. Sports* 8:58–60, 1976.

171. Wilmore JH, Ewy GA, Mortan AR, et al. The effect of beta-adrenergic blockade on submaximal and maximal exercise performance. *J. Cardiac Rehabil.* 3:30–36, 1983.

171A. Wilmore JH. Body composition in sport and exercise: directions for future research. *Med. Sci. Sports Exerc.* 15:21–31, 1983.

172. Wilmore JH, Costill DL. *Training for Sport and Activity. The Physiological Basis of the Conditioning Process*, 3rd Ed. Dubuque, IA: Wm. C. Brown, 1988, pp. 113–212.

173. Wood PD, Haskell WL, Blair SN, et al. Increased exercise level and plasma lipoprotein concentrations: a one-year, randomized, controlled study in sedentary, middle-aged men. *Metabolism* 32:31–39, 1983.

174. Zuti WB, Golding LA. Comparing diet and exercise as weight reduction tools. *Phys. Sports Med.* 4:49–53, 1976.

APPENDIX B

Individual Guidelines for Cardiovascular Exercise

1. Exercise only when feeling well.
2. Do not exercise vigorously soon after eating.
3. Adjust exercise to the weather.
4. Slow down for hills.
5. Wear proper clothing and shoes.
6. Understand personal limitations.
7. Select appropriate exercises.
8. Be alert for symptoms. If the following symptoms occur, contact a physician before continuing exercise. Although any symptom should be clarified, these are particularly important.
    a. discomfort in the upper body, including the chest, arm, neck, or jaw, during exercise
    b. faintness accompanying the exercise
    c. shortness of breath during exercise
    d. discomfort in bones or joints either during or after exercise
9. Watch for the following signs of overexercising.
    a. inability to finish training session
    b. inability to converse during the activity
    c. faintness or nausea after exercise
    d. chronic fatigue
    e. sleeplessness
    f. aches and pains in the joints
10. Start slowly and progress gradually.

Source: Reprinted with permission from G.F. Fletcher et al, Exercise Standards, A Statement for Healthcare Professionals, *Circulation*, Vol. 91, No. 2, pp. 603–604, © 1995, American Heart Association.

Appendix C

Physical Activity, Health, and Well-Being: An International Scientific Consensus Conference Consensus Statement

Physical activity positively influences physical and psychosocial health. It is important at all stages in the life cycle, from childhood to extreme old age.

A sedentary lifestyle influences the initiation, progression, and recovery from a variety of vascular and metabolic disturbances, specifically atherosclerosis, hypertension, and adult-onset diabetes mellitus. In contrast, regular physical activity decreases the risk levels for these disturbances, in part through improved weight regulation. Recent studies show a 50% reduction in the risk of dying from cardiovascular disease in men who increase physical activity and improve physical fitness, a magnitude of risk reduction comparable to smoking cessation.

Physical activity benefits most of the structural and function components of the musculoskeletal system, increasing functional capacity and hence independence and quality of life. A substantial part of the age-related decline in functional capacity is due to decreased and insufficient physical activity rather than to aging *per se.*

Physical activity decreases the risk of colon cancer and may reduce the risk of developing breast cancer.

Source: Reprinted with permission from *Research Quarterly for Exercise and Sport,* Vol. 66, No. 4, p. v, © 1995, American Alliance for Health, Physical Education, Recreation, and Dance.

Exercise has a consistent beneficial effect on mood and psychological well being, anxiety, depression, and psychological stress and may enhance cognitive functioning.

Although data from nationally representative samples are scarce, available evidence suggests that a sizeable portion of the population in industrialized countries is sedentary and unfit. Physical activity seems to be less common in developing countries, but will become an issue with continued development and urbanization. Governments and international agencies should plan for these trends and provide opportunities for their citizens of all ages to participate in physical activity, taking into account nutritional status.

Interventions to increase physical activity through worksite, community, and primary health care settings can be successful, showing a potential for change.

Promotion of physical activity for children, adolescents, young adults, the middle-aged, and older adults is one of the most effective means of improving health and enhancing function and quality of life. All governments of the world should initiate policies to increase individual participation in physical activity by creating an environment that will encourage an acceptable level of physical activity in the whole population. This will require cooperation of government agencies, scientific and professional bodies, the private sector, and other community groups.

APPENDIX D

American College of Obstetricians and Gynecologists Exercise Guidelines during Pregnancy and the Postpartum Period

Physical fitness and active recreation are integral parts of the life styles of many women. In the absence of obstetric or medical complications, pregnant women who engage in a moderate level of physical activity can maintain cardiorespiratory and muscular fitness throughout pregnancy and the postpartum period. Pregnancy-related physiologic changes, however, may interfere with the ability to engage safely in some forms of physical activities. The obstetrician is in a position to advise the pregnant patient of such physical limitations and to explain the available information regarding the effects of exercise during pregnancy as well as uncertainties in the current state of knowledge.

The American College of Obstetricians and Gynecologists has issued guidelines for women who exercise, most of which also apply to exercise during pregnancy.[1] This Technical Bulletin will outline specific recommendations and concerns unique for pregnant women and their physiologic bases.

This Technical Bulletin was developed under the direction of the Committee on Technical Bulletins of the American College of Obstetricians and Gynecologists as an educational aid to obstetricians and gynecologists. The committee wishes to thank Raul Artal, MD, for his assistance in the development of this bulletin. This Technical Bulletin does not define a standard of care, nor is it intended to dictate an exclusive course of management. It presents recognized methods and techniques of clinical practice for consideration by obstetrician–gynecologists for incorporation into their practices. Variations of practice taking into account the needs of the individual patient, resources, and limitations unique to the institution or type of practice may be appropriate.

Source: Reprinted with permission from American College of Obstetricians and Gynecologists: Exercise During Pregnancy and the Postpartum Period, Technical Bulletin No. 189, Washington, DC, ACOG, © 1994.

CARDIOVASCULAR CHANGES

Pregnancy induces profound alterations in maternal hemodynamics. Such changes include an increase in blood volume, cardiac output, and resting pulse and a decrease in systemic vascular resistance.[2-4] Hemodynamic changes are also significantly influenced by body position during pregnancy.[5] Cardiac output in third-trimester pregnancy is maximal with the subject in the left or right lateral recumbent position. In contrast, after the first trimester, the supine position results in relative obstruction of venous return by the enlarging uterus and a significant decrease in cardiac output. In some women, such decreases in cardiac output may be symptomatic, resulting in supine hypotensive syndrome. In addition, during pregnancy, motionless standing is associated with an even greater decrease in cardiac output than that seen in the supine position.[5]

Conflicting evidence exists concerning maternal heart rate response to steady-state aerobic exercise during pregnancy; both blunted and normal responses to weight-bearing and non-weight-bearing exercise have been reported.[6,7] The responses of both stroke volume and cardiac output to steady-state exercise, however, are significantly increased.[6,7] Exercise during pregnancy also induces a greater degree of hemoconcentration than does exercise in the nonpregnant state.[7] ST segment depression has been noted in 12% of patients in response to strenuous bicycle exercise both before and during pregnancy, without apparent clinical sequelae.[8] Because this depression has had no adverse clinical sequelae, it appears to be related to heart rate, not ischemia, and is similar to those effects observed with tocolytic therapy with beta-mimetics.[9]

RESPIRATORY CHANGES

During pregnancy, minute ventilation increases by almost 50%, largely as a result of increased tidal volume.[10,11]

This results in an increase in arterial oxygen tension to 106–108 mm Hg in the first trimester, decreasing to a mean of 101–106 mm Hg by the third trimester.[12] There is an associated increase in oxygen uptake, and a 10–20% increase in baseline oxygen consumption. Physiologic dead space during pregnancy remains unchanged.[11,13,14] During treadmill exercise in pregnancy, arteriovenous O_2 difference is decreased.[6] Comparative physiologic studies in pregnancy between weight-bearing and non-weight-bearing exercise indicate further hyperventilation during strenuous exercise in the latter.[15]

Because of the increased resting oxygen requirements and the increased work of breathing brought about by physical effects of the enlarged uterus on the diaphragm, there is decreased oxygen available for the performance of aerobic exercise during pregnancy. Thus, both subjective workload and maximum exercise performance are decreased.[10,16] However, in some fit women, there do not appear to be associated changes in maximum aerobic power or acid–base balance during exercise in pregnancy when compared with the nonpregnant state.[2,13,17]

MECHANICAL CHANGES

The enlargement of the uterus and breasts that occurs during normal pregnancy results in a shift in the physical center of gravity in the pregnant woman. Because balance may be affected, such changes must be kept in mind when considering physical activity in which balance is an important concern or in which loss of balance may prove dangerous.[2] While, theoretically, hormonal influences may result in generalized increases in joint laxity, predisposing the pregnant woman to mechanical trauma or sprains, this hypothesis has been substantiated by objective data only with regard to the metacarpophalangeal joints.[18]

THERMOREGULATORY CHANGES

Both basal metabolic rate and heat production increase during pregnancy.[19] Moderate aerobic exercise is associated with significant increases in core body temperature in nonpregnant individuals.[2] In one study of nonpregnant women exercising at 70% of maximal effort on a treadmill for 20 minutes, the core body temperature rose by an average of 1.5°C.

Data regarding the effects of exercise on core temperature during pregnancy are limited.[2] Fit individuals are known to thermoregulate their core temperature more efficiently. Fetal temperature remains approximately 1°C above that of the mother. In studies of pregnant animals, an increase in maternal core body temperature during embryogenesis exceeding 1.5°C has been observed to cause cessation of neuronal mitotic cell growth in the ependymal layer of the developing brain.[20] Such findings have suggested a possible maternal threshold for human teratogenesis of 39.2°C, possibly accounting for observed increases in congenital anomalies associated with hot tub use in early pregnancy.[20,21] It appears that in fit women, during pregnancy, the peak rectal temperature following exercise at an intensity of 64% of maximum oxygen consumption decreases by 0.3°C at 8 weeks and falls further at a rate of 0.1°C per month through 37 weeks of gestation.[22] Thus, the magnitude of exercise-associated thermal stress for the embryo and fetus may be reduced by maternal physiologic adaptation to pregnancy. Indeed, there has been no demonstrated increase in neural tube or other birth defects among pregnancies of women who continue to perform even vigorous exercise during early pregnancy.[2,16]

METABOLIC CHANGES

Approximately 300 extra kilocalories per day are required to meet the metabolic needs of pregnancy.[2,15,16] This caloric requirement is increased further in pregnant women who exercise regularly. Such concerns do not appear to be significant for most exercising pregnant women. Pregnant women have lower fasting blood glucose levels than do nonpregnant women. In addition, pregnant women utilize carbohydrates during exercise at a greater rate than do their nonpregnant counterparts.[23] Thus, hypoglycemia is more likely to occur both during a resting, fasting state and during exercise in pregnancy. On the cellular level, exercise induces substrate mobilization, while pregnancy is associated with increased tissue storage of fat. These opposing physiologic events could theoretically limit fetal substrate availability.[16] Thus, adequate carbohydrate intake for exercising pregnant patients is essential. In fact, the use of exercise to treat or prevent hyperglycemia in pregnancies complicated by gestational diabetes or insulin-dependent diabetes is currently being investigated.[24,25]

FETAL RESPONSE

Exercise induces significant increases in levels of both epinephrine and serum norepinephrine.[2,26] While epinephrine tends to inhibit uterine activity, norepinephrine increases both the amplitude and frequency of spontaneous uterine contractions. These changes do not necessarily negate one another, and the increased levels of norepinephrine have the potential to cause significant uterine activity or to precipitate preterm labor in individuals at risk for this complication. Although one study found an association between strenuous physical work and an increased incidence of preterm birth, effects of recreational exercise were not examined.[27] In a second study, there was a trend toward a decrease in preterm birth among women who exercised.[28] It appears that in the majority of healthy pregnant women without additional risk factors for preterm labor, exercise does not increase either baseline uterine activity or the incidence of preterm labor or delivery.[29,30]

During exercise at moderate intensity, overall visceral–splanchnic blood flow diminishes by 50%.[31] A specific 20–25% decrease in myometrial clearance of labelled sodium was noted in nonpregnant women during short-term, low-intensity bicycle ergometry.[32] During pregnancy, however, the increase in blood volume and resting cardiac output and the reduction in systemic vascular resistance may reduce the magnitude of such shunting. Such adverse effects of splanchnic shunting may also be minimized by an increase in oxygen and substrate extraction, which under normal conditions averages only 25–30% of capacity.[16] Although changes in uterine blood flow in pregnancy have been studied during exercise using Doppler wave form analysis, the results have been conflicting and no definite conclusions can be drawn in this regard.[33,34]

Several studies have suggested a decrease in birth weight among offspring of women performing heavy work in the standing position during pregnancy.[35,36] A similar decrease in birth weight has been demonstrated in some studies among offspring of women who exercise at high intensities throughout pregnancy.[37] This reduction in birth weight averaged 300–350 g and appeared to reflect primarily a decrease in subcutaneous fat in the newborn.[37] Intrauterine growth retardation and other deleterious short- or long-term effects of decreased fetal weight have not been documented.

Vigorous maternal exercise is associated with a 5–15-beats-per-minute increase in fetal heart rate.[2,16,38] Although brief periods of fetal bradycardia have been described anecdotally, such alterations may be motion-induced artifacts associated with Doppler.[2] One study using ultrasound to observe fetal heart rate during and after maternal exercise noted fetal bradycardia in less than 1% of patients during exercise. Fetal bradycardia was observed in 19% of patients within 3 minutes after cessation of maximal exercise, but in only 1% after submaximal exercise.[39] The investigators concluded that brief submaximal maternal exercise (up to approximately 70% of maternal aerobic power) does not affect fetal heart rate. Adverse fetal effects related to exercise-induced fetal heart rate changes have not been demonstrated in humans.[2,40]

DEVELOPING AN EXERCISE PROGRAM

Most women who perform regular weight-bearing exercise prior to pregnancy note a progressive decline in performance beginning in early pregnancy.[16] In one study involving runners, aerobic dancers, and cross-country skiers, 60% noted significantly decreased exercise performance in early pregnancy, and over 50% had voluntarily stopped exercise completely by the third trimester.[41] Only 10% of patients had maintained their performance at or near preconceptional levels throughout pregnancy.[42] In another study of well-conditioned runners, overall performance decreased by approximately 10% in early pregnancy followed by a gradual decline to roughly 50% of preconceptional levels by the early third trimester.[43] Aerobic capacity, however, was not the only reason for the decline in exercise performance, as many women implicated early pregnancy fatigue, nausea, vomiting, and maternal morphologic changes, especially in the third trimester. Other studies, however, suggest that women who began various forms of non-weight-bearing exercise (cycling or swimming) in early pregnancy were able to maintain a high-intensity, moderate-duration regimen of exercise training throughout the third trimester.[41,44] Thus, the maternal adaptation to both physiologic and morphologic changes appears to favor non-weight-bearing exercise over weight-bearing exercise during pregnancy.[15]

Most of the guidelines for designing a general fitness program in women outlined previously by the American College of Obstetricians and Gynecologists also apply to pregnant women.[1] An exercise prescription in pregnancy should be individualized and should include a health assessment. However, the physiologic changes occurring during pregnancy described here should lead obstetricians and pregnant women to consider several modifications of these general guidelines. It must be emphasized that none of these recommendations has a firm basis in prospective, randomized, clinical trials. These guidelines follow from a critical analysis of the available physiologic data regarding exercise and pregnancy and represent reasonable extrapolations from such knowledge.

Recommendations for Exercise in Pregnancy and Postpartum

There are no data in humans to indicate that pregnant women should limit exercise intensity and lower target heart rates because of potential adverse effects. For women who do not have any additional risk factors for adverse maternal or perinatal outcome, the following recommendations may be made:

1. During pregnancy, women can continue to exercise and derive health benefits even from mild-to-moderate exercise routines. Regular exercise (at least three times per week) is preferable to intermittent activity.
2. Women should avoid exercise in the supine position after the first trimester. Such a position is associated with decreased cardiac output in most pregnant women; because the remaining cardiac output will be preferentially distributed away from splanchnic beds (including the uterus) during vigorous exercise, such regimens are best avoided during pregnancy. Prolonged periods of motionless standing should also be avoided.

3. Women should be aware of the decreased oxygen available for aerobic exercise during pregnancy. They should be encouraged to modify the intensity of their exercise according to maternal symptoms. Pregnant women should stop exercising when fatigued and not exercise to exhaustion. Weight-bearing exercises may under some circumstances be continued at intensities similar to those prior to pregnancy throughout pregnancy. Non-weight-bearing exercises such as cycling or swimming will minimize the risk of injury and facilitate the continuation of exercise during pregnancy.
4. Morphologic changes in pregnancy should serve as a relative contraindication to types of exercise in which loss of balance could be detrimental to maternal or fetal well-being, especially in the third trimester. Further, any type of exercise involving the potential for even mild abdominal trauma should be avoided.
5. Pregnancy requires an additional 300 kcal/d in order to maintain metabolic homeostasis. Thus, women who exercise during pregnancy should be particularly careful to ensure an adequate diet.
6. Pregnant women who exercise in the first trimester should augment heat dissipation by ensuring adequate hydration, appropriate clothing, and optimal environmental surroundings during exercise.
7. Many of the physiologic and morphologic changes of pregnancy persist 4–6 weeks postpartum. Thus, prepregnancy exercise routines should be resumed gradually based on a woman's physical capability.

Contraindications to Exercise

The aforementioned recommendations are intended for women who do not have any additional risk factors for adverse maternal or perinatal outcome. A number of medical or obstetric conditions may lead the obstetrician to recommend modifications of these principles. The following conditions should be considered contraindications to exercise during pregnancy:

- Pregnancy-induced hypertension
- Preterm rupture of membranes
- Preterm labor during the prior or current pregnancy or both
- Incompetent cervix/cerclage
- Persistent second- or third-trimester bleeding
- Intrauterine growth retardation

In addition, women with certain other medical or obstetric conditions, including chronic hypertension or active thyroid, cardiac, vascular, or pulmonary disease, should be evaluated carefully in order to determine whether an exercise program is appropriate.

SUMMARY

In the absence of either obstetric or medical complications, pregnant women can continue to exercise and derive related benefits. Women who have achieved cardiovascular fitness prior to pregnancy should be able to safely maintain that level of fitness throughout pregnancy and the postpartum period. Depending on the individual's needs and the physiologic changes associated with pregnancy, women may have to modify their specific exercise regimens. Despite findings that suggest lower birth weights among offspring of women who continue to exercise vigorously throughout pregnancy, there currently are no data to confirm that, with the specific exceptions mentioned here, exercise during pregnancy has any deleterious effects on the fetus. While maternal fitness and sense of well-being may be enhanced by exercise, no level of exercise during pregnancy has been conclusively demonstrated to be beneficial in improving perinatal outcome.

REFERENCES

1. American College of Obstetricians and Gynecologists. Women and exercise. ACOG Technical Bulletin 173. Washington, DC: ACOG, 1992.
2. Artal Mittelmark R, Wiswell RA, Drinkwater BL, eds. *Exercise in Pregnancy.* 2nd ed. Baltimore: Williams and Wilkins, 1991.
3. Clark SL, Cotton DB, Lee W, Bishop C, Hill T, Southwick J, et al. Central hemodynamic assessment of normal term pregnancy. *Am J Obstet Gynecol* 1989;161:1439–1442.
4. Wolfe LA, Ohtake PJ, Mottola MF, McGrath MJ. Physiological interactions between pregnancy and aerobic exercise. *Exerc Sport Sci Rev* 1989;17:295–351.
5. Clark LS, Cotton DB, Pivarnik JM, Lee W, Hankins GDV, Benedetti TJ, et al. Position change and central hemodynamic profile during normal third-trimester pregnancy and post partum. *Am J Obstet Gynecol* 1991;164:883–887.
6. Pivarnik JM, Lee W, Clark LS, Cotton DB, Spillman HT, Miller JF. Cardiac output responses of primigravid women during exercise determined by the direct Fick technique. *Obstet Gynecol* 1990;75:954–959.
7. McMurray RG, Hackney AC, Katz VL, Gall M, Watson WJ. Pregnancy-induced changes in the maximal physiological responses during swimming. *J Appl Physiol* 1991;71:1454–1459.
8. Van Doorn MB, Lotgering FK, Struijk PC, Pool J, Wallenburg HCS. Maternal and fetal cardiovascular responses to strenuous bicycle exercise. *Am J Obstet Gynecol* 1992;166:854–859.
9. Hendricks SK, Keroes J, Katz M. Electrocardiographic changes associated with ritodrine-induced maternal tachycardia and hypokalemia. *Am J Obstet Gynecol* 1986;154:921–923.
10. Artal R, Wiswell R, Romem Y, Dorey F. Pulmonary responses to exercise in pregnancy. *Am J Obstet Gynecol* 1986;154:378–383.

11. Prowse CM, Gaensler EA. Respiratory and acid–base changes during pregnancy. *Anesthesiology* 1965;26:381–392.
12. Templeton A, Kelman GR. Maternal blood-gases, $(PA_{O_2}—Pa_{O_2})$, physiological shunt and VD/VT in normal pregnancy. *Br J Anaesth* 1976;48:1001–1004.
13. Pivarnik JM, Lee W, Spillman T, Clark SL, Cotton DB, Miller JF. Maternal respiration and blood gases during aerobic exercise performed at moderate altitude. *Med Sci Sports Exerc* 1992;24:868–872.
14. Sady SP, Carpenter MW, Thompson PD, Sady MA, Haydon B, Coustan DR. Cardiovascular response to cycle exercise during and after pregnancy. *J Appl Physiol* 1989;66:336–341.
15. Artal R, Masaki DI, Khodiguian N, Romem Y, Rutherford SE, Wiswell RA. Exercise prescription in pregnancy: weight-bearing versus non-weight-bearing exercise. *Am J Obstet Gynecol* 1989;161:1464–1469.
16. Clapp JF III. Exercise in pregnancy: a brief clinical review. *Fetal Med Rev* 1990;2:89–101.
17. Lotgering FK, Van Doorn MB, Struijk PC, Pool J, Wallenburg HCS. Maximal aerobic exercise in pregnant women: heart rate, O_2 consumption, CO_2 production, and ventilation. *J Appl Physiol* 1991;70:1016–1023.
18. Calguneri M, Bird HA, Wright V. Changes in joint laxity occurring during pregnancy. *Ann Rheum Dis* 1982;41:126–128.
19. Hytten FE. Nutrition. In: Hytten FE, Chamberlain G, eds. *Clinical Physiology in Obstetrics.* Oxford: Blackwell, 1980.
20. Edwards MJ. Hyperthermia as a teratogen: a review of experimental studies and their clinical significance. *Teratogenesis Carcinog Mutagen* 1986;6:563–582.
21. Milunsky A, Ulcickas M, Rothman KJ, Willett W, Jick SS, Jick H. Maternal heat exposure and neural tube defects. *JAMA* 1992;268:882–885.
22. Clapp JF III. The changing thermal response to endurance exercise during pregnancy. *Am J Obstet Gynecol* 1991;165:1684–1689.
23. Clapp JF III, Seaward BL, Sleamaker RH, Hiser J. Maternal physiologic adaptations to early human pregnancy. *Am J Obstet Gynecol* 1988;159:1456–1460.
24. Jovanovic-Peterson L, Durak EP, Peterson CM. Randomized trial of diet versus diet plus cardiovascular conditioning on glucose levels in gestational diabetes. *Am J Obstet Gynecol* 1989;161:415–419.
25. Bung P, Bung C, Artal R, Khodiguian N, Fallenstein F, Spätling L. Therapeutic exercise for insulin-requiring gestational diabetics: effects on the fetus—results of a randomized prospective longitudinal study. *J Perinat Med* 1993;21:125–137.
26. Artal R, Platt LD, Sperling M, Kammula RK, Jilek J, Nakamura R. Exercise in pregnancy. I. Maternal cardiovascular and metabolic responses in normal pregnancy. *Am J Obstet Gynecol* 1981;140:123–127.
27. Papiernik E, Kaminski M. Multifactorial study of the risk of prematurity at 32 weeks of gestation. I. A study of the frequency of 30 predictive characteristics. *J Perinat Med* 1974;2:30–36.
28. Berkowitz GS, Kelsey JL, Holford TR, Berkowitz RL. Physical activity and the risk of spontaneous preterm delivery. *J Reprod Med* 1983;28:581–588.
29. Veille J-C, Hohimer AR, Burry K, Speroff L. The effect of exercise on uterine activity in the last eight weeks of pregnancy. *Am J Obstet Gynecol* 1985;151:727–730.
30. Katz VL, McMurry R, Berry MJ, Cefalo RC. Fetal and uterine responses to immersion and exercise. *Obstet Gynecol* 1988;72:225–230.
31. Rowell LB. Human cardiovascular adjustments to exercise and thermal stress. *Physiol Rev* 1974;54:75–159.
32. Morris N, Osborn SB, Wright HP, Hart A. Effective uterine blood-flow during exercise in normal and pre-eclamptic pregnancies. *Lancet* 1956;2:481–484.
33. Hackett GA, Cohen-Overbeek T, Campbell S. The effect of exercise on uteroplacental Doppler waveforms in normal and complicated pregnancies. *Obstet Gynecol* 1992;79:919–923.
34. Erkkola RU, Pirhonen JP, Kivijärvi AK. Flow velocity waveforms in uterine and umbilical arteries during submaximal bicycle exercise in normal pregnancy. *Obstet Gynecol* 1992;79:611–615.
35. Naeye RL, Peters EC. Working during pregnancy: effects on the fetus. *Pediatrics* 1982;69:724–727.
36. Tafari N, Naeye RL, Gobezie A. Effects of maternal undernutrition and heavy physical work during pregnancy on birth weight. *Br J Obstet Gynecol* 1980;87:222–226.
37. Clapp JF III, Capeless EL. Neonatal morphometrics after endurance exercise during pregnancy. *Am J Obstet Gynecol* 1990;163:1805–1811.
38. Artal R, Rutherford S, Romen Y, Kammula RK, Dorey F, Wiswell RA. Fetal heart rate responses to maternal exercise. *Am J Obstet Gynecol* 1986;155:729–733.
39. Carpenter MW, Sady SP, Hoegsberg B, Sady MA, Haydon B, Cullinane EM, et al. Fetal heart rate response to maternal exertion. *JAMA* 1988;259:3006–3009.
40. Paolone AM, Shangold M, Paul D, Minnitti J, Weiner S. Fetal heart rate measurement during maternal exercise—avoidance of artifact. *Med Sci Sports Exerc* 1987;19:605–609.
41. Collings CA, Curet LB, Mullin JP. Maternal and fetal responses to a maternal aerobic exercise program. *Am J Obstet Gynecol* 1983;145:702–707.
42. Clapp JF III, Dickstein S. Endurance exercise and pregnancy outcome. *Med Sci Sports Exerc* 1984;16:556–562.
43. Clapp JF III. The effects of maternal exercise on early pregnancy outcome. *Am J Obstet Gynecol* 1989;161:1453–1457.
44. Sibley L, Ruhling RO, Cameron-Foster J, Christensen C, Bolen T. Swimming and physical fitness during pregnancy. *J Nurse-Midwif* 1981;26:3–12.

APPENDIX E

Physical Activity and Health: Summary of a Report of the Surgeon General

INTRODUCTION

This is the first Surgeon General's report to address physical activity and health. The main message of this report is that Americans can substantially improve their health and quality of life by including moderate amounts of physical activity in their daily lives. Health benefits from physical activity are thus achievable for most Americans, including those who may dislike vigorous exercise and those who may have been previously discouraged by the difficulty of adhering to a program of vigorous exercise. For those who are already achieving regular moderate amounts of activity, additional benefits can be gained by further increases in activity level.

This report grew out of an emerging consensus among epidemiologists, experts in exercise science, and health professionals that physical activity need not be of vigorous intensity for it to improve health. Moreover, health benefits appear to be proportional to amount of activity; thus, every increase in activity adds some benefit. Emphasizing the amount rather than the intensity of physical activity offers more options for people to select from in incorporating physical activity into their daily lives. Thus, a moderate amount of activity can be obtained in a 30-minute brisk walk, 30 minutes of lawn mowing or raking leaves, a 15-minute run, or 45 minutes of playing volleyball, and these activities can be varied from day to day. It is hoped that this different emphasis on moderate amounts of activity, and the flexibility to vary activities according to personal preference and life circumstances, will encourage more people to make physical activity a regular and sustainable part of their lives.

The information in this report summarizes a diverse literature from the field of epidemiology, exercise physiology, medicine, and the behavioral sciences. The report highlights what is known about physical activity and health, as well as what is being learned about promoting physical activity among adults and young people.

DEVELOPMENT OF THE REPORT

In July 1994, the Office of the Surgeon General authorized the Centers for Disease Control and Prevention (CDC) to serve as lead agency for preparing the first Surgeon General's report on physical activity and health. The CDC was joined in this effort by the President's Council on Physical Fitness and Sports (PCPFS) as a collaborative partner representing the Office of the Surgeon General. Because of the wide interest in the health effects of physical activity, the report was planned collaboratively with representatives from the Office of the Surgeon General, the Office of Public Health and Science (Office of the Secretary), the Office of Disease Prevention (National Institutes of Health [NIH]), and the following institutes from the NIH: the National Heart, Lung, and Blood Institute; the National Institute of Child Health and Human Development; the National Institute of Diabetes and Digestive and Kidney Diseases; and the National Institute of Arthritis and Musculoskeletal and Skin Diseases. CDC's nonfederal partners—including the American Alliance for Health, Physical Education, Recreation, and Dance; the American College of Sports Medicine; and the American Heart Association—provided consultation throughout the development process.

The major purpose of this report is to summarize the existing literature on the role of physical activity in preventing disease and on the status of interventions to increase physical activity. Any report on a topic this broad must restrict its scope to keep its message clear. This report focuses on disease prevention and therefore does not include the consider-

Source: Reprinted from *Physical Activity and Health: A Report of the Surgeon General Executive Summary,* 1996.

able body of evidence on the benefits of physical activity for treatment or rehabilitation after disease has developed. This report concentrates on endurance-type physical activity (activity involving repeated use of large muscles, such as in walking or bicycling) because the health benefits of this type of activity have been extensively studied. The importance of resistance exercise (to increase muscle strength, such as by lifting weights) is increasingly being recognized as a means to preserve and enhance muscular strength and endurance and to prevent falls and improve mobility in the elderly. Some promising findings on resistance exercise are presented here, but a comprehensive review of resistance training is beyond the scope of this report. In addition, a review of the special concerns regarding physical activity for pregnant women and for people with disabilities is not undertaken here, although these important topics deserve more research and attention.

Finally, physical activity is only one of many everyday behaviors that affect health. In particular, nutritional habits are linked to some of the same aspects of health as physical activity, and the two may be related lifestyle characteristics. This report deals solely with physical activity; a Surgeon General's Report on Nutrition and Health was published in 1988.

Chapters 2 through 6 of this report address distinct areas of the current understanding of physical activity and health. Chapter 2 offers a historical perspective: after outlining the history of belief and knowledge about physical activity and health, the chapter reviews the evolution and content of physical activity recommendations. Chapter 3 describes the physiologic responses to physical activity—both the immediate effects of a single episode of activity and the long-term adaptations to a regular pattern of activity. The evidence that physical activity reduces the risk of cardiovascular and other diseases is presented in Chapter 4. Data on patterns and trends of physical activity in the U.S. population are the focus of Chapter 5. Lastly, Chapter 6 examines efforts to increase physical activity and reviews ideas currently being proposed for policy and environmental initiatives.

MAJOR CONCLUSIONS

1. People of all ages, both male and female, benefit from regular physical activity.
2. Significant health benefits can be obtained by including a moderate amount of physical activity (e.g., 30 minutes of brisk walking or raking leaves, 15 minutes of running, or 45 minutes of playing volleyball) on most, if not all, days of the week. Through a modest increase in daily activity, most Americans can improve their health and quality of life.
3. Additional health benefits can be gained through greater amounts of physical activity. People who can maintain a regular regimen of activity that is of longer duration or of more vigorous intensity are likely to derive greater benefit.
4. Physical activity reduces the risk of premature mortality in general, and of coronary heart disease, hypertension, colon cancer, and diabetes mellitus in particular. Physical activity also improves mental health and is important for the health of muscles, bones, and joints.
5. More than 60 percent of American adults are not regularly physically active. In fact, 25 percent of all adults are not active at all.
6. Nearly half of American youths 12–21 years of age are not vigorously active on a regular basis. Moreover, physical activity declines dramatically during adolescence.
7. Daily enrollment in physical education classes has declined among high school students from 42 percent in 1991 to 25 percent in 1995.
8. Research on understanding and promoting physical activity is at an early stage, but some interventions to promote physical activity through schools, worksites, and health care settings have been evaluated and found to be successful.

SUMMARY

The benefits of physical activity have been extolled throughout western history, but it was not until the second half of this century that scientific evidence supporting these beliefs began to accumulate. By the 1970s, enough information was available about the beneficial effects of vigorous exercise on cardiorespiratory fitness that the American College of Sports Medicine (ACSM), the American Heart Association (AHA), and other national organizations began issuing physical activity recommendations to the public. These recommendations generally focused on cardiorespiratory endurance and specified sustained periods of vigorous physical activity involving large muscle groups and lasting at least 20 minutes on 3 or more days per week. As understanding of the benefits of less vigorous activity grew, recommendations followed suit. During the past few years, the ACSM, the CDC, the AHA, the PCPFS, and the NIH have all recommended regular, moderate-intensity physical activity as an option for those who get little or no exercise. The *Healthy People 2000* goals for the nation's health have recognized the importance of physical activity and have included physical activity goals. The 1995 *Dietary Guidelines for Americans,* the basis of the federal government's nutrition-related programs, included physical activity guidance to maintain and improve weight—30 minutes or more of moderate-intensity physical activity on all, or most, days of the week.

Underpinning such recommendations is a growing understanding of how physical activity affects physiologic function. The body responds to physical activity in ways that have important positive effects on musculoskeletal, cardiovascular, respiratory, and endocrine systems. These changes are consistent with a number of health benefits, including a reduced risk of premature mortality and reduced risks of coronary heart disease, hypertension, colon cancer, and diabetes mellitus. Regular participation in physical activity also appears to reduce depression and anxiety, improve mood, and enhance ability to perform daily tasks throughout the life span.

The risks associated with physical activity must also be considered. The most common health problems that have been associated with physical activity are musculoskeletal injuries, which can occur with excessive amounts of activity or with suddenly beginning an activity for which the body is not conditioned. Much more serious associated health problems (i.e., myocardial infarction, sudden death) are also much rarer, occurring primarily among sedentary people with advanced atherosclerotic disease who engage in strenuous activity to which they are unaccustomed. Sedentary people, especially those with preexisting health conditions, who wish to increase their physical activity should therefore gradually build up to the desired level of activity. Even among people who are regularly active, the risk of myocardial infarction or sudden death is somewhat increased during physical exertion, but their overall risk of these outcomes is lower than that among people who are sedentary.

Research on physical activity continues to evolve. This report includes both well-established findings and newer research results that await replication and amplification. Interest has been developing in ways to differentiate between the various characteristics of physical activity that improve health. It remains to be determined how the interrelated characteristics of amount, intensity, duration, frequency, type, and pattern of physical activity are related to specific health or disease outcomes.

Attention has been drawn recently to findings from three studies showing that cardiorespiratory fitness gains are similar when physical activity occurs in several short sessions (e.g., 10 minutes) as when the same total amount and intensity of activity occurs in one longer session (e.g., 30 minutes). Although, strictly speaking, the health benefits of such intermittent activity have not yet been demonstrated, it is reasonable to expect them to be similar to those of continuous activity. Moreover, for people who are unable to set aside 30 minutes for physical activity, shorter episodes are clearly better than none. Indeed, one study has shown greater adherence to a walking program among those walking several times per day than among those walking once per day, when the total amount of walking time was kept the same. Accumulating physical activity over the course of the day has been included in recent recommendations from the CDC and ACSM, as well as from the NIH Consensus Development Conference on Physical Activity and Cardiovascular Health.

Despite common knowledge that exercise is healthful, more than 60 percent of American adults are not regularly active, and 25 percent of the adult population are not active at all. Moreover, although many people have enthusiastically embarked on vigorous exercise programs at one time or another, most do not sustain their participation. Clearly, the processes of developing and maintaining healthier habits are as important to study as the health effects of these habits.

The effort to understand how to promote more active lifestyles is of great importance to the health of this nation. Although the study of physical activity determinants and interventions is at an early stage, effective programs to increase physical activity have been carried out in a variety of settings, such as schools, physicians' offices, and worksites. Determining the most effective and cost-effective intervention approaches is a challenge for the future. Fortunately, the United States has skilled leadership and institutions to support efforts to encourage and assist Americans to become more physically active. Schools, community agencies, parks, recreational facilities, and health clubs are available in most communities and can be more effectively used in these efforts.

School-based interventions for youth are particularly promising, not only for their potential scope—almost all young people between the ages of 6 and 16 years attend school—but also for their potential impact. Nearly half of young people 12–21 years of age are not vigorously active; moreover, physical activity sharply declines during adolescence. Childhood and adolescence may thus be pivotal times for preventing sedentary behavior among adults by maintaining the habit of physical activity throughout the school years. School-based interventions have been shown to be successful in increasing physical activity levels. With evidence that success in this arena is possible, every effort should be made to encourage schools to require daily physical education in each grade and to promote physical activities that can be enjoyed throughout life.

Outside the school, physical activity programs and initiatives face the challenge of a highly technological society that makes it increasingly convenient to remain sedentary and that discourages physical activity in both obvious and subtle ways. To increase physical activity in the general population, it may be necessary to go beyond traditional efforts. This report highlights some concepts from community initiatives that are being implemented around the country. It is hoped that these examples will spark new public policies and programs in other places as well. Special efforts will also be required to meet the needs of special populations, such as people with disabilities, racial and ethnic minorities, people with low income, and the elderly. Much more information about these important groups will be necessary to develop a truly comprehensive national initiative for better health through physical activity. Challenges for the future include identifying key determinants of physically active lifestyles among the diverse populations that characterize the United States (including special populations, women, and young people) and using this information to design and disseminate effective programs.

CHAPTER CONCLUSIONS

Chapter 2: Historical Background and Evolution of Physical Activity Recommendations

1. Physical activity for better health and well-being has been an important theme throughout much of western history.
2. Public health recommendations have evolved from emphasizing vigorous activity for cardiorespiratory fitness to including the option of moderate levels of activity for numerous health benefits.
3. Recommendations from experts agree that for better health, physical activity should be performed regularly. The most recent recommendations advise people of all ages to include a minimum of 30 minutes of physical activity of moderate intensity (such as brisk walking) on most, if not all, days of the week. It is also acknowledged that for most people, greater health benefits can be obtained by engaging in physical activity of more vigorous intensity or of longer duration.
4. Experts advise previously sedentary people embarking on a physical activity program to start with short durations of moderate-intensity activity and gradually increase the duration of intensity until the goal is reached.
5. Experts advise consulting with a physician before beginning a new physical activity program for people with chronic diseases, such as cardiovascular disease and diabetes mellitus, or for those who are at high risk for these diseases. Experts also advise men over age 40 and women over age 50 to consult a physician before they begin a vigorous activity program.
6. Recent recommendations from experts also suggest that cardiorespiratory endurance activity should be supplemented with strength-developing exercises at least twice per week for adults, in order to improve musculoskeletal health, maintain independence in performing the activities of daily life, and reduce the risk of falling.

Chapter 3: Physiologic Responses and Long-Term Adaptations to Exercise

1. Physical activity has numerous beneficial physiologic effects. Most widely appreciated are its effects on the cardiovascular and musculoskeletal systems, but benefits on the functioning of metabolic, endocrine, and immune systems are also considerable.
2. Many of the beneficial effects of exercise training—from both endurance and resistance activities—diminish within 2 weeks if physical activity is substantially reduced, and effects disappear within 2 to 8 months if physical activity is not resumed.
3. People of all ages, both male and female, undergo beneficial physiologic adaptations to physical activity.

Chapter 4: The Effects of Physical Activity on Health and Disease

Overall Mortality

1. Higher levels of regular physical activity are associated with lower mortality rates for both older and younger adults.
2. Even those who are moderately active on a regular basis have lower mortality rates than those who are least active.

Cardiovascular Diseases

1. Regular physical activity or cardiorespiratory fitness decreases the risk of cardiovascular disease mortality in general and of coronary heart disease mortality in particular. Existing data are not conclusive regarding a relationship between physical activity and stroke.
2. The level of decreased risk of coronary heart disease attributable to regular physical activity is similar to that of other lifestyle factors, such as keeping free from cigarette smoking.
3. Regular physical activity prevents or delays the development of high blood pressure, and exercise reduces blood pressure in people with hypertension.

Cancer

1. Regular physical activity is associated with a decreased risk of colon cancer.
2. There is no association between physical activity and rectal cancer. Data are too sparse to draw conclusions regarding a relationship between physical activity and endometrial, ovarian, or testicular cancers.
3. Despite numerous studies on the subject, existing data are inconsistent regarding an association between physical activity and breast or prostate cancers.

Non–Insulin-Dependent Diabetes Mellitus

1. Regular physical activity lowers the risk of developing non–insulin-dependent diabetes mellitus.

Osteoarthritis

1. Regular physical activity is necessary for maintaining normal muscle strength, joint structure, and joint function. In the range recommended for health, physical activity is not associated with joint damage or development of osteoarthritis and may be beneficial for many people with arthritis.
2. Competitive athletics may be associated with the development of osteoarthritis later in life, but sports-related injuries are the likely cause.

Osteoporosis

1. Weight-bearing physical activity is essential for normal skeletal development during childhood and ado-

lescence and for achieving and maintaining peak bone mass in young adults.
2. It is unclear whether resistance- or endurance-type physical activity can reduce the accelerated rate of bone loss in postmenopausal women in the absence of estrogen replacement therapy.

Falling

1. There is promising evidence that strength training and other forms of exercise in older adults preserve the ability to maintain independent living status and reduce the risk of falling.

Obesity

1. Low levels of activity, resulting in fewer kilocalories used than consumed, contribute to the high prevalence of obesity in the United States.
2. Physical activity may favorably affect body fat distribution.

Mental Health

1. Physical activity appears to relieve symptoms of depression and anxiety and improve mood.
2. Regular physical activity may reduce the risk of developing depression, although further research is needed on this topic.

Health-Related Quality of Life

1. Physical activity appears to improve health-related quality of life by enhancing psychological well-being and by improving physical functioning in persons compromised by poor health.

Adverse Effects

1. Most musculoskeletal injuries related to physical activity are believed to be preventable by gradually working up to a desired level of activity and by avoiding excessive amounts of activity.
2. Serious cardiovascular events can occur with physical exertion, but the net effect of regular physical activity is a lower risk of mortality from cardiovascular disease.

Chapter 5: Patterns and Trends in Physical Activity

Adults

1. Approximately 15 percent of U.S. adults engage regularly (3 times a week for at least 20 minutes) in vigorous physical activity during leisure time.
2. Approximately 22 percent of adults engage regularly (5 times a week for at least 30 minutes) in sustained physical activity of any intensity during leisure time.
3. About 25 percent of adults report no physical activity at all in their leisure time.
4. Physical inactivity is more prevalent among women than men, among blacks and Hispanics than whites, among older than younger adults, and among the less affluent than the more affluent.
5. The most popular leisure-time physical activities among adults are walking and gardening or yard work.

Adolescents and Young Adults

1. Only about one-half of U.S. young people (ages 12–21 years) regularly participate in vigorous physical activity. One-fourth report no vigorous physical activity.
2. Approximately one-fourth of young people walk or bicycle (i.e., engage in light to moderate activity) nearly every day.
3. About 14 percent of young people report no recent vigorous or light-to-moderate physical activity. This indicator of inactivity is higher among females than males and among black females than white females.
4. Males are more likely than females to participate in vigorous physical activity, strengthening activities, and walking or bicycling.
5. Participation in all types of physical activity declines strikingly as age or grade in school increases.
6. Among high school students, enrollment in physical education remained unchanged during the first half of the 1990s. However, daily attendance in physical education declined from approximately 42 percent to 25 percent.
7. The percentage of high school students who were enrolled in physical education and who reported being physically active for at least 20 minutes in physical education classes declined from approximately 81 percent to 70 percent during the first half of this decade.
8. Only 19 percent of all high school students report being physically active for 20 minutes or more in daily physical education classes.

Chapter 6: Understanding and Promoting Physical Activity

1. Consistent influences on physical activity patterns among adults and young people include confidence in one's ability to engage in regular physical activity (e.g., self-efficacy), enjoyment of physical activity, support from others, positive beliefs concerning the benefits of physical activity, and lack of perceived barriers to being physically active.
2. For adults, some interventions have been successful in increasing physical activity in communities, worksites, and health care settings, and at home.
3. Interventions targeting physical education in elementary school can substantially increase the amount of time students spend being physically active in physical education class.

APPENDIX F

Physical Activity and Public Health
A Recommendation From the Centers for Disease Control and Prevention and the American College of Sports Medicine

Russell R. Pate, Michael Pratt, Steven N. Blair, William L. Haskell, Caroline A. Macera, Claude Bouchard, David Buchner, Walter Ettinger, Gregory W. Heath, Abby C. King, Andrea Kriska, Arthur S. Leon, Bess H. Marcus, Jeremy Morris, Ralph S. Paffenbarger, Jr., Kevin Patrick, Michael L. Pollock, James M. Rippe, James Sallis, Jack H. Wilmore

Regular physical activity has long been regarded as an important component of a healthy lifestyle. Recently, this impression has been reinforced by new scientific evidence linking regular physical activity to a wide array of physical and mental health benefits.[1–7] Despite this evidence and the public's apparent acceptance of the importance of physical activity, millions of US adults remain essentially sedentary.[8]

If our sedentary society is to change to one that is more physically active, health organizations and educational institutions must communicate to the public the amounts and types of physical activity that are needed to prevent disease and promote health. These organizations and institutions, providers of health services, communities, and individuals must also implement effective strategies that promote the adoption of physically active lifestyles.

A group of experts was brought together by the Centers for Disease Control and Prevention (CDC) and the American College of Sports Medicine (ACSM) to review the pertinent scientific evidence and to develop a clear, concise "public health message" regarding physical activity. The panel of experts also considered the organizational initiatives that should be implemented to help US adults become more physically active.

The focus of this article is on physical activity and the health benefits associated with regular, moderate-intensity physical activity. Physical activity has been defined as "any bodily movement produced by skeletal muscles that results in energy expenditure."[9] Moderate physical activity is activity performed at an intensity of 3 to 6 METs (work metabolic rate/resting metabolic rate)—the equivalent of brisk walking at 3 to 4 mph for most healthy adults. Physical activity is closely related to, but distinct from, exercise and physical fitness. Exercise is a subset of physical activity defined as "planned, structured, and repetitive bodily movement done to improve or maintain one or more components of physical fitness."[9] Physical fitness is "a set of attributes that people have or achieve that relates to the ability to perform physical activity."[9]

This article summarizes the work of the aforementioned expert panel and has two purposes. First, we recommend the amounts and types of physical activity that are needed by adults for good health and summarize the scientific basis for this recommendation. Second, we recommend the ways that public health organizations, educational institutions, health care providers, communities, and individuals can effectively promote physical activity through more effective educational programs and the creation of programs and facilities that make it easier for people to become and remain more active. This article builds on existing recommendations, including *Healthy People 2000*,[10] the *Guide to Clinical Preventive Services*,[11] the ACSM's "Position Stand on the Recommended Quality and Quantity of Exercise for Developing and Maintaining Cardiorespiratory and Muscular Fitness in Healthy Adults,"[12] and the American Heart Association's recent "Statement on Exercise."[13] This article is not meant to be a definitive review of the many health aspects of physical activity; a thorough discussion can be found elsewhere.[14]

RELATIONSHIP BETWEEN PHYSICAL ACTIVITY AND HEALTH

Cross-sectional epidemiologic studies[15,16] and controlled, experimental investigations[12] have demonstrated that physically active adults, as contrasted with their sedentary counterparts, tend to develop and maintain higher levels of physical fitness. Epidemiologic research has demonstrated

Source: Reprinted from R.R. Pate et al., *Physical Activity and Public Health*. A Recommendation from the Centers for Disease Control and Prevention and the American College of Sports Medicine.

protective effects of varying strength between physical activity and risk for several chronic diseases, including coronary heart disease (CHD),[1-3,17,18] hypertension,[4,19-21] non-insulin-dependent diabetes mellitus,[22-24] osteoporosis,[7,25,26] colon cancer,[27] and anxiety and depression.[5,28]

Other epidemiologic studies have shown that low levels of habitual physical activity and low levels of physical fitness are associated with markedly increased all-cause mortality rates.[1,29] A midlife increase in physical activity is associated with a decreased risk of mortality.[30] It has been estimated that as many as 250,000 deaths per year in the United States, approximately 12% of the total, are attributable to a lack of regular physical activity.[31,32]

The conclusions of these epidemiologic studies are supported by experimental studies showing that exercise training improves CHD risk factors and other health-related factors, including blood lipid profile,[33] resting blood pressure in borderline hypertensives,[4,34-36] body composition,[37-39] glucose tolerance and insulin sensitivity,[40,41] bone density,[42] immune function,[43,44] and psychological function.[45]

Epidemiologic criteria used to establish causal relationships can be applied to the association between physical activity and CHD.[46] The following principles of causality appear to have been met: Consistency: The association of physical inactivity and risk of CHD is observed in a number of settings and populations, with the better-designed studies showing the strongest associations. Strength: The relative risk of CHD associated with physical inactivity ranges from 1.5 to 2.4, an increase in risk comparable with that observed for hypercholesterolemia, hypertension, and cigarette smoking.[3,47] Temporal sequencing: The observation of physical inactivity predates the diagnosis of CHD. Dose response: Most studies demonstrate that the risk of CHD increases as physical activity decreases. Plausibility and coherence: Physical activity reduces the risk of CHD through a number of physiological and metabolic mechanisms. These include the potential for increasing the level of high-density lipoprotein cholesterol; reducing serum triglyceride levels; reducing blood pressure; enhancing fibrinolysis and altering platelet function, thereby reducing the risk of acute thrombosis; enhancing glucose tolerance and insulin sensitivity; and reducing the sensitivity of the myocardium to the effects of catecholamines, thereby reducing the risk of ventricular arrhythmias.[4,33,40,48,49]

DESCRIPTIVE EPIDEMIOLOGY OF PHYSICAL ACTIVITY

Physical activity recommendations in *Healthy People 2000*[10] are to "[i]ncrease to at least 30 percent the proportion of people aged 6 and older who engage regularly, preferably daily, in light to moderate physical activity for at least 30 minutes per day." However, only about 22% of adults are active at this level recommended for health benefits, 54% are somewhat active but do not meet this objective, and 24% or more are completely sedentary (ie, reporting no leisure-time physical activity during the past month). Participation in regular physical activity gradually increased during the 1960s, 1970s, and early 1980s, but seems to have plateaued in recent years.[50]

Patterns of physical activity vary with demographic characteristics (Table 1). Men are more likely than women to engage in regular activity,[51] in vigorous exercise, and sports.[52] The total amount of time spent engaging in physical activity declines with age.[53,54] Adults at retirement age (65 years) show some increased participation in activities of light to moderate intensity, but, overall, physical activity declines continuously as age increases.[53,55] African Americans and other ethnic minority populations are less active than white Americans,[51,55,56] and this disparity is more pronounced for women.[56] People with higher levels of education participate in more leisure-time physical activity than do people with less education.[51] Differences in education and socioeconomic status account for most, if not all, of the differences in leisure-time physical activity associated with race/ethnicity.[57]

Table 1 Proportion of Adults Reporting No Leisure-Time Physical Activity Within the Last Month, 1991 Behavioral Risk Factor Surveillance System*

Demographic Group	Sedentary, % (95% CI)
Sex	
Male	27.89 (27.18–28.60)
Female	31.48 (30.85–32.11)
Race	
White	27.75 (27.24–28.26)
Nonwhite	37.52 (36.27–38.77)
Age, y	
18–34	23.77 (23.01–24.53)
35–54	29.50 (28.70–30.30)
≥55	38.00 (37.10–38.90)
Annual Income, $	
≤14,999	40.14 (39.06–41.22)
15,000–24,999	32.00 (30.90–33.10)
25,000–50,000	25.43 (24.63–26.23)
>50,000	18.64 (17.60–19.68)
Education	
Some high school	48.06 (46.75–49.37)
High school/ tech school graduate	33.57 (32.79–34.35)
Some college/ college graduate	20.16 (19.55–20.77)

*A population-based random-digit-dial telephone survey with 87,433 respondents aged 18 years and older from 47 states and the District of Columbia. Data are weighted, and point estimates and confidence intervals (CIs) are calculated using the SESUDAAN procedure to adjust for the complex sampling frame.[10]

DETERMINANTS OF PARTICIPATION IN PHYSICAL ACTIVITY

Physiological, behavioral, and psychological variables are related to physical activity.[58-60] A lack of time is the most commonly cited barrier to participation in physical activity,[61] and injury is a common reason for stopping regular activity. Cigarette smoking is only weakly inversely related to participation in physical activity, but smokers are more likely than nonsmokers to drop out of exercise programs.[62] Body composition (percentage of body fat) is not a powerful predictor of physical activity habits; however, persons who are obese are usually inactive.[37]

An intention to exercise and awareness of the benefits of exercise are weakly related to participation in physical activity.[63] Confidence in the ability to be physically active, perceived barriers to activity, and enjoyment of activity are strongly related to participation.[64] Low- to moderate-intensity physical activities are more likely to be continued than high-intensity activities.[65] Self-regulatory skills, such as goal setting, self-monitoring progress, and self-reinforcement, contribute to continued physical activity.[66]

A number of physical and social environmental factors can affect physical activity behavior.[59] Family and friends can be role models, provide encouragement, or be companions during physical activity. The environment often presents important barriers to participation in physical activity, including a lack of bicycle trails and walking paths away from traffic, inclement weather, and unsafe neighborhoods.[67] Excessive television viewing may also deter persons from being physically active.[68]

PHYSICAL ACTIVITY RECOMMENDATION FOR ADULTS

The current low-participation rate may be due in part to the misperception of many people that to reap health benefits they must engage in vigorous, continuous exercise. The scientific evidence clearly demonstrates that regular, moderate-intensity physical activity provides substantial health benefits. After review of physiological, epidemiologic, and clinical evidence, an expert panel formulated the following recommendation:

Every US adult should accumulate 30 minutes or more of moderate-intensity physical activity on most, preferably all, days of the week.

This recommendation emphasizes the benefits of moderate-intensity physical activity and of physical activity that can be accumulated in relatively short bouts. Adults who engage in moderate-intensity physical activity—ie, enough to expend approximately 200 calories per day—can expect many of the health benefits described herein. To expend these calories, about 30 minutes of moderate-intensity physical activity should be accumulated during the course of the day. One way to meet this standard is to walk 2 miles briskly. Table 2 provides examples of moderate-intensity physical activities.

Intermittent activity also confers substantial benefits.[1,17,72,73] Therefore, the recommended 30 minutes of ac-

Table 2 Examples of Common Physical Activities for Healthy US Adults by Intensity of Effort Required in MET Scores and Kilocalories per Minute*

Light (<3.0 METs or <4 kcal · min^{-1})	Moderate (3.0–6.0 METs or 4–7 kcal · min^{-1})	Hard/Vigorous (>6.0 METs or >7 kcal · min^{-1})
Walking, slowly (strolling) (1–2 mph)	Walking, briskly (3–4 mph)	Walking, briskly uphill or with a load
Cycling, stationary (<50W)	Cycling for pleasure or transportation (≤10 mph)	Cycling, fast or racing (>10 mph)
Swimming, slow treading	Swimming, moderate effort	Swimming, fast treading or crawl
Conditioning exercise, light stretching	Conditioning exercise, general calisthenics	Conditioning exercise, stair ergometer, ski machine
. . .	Racket sports, table tennis	Racket sports, singles tennis, racketball
Golf, power cart	Golf, pulling cart or carrying clubs	. . .
Bowling	. . .	
Fishing, sitting	Fishing, standing/casting	Fishing in stream
Boating, power	Canoeing, leisurely (2.0–3.9 mph)	Canoeing, rapidly (≥4 mph)
Home care, carpet sweeping	Home care, general cleaning	Moving furniture
Mowing lawn, riding mower	Mowing lawn, power mower	Mowing lawn, hand mower
Home repair, carpentry	Home repair, painting	. . .

*Data from Ainsworth et al,[69] Leon,[70] and McCardle et al.[71] The METs (work metabolic rate/resting metabolic rate) are multiples of the resting rate of oxygen consumption during physical activity. One MET represents the approximate rate of oxygen consumption of a seated adult at rest, or about 3.5 mL · min^{-1} · kg^{-1}. The equivalent energy cost of 1 MET in kilocalories · min^{-1} is about 1.2 for a 70-kg person, or approximately 1 kcal · kg^{-1} · hr^{-1}.

tivity can be accumulated in short bouts of activity: walking up the stairs instead of taking the elevator, walking instead of driving short distances, doing calisthenics, or pedaling a stationary cycle while watching television. Gardening, housework, raking leaves, dancing, and playing actively with children can also contribute to the 30-minute-per-day total if performed at an intensity corresponding to brisk walking. Those who perform lower-intensity activities should do them more often, for longer periods of time, or both.

People who prefer more formal exercise may choose to walk or participate in more vigorous activities, such as jogging, swimming, or cycling for 30 minutes daily. Sports and recreational activities, such as tennis or golf (without riding a cart), can also be applied to the daily total.

Because most adults do not currently meet the standard described herein, almost all should strive to increase their participation in physical activity that is of at least moderate intensity. Those who do not engage in regular physical activity should begin by incorporating a few minutes of increased activity into their day, building up gradually to 30 minutes per day of physical activity. Those who are active on an irregular basis should strive to adopt a more consistent activity pattern.

The health benefits gained from increased physical activity depend on the initial activity level (Figure 1). Sedentary individuals are expected to benefit most from increasing their activity to the recommended level. People who are physically active at a level below the standard would also benefit from reaching the recommended level of physical activity. People who already meet the recommendation are also likely to derive some additional health and fitness benefits from becoming more physically active.

Most adults do not need to see their physician before starting a moderate-intensity physical activity program.[74] However, men older than 40 years and women older than 50 years who plan a vigorous program (intensity >60% individual maximum oxygen consumption; Table 1) or who have either chronic disease or risk factors for chronic disease should consult their physician to design a safe, effective program.[74]

PREVIOUS EXERCISE RECOMMENDATIONS

The recommendation presented in this article is intended to complement, not supersede, previous exercise recommendations. In the past, exercise recommendations (including those from the ACSM) were based on scientific studies that investigated dose-response improvements in performance capacity after exercise training, especially the effects of endurance exercise training on maximal aerobic power (maximum oxygen consumption). The recommendations usually involved 20 to 60 minutes of moderate- to high-intensity endurance exercise (60% to 90% of maximum heart rate or 50% to 85% of maximal aerobic power) performed three or more times per week.

Although the earlier exercise recommendations were based on documented improvements in fitness, they probably provide most of the disease prevention benefits associated with an increase in physical activity. However, it now appears that the majority of these health benefits can be gained by performing moderate-intensity physical activities outside of formal exercise programs.

UNIQUE ASPECTS OF THE NEW RECOMMENDATION

The new recommendation extends the traditional exercise-fitness model to a broader physical activity-health paradigm. The recommendation is distinct in two important ways. First, the health benefits of moderate-intensity physical activity are emphasized. Second, accumulation of physical activity in intermittent, short bouts is considered an appropriate approach to achieving the activity goal. These unique elements of the recommendation are based on mounting evidence indicating that the health benefits of physical activity are linked principally to the total amount of physical activity performed. This evidence suggests that amount of activity is more important than the specific manner in which the activity is performed (ie, mode, intensity, or duration of the activity bouts).

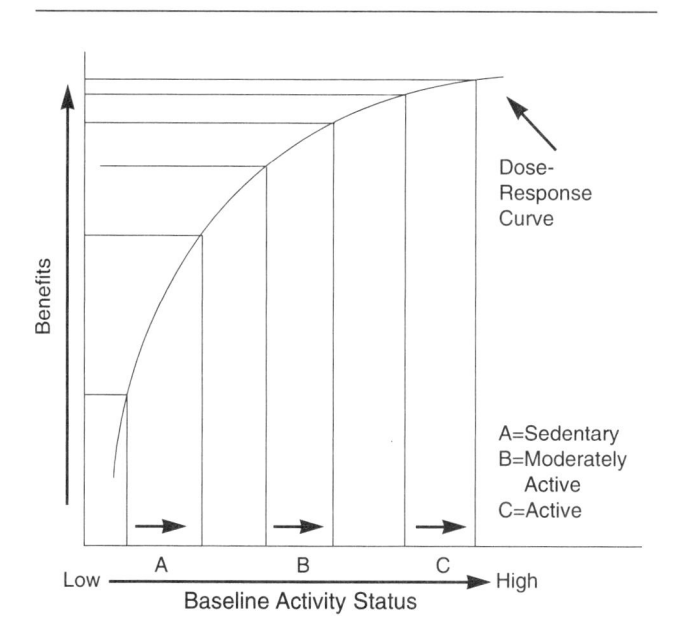

Figure 1 The dose-response curve represents the best estimate of the relationship between physical activity (dose) and health benefit (response). The lower the baseline physical activity status, the greater will be the health benefit associated with a given increase in physical activity (arrows A, B, and C).

The health benefits of physical activity appear to accrue in approximate proportion to the total amount of activity performed, measured as either caloric expenditure or minutes of physical activity (Figure 2). For example, observational studies have shown a significantly lower death rate from CHD in people who perform an average of 47 minutes vs 15 minutes of activity per day,[17] and in men who expend an estimated 2000 or more calories per week vs those who expend 500 or fewer calories per week.[1] Five of the six studies shown in Figure 2 included men only; however, the relationship between physical fitness and cardiovascular disease mortality was identical for men and women in the one study that included both.[29]

There is a clear association between total daily or weekly caloric expenditure and cardiovascular disease mortality. In most of the epidemiologic studies that have demonstrated this association, physical activity was assessed by questionnaires, and total activity was summed during periods ranging from 1 day to 1 year and then reported as average daily or weekly levels of physical activity. For example, among Harvard alumni the summed activity consisted of blocks walked, flights of stairs climbed, and moderate and vigorous sports play.[1] In the Multiple Risk Factor Intervention Trial,[17] the most frequently reported activities were lawn and garden work (80% of men), walking (65%), and home repairs (67%). It is not possible to ascertain with certainty whether the activity reported in these studies was performed in single, continuous daily bouts or was accumulated in multiple episodes. However, the nature of the most frequently reported activities suggests that it is unlikely that most of the activity was performed continuously. It is more likely that the daily or weekly caloric expenditures reflect accumulation of activity, most of which was performed intermittently. Also, the activities most commonly reported in these studies (eg, walking, lawn work, and gardening) typically are performed at moderate intensity (Table 2).

Two published experimental studies have addressed the effects of continuous vs intermittent activity on fitness.[72,73] DeBusk et al[72] examined the effects of three 10-minute bouts of moderate to vigorous activity daily compared with a single 30-minute daily period of exercise of equal intensity in men. Ebisu[73] studied the effects of running on fitness and blood lipids in three groups of men. Subjects were divided into three exercise groups and one inactive control group. Each exercise group ran the same total distance, but in one, two, or three sessions daily. In both studies, fitness (measured as maximal oxygen uptake) increased significantly in all exercise groups, and the differences in fitness across the exercising groups were not significant. In the latter study, high-density lipoprotein cholesterol levels increased significantly only in the group that exercised three times per day.[73]

Although more research is needed to better elucidate the health effects of moderate- vs high-intensity activity and intermittent vs continuous activity, clinicians and public health practitioners must rely on the most reasonable interpretation of existing data to guide their actions. We believe that the most reasonable interpretation of the currently available data is the (1) caloric expenditure and total time of physical activity are associated with reduced cardiovascular disease incidence and mortality; (2) there is a dose-response relationship for this association; (3) regular moderate physical activity provides substantial health benefits; and (4) intermittent bouts of physical activity, as short as 8 to 10 minutes, totaling 30 minutes or more on most days provide beneficial health and fitness effects.

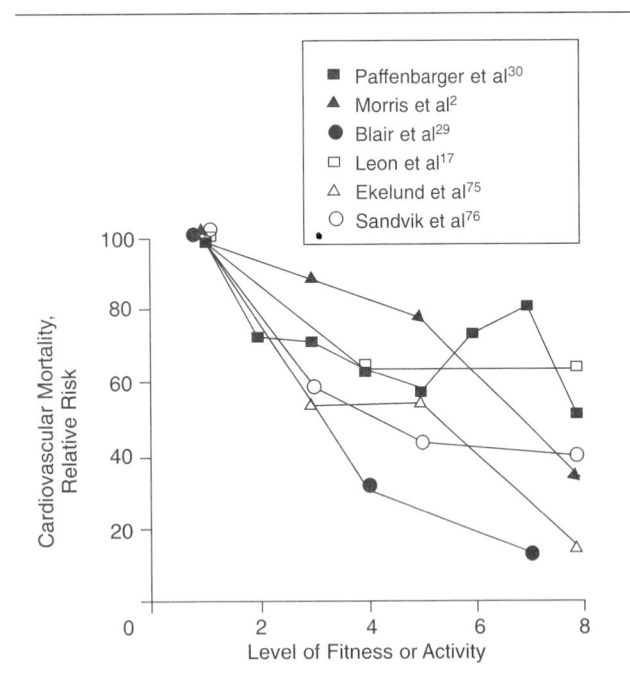

Figure 2 The relationship between level of physical activity (Paffenbarger et al,[30] Morris et al,[2] and Leon et al[17]) or exercise capacity (Blair et al,[29] Ekelund et al,[75] and Sandvik et al[76]) and coronary heart disease mortality. Values for more active or fit persons are expressed as the ratio of the event rate for more active or fit divided by the event rate for least active or fit.

MUSCULAR STRENGTH AND FLEXIBILITY

The preceding recommendation addresses the role of endurance exercise in preventing chronic diseases. However, two other components of fitness—flexibility and muscular strength—should not be overlooked. Clinical experience and limited studies suggest that people who maintain or improve their strength and flexibility may be better able to perform daily activities, may be less likely to develop back pain, and may be better able to avoid disability, especially as they advance into older age. Regular physical activity also may contribute to better balance, coordination, and agility, which in turn may help prevent falls in the elderly.[77]

CALL TO ACTION

Successfully changing our sedentary society into an active one will require effective dissemination and acceptance of the message that moderate physical activity confers health benefits.

Public Health Agencies

The public health community will need to strengthen its leadership role if improvement in population levels of physical activity is to occur. The CDC, the ACSM, the President's Council on Physical Fitness and Sports, and the American Heart Association have been leaders in promoting physical activity and will continue to be crucial in this effort. However, new partners must also be enlisted. State and local health departments, departments of public transportation and planning, parks and recreation associations, state and local councils on physical fitness, environmental groups, and the sports and recreation industry all have interests that coincide with the public health goal of making our society more active.

Health Professionals

Physicians and other health professionals should routinely counsel patients to adopt and maintain regular physical activity. Physicians can be effective proponents of physical activity because patients respect physicians' advice and change their exercise behaviors as a result.[78] The large number of primary care physicians and the frequency with which Americans visit them[79] suggest that even modestly effective physician counseling would have a substantial public health impact.

Inadequate reimbursement, limited physician knowledge of the benefits of physical activity, lack of training in physical activity counseling, and inadequate knowledge of effective referral are barriers to achieving these goals. While policymakers work to improve reimbursement for preventive services, educators of physicians and other health professionals should develop effective ways to teach physical activity counseling and incorporate them into curricula for health professionals. In response to this need, the PACE (Physical Activity Counseling and Evaluation) program was recently developed. This approach relies on providing specific counseling protocols matched to the patient's level of activity and readiness to change.[80] Preliminary evidence indicates that the PACE program is practical and effective in increasing physical activity among patients counseled in the primary care setting.[81]

The personal physical activity practices of health professionals should not be overlooked. Health professionals should be physically active not only to benefit their own health but to make more credible their endorsement of an active lifestyle.

Special Populations

Special efforts will be required to target populations in which physical inactivity is particularly prevalent. These groups include the socioeconomically disadvantaged, the less educated, persons with disabilities, and older adults.

Interventions should be designed with input from the target population. Physical activity promotional efforts targeted to people with disabilities, or chronic disease, or to older adults should emphasize the importance of being physically active by routinely carrying out their daily activities with a minimum of assistance. There is clear evidence demonstrating that physiological and performance capacities can be improved by regular physical activity in older adults[82-84] and in persons with disabilities and/or chronic disease.[85]

Communities

Institutions such as schools, worksites, and the medical community are specifically targeted in *Healthy People 2000*[10] because they offer the means to reach most of the US population. Facilities in these institutions and the broader community can be used to a much greater extent. Corporate, government, school, and hospital policies should be restructured to encourage individuals to be active by making time and facilities available.

Organized programs emphasizing lifelong physical activity should be promoted in schools, worksites, and community organizations. Efforts should be made to develop walking trails and other exercise facilities, and to encourage walking and bicycling for transportation.

Educators

Schools should deliver comprehensive health and physical education programs that provide and promote physical activity at every opportunity.

Physical education curricula should be developmentally appropriate, provide youngsters with enjoyable experiences that build exercise self-efficacy, provide significant amounts of physical activity, and promote cognitive learning related to lifelong participation in physical activity. These curricula also should acquaint youngsters with physical activity resources in their community. The school environment should encourage physical activity for all students and promote development of physically active lifestyles. Educators at all levels should be good models of physical activity behavior.

Individuals and Families

Individuals can make modest adaptations in their physical and social environment to enhance their participation in physical activity. Parents should be physical activity role models for their children and support their children's participation in enjoyable physical activities.

CONCLUSIONS

If Americans who lead sedentary lives would adopt a more active lifestyle, there would be enormous benefit to the public's health and to individual well-being. An active lifestyle does not require a regimented, vigorous exercise program. Instead, small changes that increase daily physical activity will enable individuals to reduce their risk of chronic disease and may contribute to enhanced quality of life.

We wish to acknowledge the many helpful comments received from the participants at the Workshop on Physical Activity and Public Health and from the individual reviewers. Special thanks to Marjorie Speers, director, and John Livengood, associate director for science, Division of Chronic Disease Control and Community Intervention, National Center for Chronic Disease Prevention and Health Promotion, Centers for Disease Control and Prevention, and to James Whitehead, executive vice president, American College of Sports Medicine, for their personal and organizational support. Thanks are also due to representatives of the following organizations for their critical comments and review of this document: American Heart Association; American Alliance for Health, Physical Education, Recreation, and Dance; Association of State and Territorial Directors of Health Promotion and Public Health Education; Association of Governor's Councils on Physical Fitness and Sports; National Recreation and Parks Association; National Cancer Institute; National Heart, Lung, and Blood Institute; National Institute on Aging; National Institute of Diabetes and Digestive and Kidney Diseases; Office of Disease Prevention and Health Promotion; and The President's Council on Physical Fitness and Sports.

REFERENCES

1. Paffenbarger RS, Hyde RT, Wing AL, Hsieh C-C. Physical activity, all-cause mortality, and longevity of college alumni. *N Engl J Med.* 1986; 314:605–613.
2. Morris JN, Clayton DG, Everitt MG, Semmence AM, Burgess EH. Exercise in leisure time: coronary attack and death rates. *Br Heart J.* 1990; 63:325–334.
3. Powell KE, Thompson PD, Casperson CJ, Ford ES. Physical activity and the incidence of coronary heart disease. *Annu Rev Public Health.* 1987;8:253–287.
4. Hagberg JM. Exercise, fitness, and hypertension. In: Bouchard C, Shephard RJ, Stephens T, Sutton JR, McPherson BD, eds. *Exercise, Fitness, and Health.* Champaign, Ill: Human Kinetics Publishers; 1990:455–566.
5. King AC, Taylor CB, Haskell WL, DeBusk RF. Influence of regular aerobic exercise on psychological health. *Health Psychol.* 1989; 8:305–324.
6. Dishman RK. Psychological effects of exercise for disease resistance and health promotion. In: Watson RR, Eisinher M, eds. *Exercise and Disease.* Boca Raton, Fla: CRC Press; 1992:179–207.
7. Marcus R, Drinkwater B, Dalsky G, et al. Osteoporosis and exercise in women. *Med Sci Sports Exerc.* 1992;24(suppl):S301–S307.
8. Centers for Disease Control and Prevention. Prevalence of sedentary lifestyle—behavioral risk factor surveillance system, United States, 1991. *MMWR Morb Mortal Wkly Rep.* 1993;42:576–579.
9. Caspersen GJ, Powell KE, Christenson GM. Physical activity, exercise, and physical fitness. *Public Health Rep.* 1985;100:125–131.
10. US Dept of Health and Human Services. *Healthy People 2000: National Health Promotion and Disease Prevention Objectives.* Washington, DC: US Dept of Health and Human Services; 1991. DHHS publication PHS 91-50212.
11. Fisher M, Eckhart C, eds. *Guide to Clinical Preventive Services: An Assessment of the Effectiveness of 169 Interventions.* Baltimore, Md: Williams & Wilkins; 1989.
12. American College of Sports Medicine. Position stand on the recommended quantity and quality of exercise for developing and maintaining cardiorespiratory and muscular fitness in healthy adults. *Med Sci Sports Exerc.* 1990;22:265–274.
13. Fletcher GF, Blair SN, Blumenthal J, et al. AHA medical/scientific statement on exercise. *Circulation.* 1992;86:340–344.
14. Bouchard C, Shephard RJ, Stephens T, eds. *Physical Activity, Fitness, and Health.* Champaign, Ill: Human Kinetics Publishers; 1994.
15. Kohl HW, Blair SN, Paffenbarger RS, Macera CA, Kronenfeld JJ. A mail survey of physical activity habits as related to measured physical fitness. *Am J Epidemiol.* 1988;127:1228–1239.
16. Taylor HL, Jacobs DR, Schucker B, Knudsen J, Leon AS, Debacker G. A questionnaire for the assessment of leisure time physical activities. *J Chronic Dis.* 1978;31:741–755.
17. Leon AS, Connett J, Jacobs DR Jr, Rauramaa R. Leisure-time physical activity levels and risk of coronary heart disease and death: the Multiple Risk Factor Intervention Trial. *JAMA.* 1987;258:2388–2395.
18. Morris JN, Kagan A, Pattison DC, Chave SPW, Semmence AM. Incidence and prediction of ischemic heart disease in London busman. *Lancet.* 1966;2:533–559.
19. Blair SN, Goodyear NN, Gibbons LW, Cooper KH. Physical fitness and incidence of hypertension in healthy normotensive men and women. *JAMA.* 1984;252:487–490.
20. Paffenbarger RS, Wing AL, Hyde RT, Jung DL. Physical activity and incidence of hypertension in college alumni. *Am J Epidemiol.* 1983; 117:245–257.
21. American College of Sports Medicine. Position stand: physical activity, physical fitness, and hypertension. *Med Sci Sports Exerc.* 1993;10:i–x.
22. Helmrich SP, Ragland DR, Leung RW, Paffenbarger RS. Physical activity and reduced occurrence on non–insulin-dependent diabetes mellitus. *N Engl J Med.* 1991;325:147–152.
23. Manson JE, Nathan DM, Krolewski AS, Stampfer MJ, Willett WC, Hennekens CH. A prospective study of exercise and incidence of diabetes among US male physicians. *JAMA.* 1992;268:63–67.
24. Manson JE, Rimm EB, Stampfer MJ, et al. Physical activity and incidence of non–insulin-dependent diabetes mellitus in women. *Lancet.* 1991;338:774–778.
25. Cummings SR, Kelsey JL, Nevitt MD, O'Dowd KJ. Epidemiology of osteoporosis and osteoporotic fractures. *Epidemiol Rev.* 1985;7: 178–208.

26. Snow-Harter C, Marcus R. Exercise, bone mineral density, and osteoporosis. *Exerc Sport Sci Rev.* 1991;19:351–388.
27. Lee I, Paffenbarger RS, Hsieh C. Physical activity and risk of developing colorectal cancer among college alumni. *J Natl Cancer Inst.* 1991;83:1324–1329.
28. Taylor CB, Sallis JF, Needle R. The relationship of physical activity and exercise to mental health. *Public Health Rep.* 1985;100:195–201.
29. Blair SN, Kohl HW, Paffenbarger RS, Clark DG, Cooper KH, Gibbons LW. Physical fitness and all-cause mortality. *JAMA.* 1989;262:2395–2401.
30. Paffenbarger RS, Hyde RT, Wing AL, Lee I, Jung DL, Kampert JB. The association of changes in physical-activity level and other lifestyle characteristics with mortality among men. *N Engl J Med.* 1993;328:538–545.
31. Hahn RA, Teutsch SM, Rothenberg RB, Marks JS. Excess deaths from nine chronic diseases in the United States. *JAMA.* 1986;264:2654–2659.
32. McGinnis JM, Foege WH. Actual causes of death in the United States. *JAMA.* 1993;270:2207–2212.
33. Haskell WL. The influence of exercise training on plasma lipids and lipoproteins in health and disease. *Acta Med Scand.* 1986;711(suppl):25–37.
34. Duncan JJ, Farr JE, Upton SJ, Hagan RD, Oglesby ME, Blair SN. The effects of aerobic exercise on plasma catecholamines and blood pressure in patients with mild essential hypertension. *JAMA.* 1985;254:2609–2613.
35. Hagberg JM, Montain SJ, Martin WH, et al. Effect of exercise training on 60–69 year old persons with essential hypertension. *Am J Cardiol.* 1989;64:348–353.
36. Tipton CM. Exercise training and hypertension: an update. *Exerc Sports Sci Rev.* 1991;19:447–505.
37. Bouchard C, Depres JP, Tremblay A. Exercise and obesity. *Obesity Res.* 1993;1:133–147.
38. Pavlou K, Krey S, Steffee WP. Exercise as an adjunct to weight loss and maintenance in moderately obese subjects. *Am J Clin Nutr.* 1989;49:1115–1123.
39. Wood PD, Stefanick ML, Williams PT, Haskell WL. The effects on plasma lipoproteins of prudent weight-reducing diet, with or without exercise, in overweight men and women. *N Engl J Med.* 1991;325:461–466.
40. Ivy JL. The insulin-like effect of muscle contraction. *Exerc Sports Sci Rev.* 1987;15:29–51.
41. Koivisto VA, Yki-Jarvinen H, DeFronzo RA. Physical training and insulin sensitivity. *Diabetes Metab Rev.* 1986;1:445–481.
42. Dalsky GP, Stoke KS, Ehsani AA, Slatopolsky E, Lcc WC, Birge SJ. Weight-bearing exercise training and lumbar bone mineral content in postmenopausal women. *Ann Intern Med.* 1988;108:824–828.
43. Nehlsen-Cannarella SL, Niemann DC, Balk-Lamberton AJ, et al. The effects of moderate exercise training on immune response. *Med Sci Sports Exerc.* 1991;28:64–70.
44. Nieman DC. Physical activity, fitness, and infection. In: Bouchard C, Shephard RJ, Stephens T, eds. *Physical Activity, Fitness, and Health.* Champaign, Ill: Human Kinetics Publishers; 1994:796–813.
45. King AC, Taylor CB, Haskell WL. Effects of differing intensities and formats of 12 months of exercise training on psychological outcomes in older adults. *Health Psychol.* 1993;12:292–300.
46. Hill AB. The environment and disease: association or causation? *Proc R Soc Med.* 1965;58:295–300.
47. Centers for Disease Control and Prevention. Public health focus: physical activity and the prevention of coronary heart disease. *MMWR Morb Mortal Wkly Rep.* 1993;42:669–672.
48. Rauramaa R, Salonen JT. Physical activity, fibrinolysis, and platelet aggregability. In: Bouchard C, Shepard RJ, Stephens T, eds. *Physical Activity, Fitness, and Health.* Champaign, Ill: Human Kinetics Publishers; 1994:471–479.
49. Moore S. Physical activity, fitness, and atherosclerosis. In: Bouchard C, Shepard RJ, Stephens T, eds. *Physical Activity, Fitness, and Health.* Champaign, Ill: Human Kinetics Publishers; 1994:570–578.
50. Stephens T. Secular trends in adult physical activity. *Res Q Exerc Sport.* 1987;58:94–105.
51. Caspersen CJ, Christenson GM, Pollard RA. The status of the 1990 Physical Fitness Objectives—evidence from NHIS 85. *Public Health Rep.* 1986;101:587–592.
52. Stephens T, Jacobs DR, White CC. A descriptive epidemiology of leisure-time physical activity. *Public Health Rep.* 1985;100:147–158.
53. Caspersen CJ, Pollard RA, Pratt SO. Scoring physical activity data with special consideration for elderly population. In: *Proceedings of the 21st National Meeting of the Public Health Conference on Records and Statistics: Data for an Aging Population.* Washington, DC: Public Health Service; July 13–15, 1987:30–34. DHHS publication PHS 88-1214.
54. Schoenborn CA. Health habits of US adults, 1985: the 'Alameda 7' revisited. *Public Health Rep.* 1986;101:571–580.
55. Caspersen CJ, Merritt RK. Trends in physical activity patterns among older adults: the Behavioral Risk Factor Surveillance System, 1986–1990. *Med Sci Sports Exerc.* 1992;24(suppl):S26.
56. DiPietro L, Caspersen C. National estimates of physical activity among white and black Americans. *Med Sci Sports Exerc.* 1991;23(suppl):S105.
57. White CC, Powell KE, Goelin GC, Gentry EM, Forman MR. The behavioral risk factor surveys, IV: the descriptive epidemiology of exercise. *Am J Prev Med.* 1987;3:304–310.
58. Dishman RK, ed. *Exercise Adherence.* Champaign, Ill: Human Kinetics Publishers; 1988.
59. Sallis JF, Hovell MF, Hofstetter CR. Predictors of adoption and maintenance of vigorous physical activity in men and women. *Prev Med.* 1992;21:237–251.
60. Sallis JF, Hovell MF. Determinants of exercise behavior. *Exerc Sport Sci Rev.* 1990;18:307–330.
61. Martin JE, Dubbert PM. Exercise applications and promotion in behavioral medicine. *J Consult Clin Psychol.* 1982;50:1004–1017.
62. Dishman RK, Sallis JF. Determinants and interventions for physical activity and exercise. In: Bouchard C, Shepard RJ, Stephens T, eds. *Physical Activity, Fitness, and Health.* Champaign, Ill: Human Kinetics Publishers; 1994:214–238.
63. Godin G, Valois P, Shephard RJ, Desharnais R. Prediction of leisure-time exercise behavior: a path analysis (LISREL V) model. *J Behav Med.* 1987;10:145–158.
64. Sallis JF, Hovell MF, Hofstetter CR, et al. A multivariate study of determinants of vigorous exercise in a community sample. *Prev Med.* 1989;18:20–34.
65. Pollock ML. Prescribing exercise for fitness and adherence. In: Dishman RK, ed. *Exercise Adherence.* Champaign, Ill: Human Kinetics Publishers; 1988:259–277.
66. Dishman RK. Compliance/adherence in health-related exercise. *Health Psychol.* 1982;1:237–267.

67. Sallis JF, Hovell MF, Hofstetter CR, et al. A multivariate study of determinants of vigorous exercise in a community sample. *Prev Med.* 1989;18:20–34.
68. Tucker LA. Television viewing and physical fitness in adults. *Res Q Exerc Sport.* 1990;61:315–320.
69. Ainsworth BE, Haskell WL, Leon AS, et al. Compendium of physical activities. *Med Sci Sports Exerc.* 1993;25:71–80.
70. Leon AS. Physical fitness. In: Wyinder EL, ed. *American Health Foundation, The Book of Health.* New York, NY: Franklin Watts; 1981:293.
71. McCardle WD, Katch FI, Katch VL. *Exercise Physiology, Energy Nutrition Performance.* 2nd ed. Philadelphia, Pa: Lea & Febiger; 1986:642.
72. DeBusk RF, Stenestrand U, Sheehan M, Haskell WL. Training effects of long versus short bouts of exercise in health subjects. *Am J Cardiol.* 1990;65:1010–1013.
73. Ebisu T. Splitting the distance of endurance running: on cardiovascular endurance and blood lipids. *Jpn J Phys Educ.* 1985;30:37–43.
74. American College of Sports Medicine. *Guidelines for Exercise Testing and Prescription.* 4th ed. Philadelphia, Pa: Lea & Febiger; 1991.
75. Ekelund LG, Haskell WL, Johnson JL, Wholey FS, Criqui MH, Sheps DS. Physical fitness as a prevention of cardiovascular mortality in asymptomatic North American men. *N Engl J Med.* 1988;319:1379–1384.
76. Sandvik L, Erikssen J, Thaulow E, Erikssen G, Mundal R, Rodhal K. Physical fitness as a predictor of mortality among healthy, middle-aged Norwegian men. *N Engl J Med.* 1993;328:533–537.
77. Parsons D, Foster V, Harman F, Dickinson A, Westerlind K. Balance and strength changes in elderly subjects after heavy-resistance strength training. *Med Sci Sports Exerc.* 1992;24(suppl):S21.
78. Lewis BS, Lynch WD. The effect of physician advise on exercise behavior. *Prev Med.* 1993;22:110–121.
79. US Dept of Health and Human Services. *Physician Visits: Volume and Interval Since Last Visit, United States, 1980.* Hyattsville, Md: National Center for Health Statistics; June 1983. DHHS publication PHS 83-1572.
80. Centers for Disease Control. *Project PACE: Physician's Manual: Physician-Based Assessment and Counseling for Exercise.* Atlanta, Ga: Centers for Disease Control; 1992.
81. Long BJ, Calfas KJ, Sallis JF, et al. Evaluation of patient physical activity after counseling by primary care providers. *Med Sci Sports Exerc.* 1994;26(suppl):S4.
82. Kohrt WM, Malley MT, Coggan AR, et al. Effects of gender, age, and fitness levels on response of $\dot{V}O_{2max}$ to training to 60–71 year olds. *J Appl Physiol.* 1991;71:2004–2011.
83. Meredith C, Frontera W, Fisher E, et al. Peripheral effects of endurance training in young and old subjects. *J Appl Physiol.* 1989;66:2844–2849.
84. Roger MA, Evans WJ. Changes in skeletal muscle with aging: effects of exercise training. *Exerc Sport Sci Rev.* 1993;21:365–379.
85. Pollock ML, Miller HA, Linnerud AC, et al. Arm pedaling as an endurance training regimen for the disabled. *Arch Phys Med Rehabil.* 1974;55:418–424.

Appendix G

Sample Exercise Programs

PROGRAM A

Monday	Tuesday	Wednesday	Thursday	Friday	Saturday	Sunday
RESISTIVE	RECOVERY	RESISTIVE	RECOVERY	RESISTIVE	RECOVERY	RECOVERY
4-way neck	walk	leg extension	walk	4-way neck	walk	
leg press	(optional)	seated leg curl	(optional)	dumbbell lunge	(optional)	
leg curl		low back machine		standing leg curl		
prone back extension		heels up		prone back extension		
abdominal curl		calf raise		abdominal curl		
pullup		supraspinatus raise		dumbbell row		
posterior deltoid		bench press		machine tricep extension		
machine chest fly		posterior deltoid		dumbbell incline press		
lateral raise		lat rowing		ankle dorsiflexion		
dumbbell tricep extension		dumbbell bicep curl		shoulder rotators		
AEROBIC		AEROBIC		AEROBIC		
bike		upper extremity ergometer		swim—intervals		
RANGE OF MOTION		RANGE OF MOTION		RANGE OF MOTION		

EXERCISE TIME		EXERCISE TIME		EXERCISE TIME	
Resistive Exercise =	27 minutes	Resistive Exercise =	27 minutes	Resistive Exercise =	27 minutes
Aerobic Exercise =	20 minutes	Aerobic Exercise =	20 minutes	Aerobic Exercise =	20 minutes
Range of Motion =	10 minutes	Range of Motion =	10 minutes	Range of Motion =	10 minutes
Total Time	**57 minutes**	**Total Time**	**57 minutes**	**Total Time**	**57 minutes**

Total Weekly Exercise Time = 57 minutes × 3 = 171 minutes = 2 hours, 51 minutes.

RESISTIVE EXERCISE: 1–2 sets per movement
8–12 repetitions per set

RESISTIVE EXERCISE TIME IS BASED ON THE FOLLOWING:
- Time to complete 1 repetition = approximately 6 seconds
- Time to complete 1 set = 6 seconds × 12 repetitions = approximately 72 seconds
- Recovery time = 90 seconds
- Time to complete 1 set + recovery time for that set = 72 + 90 = 162 seconds = 2.7 minutes
- Time to complete 10 sets of resistive exercise + recovery time = 2.7 minutes/set × 10 sets = approximately 27 minutes

Note: If 2 sets per movement are performed, add an additional 27 minutes to each exercise session. Precede each session with a 5-minute warm-up. Conclude each session with a 5-minute cool-down.

PROGRAM B

Monday	Tuesday	Wednesday	Thursday	Friday	Saturday	Sunday
RESISTIVE	AEROBIC	RECOVERY	RESISTIVE	AEROBIC	RECOVERY	RECOVERY
leg press	stepper	walk (optional)	seat leg curl	low impact class	walk (optional)	
leg curl	—intervals		leg extension			
low back machine			prone back extension			
abdominal machine			side bends			
wide grip lat pulldown			pullup			
front raise			posterior deltoid			
dumbbell incline press			machine chest fly			
bar bicep curl			reverse curl			
dumbbell tricep extension			machine tricep extension			
RANGE OF MOTION			RANGE OF MOTION			
EXERCISE TIME	EXERCISE TIME		EXERCISE TIME	EXERCISE TIME		
Resistive Exercise = 25 minutes			Resistive Exercise = 25 minutes			
Range of Motion = 10 minutes	Aerobic Exercise = 20 minutes		Range of Motion = 10 minutes	Aerobic Exercise = 20 minutes		
Total Time 35 minutes	**Total Time 20 minutes**		**Total Time 35 minutes**	**Total Time 20 minutes**		

Total Weekly Exercise Time = (35 minutes × 2) + (20 minutes × 2) = 70 minutes + 40 minutes = 1 hour, 50 minutes

RESISTIVE EXERCISE: 1–2 sets per movement
8–12 repetitions per set

RESISTIVE EXERCISE TIME IS BASED ON THE FOLLOWING:
- Time to complete 1 repetition = approximately 6 seconds
- Time to complete 1 set = 6 seconds × 12 repetitions = approximately 72 seconds
- Recovery time = 90 seconds
- Time to complete 1 set + recovery time for that set = 72 + 90 = 162 seconds = 2.7 minutes
- Time to complete 9 sets of resistive exercise + recovery time = 2.7 minutes/set × 9 sets = 24.3 = approximately 25 minutes

Note: If 2 sets per movement are performed, add an additional 25 minutes to each exercise session. Precede each session with a 5-minute warm-up. Conclude each session with a 5-minute cool-down.

PROGRAM C

Monday	Tuesday	Wednesday	Thursday	Friday	Saturday	Sunday
RESISTIVE	RECOVERY	RESISTIVE	RECOVERY	RESISTIVE	AEROBIC	RECOVERY
4-way neck	walk (optional)	leg extension	walk (optional)	prone back	swim	
leg press		seated leg curl		extension		
leg curl		low back machine		hip extension		
prone back		twisting abdominal		leg curl		
extension		curl		manual row		
abdominal curl		calf raise		side bends		
pullup		supraspinatus raise		dumbbell scapular		
posterior deltoid		bench press		protraction		
machine chest fly		manual posterior		dumbbell incline		
manual lateral raise		deltoid		press		
shoulder rotators		narrow grip lat		lat rowing—arms		
		pulldown		horizontal		
AEROBIC		dumbbell bicep curl		dumbbell shrug		
treadmill				shoulder rotators		
		AEROBIC				
		upper extremity				
		ergometer—intervals				
RANGE OF		RANGE OF			RANGE OF	
MOTION		MOTION			MOTION	

EXERCISE TIME		EXERCISE TIME		EXERCISE TIME	EXERCISE TIME	
Resistive		Resistive				
Exercise = 27 minutes		Exercise = 27 minutes				
Aerobic		Aerobic			Aerobic	
Exercise = 20 minutes		Exercise = 20 minutes			Exercise = 20 minutes	
Range of		Range of		Resistive	Range of	
Motion = 10 minutes		Motion = 10 minutes		Exercise = 27 minutes	Motion = 10 minutes	
Total Time 57 minutes		**Total Time 57 minutes**		**Total Time 27 minutes**	**Total Time 30 minutes**	

Total Weekly Exercise Time = 57 + 57 + 27 + 30 = 171 minutes = 2 hours, 51 minutes

RESISTIVE EXERCISE: 1–2 sets per movement
                                  8–12 repetitions per set

RESISTIVE EXERCISE TIME IS BASED ON THE FOLLOWING:
- Time to complete 1 repetition = approximately 6 seconds
- Time to complete 1 set = 6 seconds × 12 repetitions = approximately 72 seconds
- Recovery time = 90 seconds
- Time to complete 1 set + recovery time for that set = 72 + 90 = 162 seconds = 2.7 minutes
- Time to complete 10 sets of resistive exercise + recovery time = 2.7 minutes/set × 10 sets = approximately 27 minutes

Note: If 2 sets per movement are performed, add an additional 27 minutes to each exercise session. Precede each session with a 5-minute warm-up. Conclude each session with a 5-minute cool-down.

APPENDIX H

Recording Sheet

Exercise Record

Name _____

Precautions _____

Contraindications _____

Comments _____

DIFFICULTY SCALE
E easy
M moderate
D difficult

	Date R r D	Date R r D	Date R r D	Date R r D	Date R r D
Pre-ex HR					
Resistive Exercise					
(Perform 8–12 of the above movements. Address each major muscle group.)					
Aerobic Exercise	Duration/Difficulty				
Flexibility (check when completed)					

Copyright © 1997, Aspen Publishers, Inc.
Exercises for Health Promotion

Index

A

Abdominal curl, 89
   manual resistive, 172
   twisting, 93
Activity-specific stretches, 181–86
   ball sports, 40, 181
   cycling, 40, 181
   golf, 40, 181
Adaptation, physiological, exercise and, 13
Adolescence, defined, 55
Aerobic exercise, 31–37
   benefits of, 31
   duration of, 33–34
   heart rate
      recording sheet, 33
      target, 32–33
   at home, 71
   intensity, 32
   longevity factors, 36
   metabolic pathways, 31–32
   overtraining, 51–52
   overview, 36
   perceived exertion scale, ratings, 33
   research on, 36
   weather, 34
Aerobics, 4
Aged. *See* Older persons
Agonist, defined, 88
American Alliance of Health, Physical Education, and Recreation, establishment of, 4
American College of Obstetricians and Gynecologists, pregnancy, postpartum, exercise guidelines, 200–204
American College of Sports Medicine
   formation of, 4
   recommendations, 187
American Heart Association Guidelines for Cardiovascular Exercise in Apparently Healthy Individuals, 1995, 50
Amount of exercise, client education and, 10
Angular velocity spectrum, 12
Ankle dorsiflexion, with elastic band/tubing, 124
Ankle eversion, with elastic band/tubing, 125
Ankle inversion, with elastic tubing/resistance, 126
Antagonist, defined, 88
Arm, defined, 88
Augmented feedback. *See* Extrinsic feedback

B

Back extension
   on machine, 96
   manual resistive, 171
   prone, 95
Ball sports
   flexibility and, 40
   stretching, 181
Bench press, 138
Benefits of exercise, 5
   in workplace, 5
Biomechanical model, resistive exercise, 73–83
   cervical flexion, 81
   elbow, flexion, extension, 80
   hip extension, 79
   movement derivative model, 74–77
   purpose, 73
   shoulder transverse abduction, 78
Body composition, weight control and, 191
Body weight, gain in, resistance, repetitions and, 12
Bodybuilding, defined, 88

C

Cancer, exercise and, 209
Cardiovascular fitness
   American College of Sports Medicine recommendations, 187–97
   exercise and, 198, 208
Cascade, of exercise, 6
CDC. *See* Centers for Disease Control and Prevention
Centers for Disease Control and Prevention, 205
Cervical extension
   manual resistive, 177
   with strap, 163
Cervical flexion
   lateral
      manual resistive, 178
      with strap, 164
   manual resistive, 176
   resistive, 81
   with strap, 162
Children, exercise for, 55–62
   activities, injury trends, 56–57
   adolescence, defined, 55
   benefits of, 55–56
      research on, 56–57
   injuries
      case reports, 58
      cohort studies, 59
   knee joint angle, muscle condition, relationship between, 61
   knee resistance, 60
   overview, 55, 61
   patellofemoral joint
      dysfunction, prevention of, 58–61
      reaction force, 60
      stress at flexion angles, 61
   prepubescence, defined, 55
   recommendations, 57–58
   variables, recommended, 59
Client compliance
   facilitation of, 21–22
   research literature, 22

Client education, 9–20
  amount of exercise, 10
  angular velocity spectrum, 12
  body weight, gain in, resistance, repetitions and, 12
  client interview, 9–10
    goals, identifying, 10
    questions/answers, 10
  Commonwealth of Independent States, training methods, 14
  complexity, of exercise, 12–13
  Eastern Europen training methods, 14
  equipment, importance of, 10
  gender and, 14
  masculinization of female, 12
  medical approval to exercise, 14
  misconceptions, 10–14
  motor learning
    constant practice, 14
    distributed practice, 14
    extrinsic feedback, 14
    facilitation of, 14–15
    feedback, 14–15
      amount, frequency of, 15
    intrinsic feedback, 14
    knowledge of performance, 15
    knowledge of results, 15
    massed practice, 14
    practice, 14
    strategies, practical application of, 15
    transfer of learning, 15
    variable practice, 14
  muscle contraction, following rapid stretch, 17–19
  overview, 19
  physiological adaptation, 13
  plyometrics, defined, 17
  prescription schema for exercise, 13
  progress, evaluation of, 13–14
  recording, exercise data, 16, 17, 18
  resistive exercise
    explosive, sport skill development and, 10–12
    intensity, 16–17
    range of motion and, 12
    resistance, 16
    scale, 16
    speed of movement, in sport skills and, 14
  specificity, 15–16
    simulation, distinguished, 16
  speed of movement, during resistive exercise, research, 11
  speed training methods, 14
  split-routines, 12
  spot reduction, 13
  strength, defining, 10

Client interview, 9–10
  goals, identifying, 10
  questions/answers, 10
Commonwealth of Independent States, training method, rating of, 14
Competitive sports, growth of, 4
Complexity, of exercise, client education, 12–13
Compliance of client
  facilitation of, 21–22
  research literature, 22
Concentric muscle action, defined, 88
Cool-down, after resistive exercise, 28
Cooper, Kenneth, 4
Corner stretch, 186
Cost-effectiveness, of exercise, 5
Cycling, flexibility and, 40, 181

D

Dependence, on exercise, 53–54
  defined, 53–54
  diagnostic criteria, 53
  exercise continuum, 54
  intervention, 54
Diabetes mellitus, non-insulin-dependent, exercise and, 208
Difficulty, of resistive exercise. See Intensity
Distributed practice, motor learning and, 14
Documentation, of resistive exercise, 27
Dumbbell bench press, 136
Dumbbell incline press, 137
Dumbbell lunge, 98
Duration, of resistive exercise, 26

E

Eastern Europen training methods, rating of, 14
Eccentric muscle action, defined, 88
Elbow extension
  with dumbbell, 156
  resistive, 80
Elbow flexion
  with dumbbell, 152
  on machine, 153, 155
  manual resistive, 180
  pronated, 154
  resistive, 80
Elderly. See Older persons
Electrical analogy, of overtraining, 51
Epidemiology, physical activity, 211
Evaluation of progress, 13–14
Evolution, of exercise, 4–5
Exercise cascade, 6

Exercise continuum, exercise dependence and, 54
Exercise data, recording of, 16, 17, 18
  sheet for, 223
Exercise dependence, 53–54
  defined, 53–54
  diagnostic criteria, 53
  exercise continuum, 54
  intervention, 54
Exercise equipment
  importance of, 10
  posture and, 44
  safety, 48
Exercise facility, safety, 48
Explosive resistive exercise, sport skill development and, 10–12
Extrinsic feedback, motor learning and, 14

F

Facility, for exercise, safety, 48
Falling, prevention, exercise and, 209
  in older persons, 65–66
Feedback
  motor learning, 14–15
    amount, frequency of, 15
Female, masculinization of, 12
Fetal response, in exercise regimen, 201–2
Fitness, health benefits of exercise, contrasted, 188
Flexibility, 39–41, 181–86
  activity-specific stretches, 181–86
    ball sports, 181
    cycling, 181
    golf, 181
  corner stretch, 186
  flexibility program, 181
  flexor stretch, 184
  gastrocnemius/soleus stretch, 185
  hamstring stretch, 184
  hanging stretch, 185
  heel sit, 182
  knee to chest, 182
  piriformis stretch, 183
  press up, prone, 183
  research, 40–41
  wall stretch, 186
Flexor stretch, 184
Forearm, defined, 88
Forearm pronation, supination, with dumbbell, 157
Form, in performance of resistive exercise, 25
Framingham studies, 3
Frequency, of resistive exercise, 26
Full-body extension, 102
Full-body resistive exercise, 25
Functional independence, defined, 63

G

Galen, 4
Gastrocnemius/soleus stretch, 185
Gender, exercise and, 14
Golf, flexibility and, 40, 181
Guidance, in resistive exercise, 24

H

Hamstring stretch, 184
Hanging stretch, 185
Health benefits of exercise, fitness, contrasted, 188
Healthy People 2000, 211
Heart rate, 187–89
    American College of Sports Medicine, recommendations, 187–89
    recording sheet, aerobic exercise and, 33
    target
        aerobic exercise, 32–33
        safety, 48
Heel raise
    with bodyweight/dumbbell, 121
    on leg press machine, 122
    seated, 123
Heel sit, flexibility exercise, 182
Heels up exercise, 90
Herodicus, 4
Hip abduction
    on abduction machine, 107
    with cuff weight, 110
    manual resistive, 169
    with multi-hip machine, 109
Hip adduction
    on adduction machine, 104
    with cuff weight, 106
    manual resistive, 170
    on multi-hip machine, 105
Hip extension
    on multi-hip machine, 99
    prone, 101
    resistive, 79
Hip flexion, on multi-hip machine, 103
Hip lateral rotation
    with elastic band/tubing, standing, 115
    in side-lying position, with cuff weight, 114
Hip medial rotation
    with elastic band/tubing
        seated, 113
        standing, 112
    in side-lying position with cuff weight, 111
Hippocrates, 4
Home exercise, 71–72
    aerobic exercise, 71
    overview, 72
    safety, 72
    strength training, 71–72
    stretches, 72

I

Independence
    loss of, elderly and, 66
    quality, defined, 63
Injury
    of children
        activities, 56–57
        case reports, 58
        cohort studies, 59
    prevention, resistive exercise, 24
Intensity
    of aerobic exercise, 32
    classification of, 189
    of resistive exercise, 16–17
    scale, 16
Interscholastic sports, proliferation of, 4
Intervention, for exercise dependence, 54
Intrinsic feedback, motor learning, 14
Inversion injury prevention, resistive exercise and, 82
Isometric muscle action, defined, 88

K

Knee extension, 120
    manual resistive, 167
Knee flexion
    with cuff weight, standing, 119
    manual resistive, 166
    prone, 116
    seated, 117
    standing, 118
Knee joint angle, muscle condition, relationship between, 61
Knee resistance, in children, 60
Knee to chest, flexibility exercise, 182
Knowledge of performance, motor learning and, 15

L

Leg, defined, 88
Leg press, 97
Leg squat, single, manual resistive, 168
Lifting object from floor, body mechanics, 27–28
Longevity, aerobic exercise, 36
Lunge, lateral, 107

M

Manual resistive exercise, 165–80
    abdominal curl, 172
    back extension, 171
    cervical extension, 177
    cervical flexion, 176
        lateral, 178
    elbow flexion, 180
    guidelines, 165
    hip abduction, 169
    hip adduction, 170
    knee extension, 167
    knee flexion, 166
    leg squat, single, 168
    shoulder extension, 173
    shoulder transverse abduction, 175
    shoulder transverse adduction, 174
    tricep extension, 179
Masculinization, of female, 12
Massed practice, motor learning and, 14
Medical approval to exercise, 14
Mental health, exercise and, 209
Metabolic pathways, aerobic exercise, 31–32
Misconceptions about exercise, 10–14
Motivation, of client, 21
    research literature, 22
Motor learning
    facilitation of, 14–15
    feedback
        amount, frequency of, 15
        extrinsic, 14
        intrinsic, 14
    knowledge of performance, 15
    knowledge of results, 15
    massed practice, 14
    practice, 14
    transfer, 15
    variable practice, 14
Movement derivative model, resistance exercise, 74–77
Movements per session, number of, resistive exercise, 26
Muscle condition, knee joint angle, relationship between, 61
Muscle contraction, following rapid stretch, 17–19
Muscles for posture, 43
Muscular fitness, exercise recommendations, American College of Sports Medicine, 187–97

N

National Athletic Trainers Association, formation of, 4
Non-insulin-dependent diabetes mellitus, exercise and, 208

O

Obesity, exercise and, 158–59, 188–91, 209

Older persons, 63–70
  benefits of exercise, 63–65
  exercise programming, 68
  falling, 65–66
  function, effects of exercise on, 67
  independence
    functional, defined, 63
    loss of, 66
  overview, 68–69
  posture and, 44
  quality independence, defined, 63
  research, 63, 64–65
  resistance training, conditioning data, 66
  self-efficacy, 68
Olympic weightlifting, defined, 87
Osteoarthritis, exercise and, 208
Osteoporosis, exercise and, 208–9
Overload, resistive exercise, 25
Overtraining, 49–52
  1995 American Heart Association Guidelines for Cardiovascular Exercise in Apparently Healthy Individuals, 50
  aerobic activities, 51–52
  electrical analogy, 51
  symptoms of, 49–50
  terminology, 50
Oxygen uptake, 187–89
  American College of Sports Medicine, recommendations, 187–89

P

Pain reduction, exercise and, 5
Pan Hellenic Games, 4
Patellofemoral joint
  dysfunction, prevention of, in children, 58–61
  reaction force, 60
  stress, at flexion angles, 61
PCPFS. *See* President's Council on Physical Fitness and Sports
Perceived exertion scale, ratings, aerobic exercise and, 33
Physical examination, as prerequisite to resistive exercise, 24
Physiological adaptation, exercise and, 13
Piriformis stretch, 183
Plyometrics, defined, 17
Postpartum period, American College of Obstetricians and Gynecologists, exercise guidelines, 200–204
Posture, 43–45
  aging and, 44
  control of, 44
  exercise equipment, 44
  exercises, 44–45
  muscles, 43
  overview, 45
  postural base for exercise, 43–44
  resistive exercise, 24–25, 45
Powerlifting, defined, 87
Practice
  massed, motor learning and, 14
  motor learning and, 14
  variable, 14
Pregnancy, American College of Obstetricians and Gynecologists, exercise guidelines, 200–204
Prepubescence, defined, 55
Prescription schema, for exercise, 13
President's Council on Physical Fitness and Sports, 205
President's Council on Youth Fitness, formation of, 4
President's Physical Fitness Awards Program, 4
Press up, prone, flexibility exercise, 183
Preventive exercise, 3–8
  Aerobics, 4
  American Alliance of Health, Physical Education, and Recreation, establishment of, 4
  American College of Sports Medicine, formation of, 4
  benefits of, 5
    in workplace, 5
  cascade, exercise, 6
  competitive sports, growth of, 4
  Cooper, Kenneth, 4
  cost-effectiveness, 5
  evolution of, 4–5
  Framingham studies, 3
  Galen, 4
  Herodicus, 4
  Hippocrates, 4
  interscholastic sports, proliferation of, 4
  National Athletic Trainers Association, formation of, 4
  overview, 3–4, 5
  pain reduction, exercise and, 5
  Pan Hellenic Games, 4
  President's Council on Youth Fitness, formation of, 4
  President's Physical Fitness Awards Program, 4
  Renaissance, interest in sports, 4
  Roman Empire, interest in sports, 4
  TENS, in addition to exercise program, 5
Principles of resistive exercise, 24–28
Productivity, resistive exercise and, 23
Progress, evaluation of, 13–14
Progression, in resistive exercise, 25
Public health, physical activity and, 210–18
Pull up, 128
  with wide, pronated grip, 132
Push up, 139

Q

Quality of exercise, recommendations, American College of Sports Medicine, 187–97
Quality of life, exercise and, 209
Quantity of exercise, recommendations, quality of exercise, American College of Sports Medicine, 187–97

R

Radial deviation, with dumbbell, 160
Range of motion, resistive exercise, 12
Rapid stretch, muscle contraction following, 17–19
Recommendations, quantity, quality of exercise, American College of Sports Medicine, 187–97
Recording, of exercise data, 16–18
  sheet for, 223
Recovery from exercise, 49–52
  1995 American Heart Association Guidelines for Cardiovascular Exercise in Apparently Healthy Individuals, 50
  sets, 50–51
Renaissance, interest in sports, 4
Repetitions, in resistive exercise, 25–26, 50–51
Research literature
  aerobic exercise, 36
  children, exercise and, 56–57
  client education, speed of movement, during resistive exercise, 11
  client motivation, 22
  flexibility, 40–41
  knowledge of, safety and, 48
  older persons, exercise and, 63, 64–65
  remaining current in, 48
Resistive exercise, 23–29, 87–180
  abdominal curl, 89
    twisting, 93
  agonist, defined, 88
  ankle dorsiflexion, with elastic band/tubing, 124
  ankle eversion, with elastic band/tubing, 125
  ankle inversion, with elastic tubing/resistance, 126
  antagonist, defined, 88
  arm, defined, 88
  back extension
    on machine, 96
    prone, 95

bench press, 138
  dumbbell, 136
biomechanical model, 73–83
  cervical flexion, 81
  elbow, flexion, extension, 80
  hip extension, 79
  inversion injury, prevention, 82
  movement derivative model, 74–77
  purpose, 73
  shoulder transverse abduction, 78
body weight exercises, 27
bodybuilding, defined, 88
breathing, 24–25
case study, 28–29
cervical extension, with strap, 163
cervical flexion, with strap, 162, 164
characteristics of, 23
  productivity, 23
  safety, 23
  time efficiency, 23
concentric muscle action, defined, 88
conditioning data, older persons, 66
cool-down, 28
defined, 87
documentation, 27
dumbbell bench press, 136
dumbbell incline press, 137
dumbbell lunge, 98
duration, 26
eccentric muscle action, defined, 88
education, 24
elbow extension, with dumbbell, 156
elbow flexion
  with dumbbells, 152
  on machine, 153, 155
  pronated, 154
explosive, sport skill development and, 10–12
forearm
  defined, 88
  pronation, supination, with dumbbell, 157
form, 25
frequency of, 26
full-body exercise, 25
full-body extension, 102
guidance, 24
heel raise
  with bodyweight/dumbbell, 121
  on leg press machine, 122
  seated, 123
heels up, 90
hip abduction
  on abduction machine, 107
  with cuff weight, 110
  with multi-hip machine, 109
hip adduction
  on adduction machine, 104
  with cuff weight, 106
  on multi-hip machine, 105
hip extension
  on multi-hip machine, 99
  prone, 101
hip flexion, on multi-hip machine, 103
hip lateral rotation
  with elastic band/tubing, standing, 115
  in side-lying position, with cuff weight, 114
hip medial rotation
  with elastic band/tubing
    seated, 113
    standing, 112
  in side-lying position with cuff weight, 111
incline press, dumbbell, 137
injury prevention, 24
intensity, 16–17
inversion injury prevention, 82
isometric muscle action, defined, 88
knee extension, 120
knee flexion
  with cuff weight, standing, 119
  prone, 116
  seated, 117
  standing, 118
leg, defined, 88
leg press, 97
lifting object from floor, correct body mechanics, 27–28
lunge, lateral, 107
manual resistive exercise, 165–80
  abdominal curl, 172
  back extension, 171
  cervical extension, 177
  cervical flexion, 176, 178
  elbow flexion, 180
  guidelines, 165
  hip abduction, 169
  hip adduction, 170
  knee extension, 167
  knee flexion, 166
  leg squat, single, 168
  shoulder extension, 173
  shoulder transverse abduction, 175
  shoulder transverse adduction, 174
  tricep extension, 179
movement derivative model, 74–77
movements per session, number of, 26
Olympic weightlifting, defined, 87
overload, 25
overview, 29
physical examination, 24
posture, 24–25, 45

powerlifting, defined, 87
principles of, 24–28
progression, 25
pull up, 128
  with wide, pronated grip, 132
push up, 139
radial deviation, with dumbbell, 160
range of motion and, 12
repetitions, 25–26, 50–51
resistance, 16
rest duration, between movements, sets, 26
resting time, graph, 27
safety, 23
sample exercise program, 28
scale, 16
scapular protraction, 145
scapular retraction
  shoulder elevation, combined, 147
  using lat rowing machine, 146
sets, 25–26, 50–51
shoulder abduction, 130
shoulder adduction, on lat pulldown machine, 131
shoulder depression
  using dip bars, 143
  using overhead bar, 142
  using weight bench, 144
shoulder elevation, 141
shoulder extension, on lat row machine, 127
shoulder flexion, 129
shoulder lateral rotation
  with dumbbell, 150
  with elastic/cable, 151
shoulder medial rotation
  with dumbbell, 148
  with elastic/cable resistance, 149
shoulder transverse abduction, 140
shoulder transverse adduction
  on chest fly machine, 134
  with pulleys/cables, 135
side bends, standing, 91
side-lying lateral curl, 92
speed of movement
  during, research, 11
  in sport skills and, 14
squat, 100
supervision, 24
supraspinatus raise, 133
terminology, 87
thigh, defined, 88
time
  graph, 26
  resting, graph, 27
  set-repetition protocols, 26
time-efficiency index, 27

torso, defined, 88
trunk rotation, on machine, 94
ulnar deviation, with dumbbell, 161
variety of, 27
volume-intensity relationship, 25
warm-up, 28
wrist
    extension, with bar/dumbbells, 159
    flexion, with bar/dumbbells, 158
Respiratory fitness, exercise recommendations, American College of Sports Medicine, 187–97
Resting time
    graph, 27
    between movements, 26
Roman Empire, interest in sports, 4

S

Safety, 47–48
    equipment, 48
    exercise facilities, 48
    guidelines, 48
    in home exercise, 72
    overview, 48
    research on, 48
    resistive exercise, 23
    target heart range, 48
    warm-up, 48
Sample exercise programs, 28, 219–21
Scapular protraction, 145
Scapular retraction
    shoulder elevation, combined, 147
    using lat rowing machine, 146
Self-efficacy, of elderly, exercise and, 68
Set-repetition protocols, 26
Sets
    recovery from exercise and, 50–51
    in resistive exercise, 25–26, 50–51
Shoulder abduction, 130
Shoulder adduction, on lat pulldown machine, 131
Shoulder depression
    with dip bars, 143
    with overhead bar, 142
    with weight bench, 144
Shoulder elevation, 141
Shoulder extension
    on lat row machine, 127
    manual resistive, 173
Shoulder flexion, 129
Shoulder lateral rotation
    with dumbbell, 150
    with elastic/cable, 151
Shoulder medial rotation
    with dumbbell, 148
    with elastic/cable resistance, 149
Shoulder transverse abduction, 140
    manual resistive, 175
    resistive, 78
Shoulder transverse adduction
    on chest fly machine, 134
    manual resistive, 174
    with pulleys/cables, 135
Side bends, standing, 91
Side-lying lateral curl, 92
Simulation, specificity, distinguished, 15–16
Specificity, simulation, distinguished, 15–16
Speed
    during resistive exercise, research, 11
    in sport skills, resistive exercise and, 14
Speed training methods, 14
Split-routines, 12
Sports
    competitive, growth of, 4
    interscholastic, proliferation of, 4
    skills
        development, explosive resistive exercise and, 10–12
        speed in, resistive exercise and, 14
Spot reduction, 13
Squat, 100
Standardization of procedures, need for, American College of Sports Medicine, 188
Strength, defining, 10
Strength training, at home, 71–72
Stretches
    ball sports, 40, 181
    corner, 186
    cycling, 40, 181
    flexibility and, 40
        overview, 41
        physiology of, 39–40
    flexor, 184
    gastrocnemius/soleus, 185
    golf, 40, 181
    hamstring, 184
    hanging, 185
    at home, 72
    physiology of, 39–40
    piriformis, 183
    rapid, muscle contraction following, 17–19
    research on, 40–41
    wall, 186
Supervision, of resistive exercise, 24
Supraspinatus raise, 133
Surgeon General's Report, physical activity, health, 205–9

T

Target heart rate, 32–33, 48
TENS, in addition to exercise program, 5
Thigh, defined, 88
Time, resistive exercise
    graph, 26
    resting, 27
    set-repetition protocols, 26
Time-efficiency index, resistive exercise, 23
Torso, defined, 88
Transcutaneous electrical nerve stimulation. See TENS
Transfer, motor learning, 15
Tricep extension, manual resistive, 179
Trunk rotation, on machine, 94

U

Ulnar deviation, with dumbbell, 161

V

Variable practice, motor learning and, 14
Variety, in resistive exercise, 27
Volume–intensity relationship, resistive exercise, 25

W

Wall stretch, 186
Warm-up, 48
    resistive exercise, 28
Weather, aerobic exercise and, 34
Weight control
    American College of Sports Medicine recommendations, 188–91
    body composition and, 191
Wrist
    extension, with bar/dumbbells, 159
    flexion, with bar/dumbbells, 158

Y

Youth. See Children

About the Authors

David Ash, MPT, ATC, CSCS, has ten years of experience prescribing preventive exercise programs as a Division I University Conditioning Specialist at George Mason University, The University of Kentucky, and The University of Iowa. With over twenty years of personal experience in resistive and aerobic exercise, Mr. Ash has designed, implemented, and supervised exercise programs for individuals of all ages, abilities, and experience levels.

Caren J. Werlinger, PT, is Partner and Director of Clinical Services at the Physical Evaluation and Rehabilitation Center in Winchester, Virginia. She is a 1989 graduate of the West Virginia University Physical Therapy Program. Ms. Werlinger has served as adjunct instructor for the SU-WMC Program in Physical Therapy since 1990. Her teaching experience includes orthopedics, evaluation and treatment, and prosthetics and orthotics. She has over twelve years of personal experience in resistive exercise, bicycling, and running.